FINANCIAL MANAGEMENT FOR MEDICAL GROUPS

A Resource for New and Experienced Managers

Third Edition

MGMA-ACMPE
104 Inverness Terrace East
Englewood, CO 80112-5306
877.275.6462
mgma.com

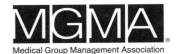

Medical Group Management Association

MGMA publications are intended to provide current and accurate information and are designed to assist readers in becoming more familiar with the subject matter covered. Such publications are distributed with the understanding that MGMA does not render any legal, accounting, or other professional advice that may be construed as specifically applicable to individual situations. No representations or warranties are made concerning the application of legal or other principles discussed by the authors to any specific factual situation, nor is any prediction made concerning how any particular judge, government official, or other person will interpret or apply such principles. Specific factual situations should be discussed with professional advisors.

Production Credits
Senior Knowledge Advisors: Marilee Aust and Craig Wiberg
Editorial and Production Management: Erica Nikolaidis
Compositor: Virginia Howe
Proofreader: Mary Kay Kozrya
Indexer: Sara Lynn Eastler

Library of Congress Control Number: 2013938554

Item 8428
ISBN: 978-1-56829-395-0

10 9 8 7 6 5 4 3

About the Contributors

Dr. Pawan Arya, MD, MBA-HCM, MCMC, CMPE, CPC, CPC-H, is a foreign medical graduate with more than 15 years of medical practice experience in India. He also has an MBA in healthcare management from Phoenix University. He is an accomplished administrator, and his forte is operational and financial benchmarking, process redesign and improvement, quality management, and compliance. Dr. Arya is a current member of MGMA-ACMPE's Patient Safety and Quality of Care Advisory Committee and a former member of MGMA-ACMPE's Government Affairs Committee. He is also a member of the American Academy of Professional Coders (AAPC), the American Institute of Healthcare Compliance (AIHC), and the Gastroenterology Administration Assembly (GAA). Dr. Arya has a rich and diverse management experience. He is currently the CEO for Digestive Disease & Nutrition Center of Westchester and New York Endoscopy. In the past, Dr. Arya has managed a cancer center and acted as director of operations for a multispecialty group practice.

James D. Barrett, MS, FACMPE, has more than 16 years of medical management experience. He has been instrumental in expanding his current practice as well as that of his previous employer. He has a master's degree in health administration from the Rochester Institute of Technology and a bachelor's degree in finance from Syracuse University. Mr. Barrett is a fellow at MGMA-ACMPE and also serves as chair of the organization's steering committee. He is the COO at Anne Arundel Eye Center in Annapolis, Md.

Owen Dahl, FACHE, CHBC, LSSMBB, has more than 40 years of experience in managing medical practices and healthcare consulting. While working in administration, Dahl was CEO for a physician practice management company with combined revenues of more than $75 million and 18 groups under contract. Dahl also acted as CEO for a merged hospital with a 300-bed facility and as president of a physician practice management and billing company.

Nancy Enos, FACMPE, CPMA, CEMC, CPC-I, CPC, is an independent consultant and coding instructor. She has 35 years of operations experience in the practice management field, managing an orthopedic practice for 13 years before joining LighthouseMD, a medical billing company in Providence, RI, and served as the director of physician services until July 2008. In 2009, Nancy opened an independent consulting practice.

As an approved PMCC instructor of the American Academy of Professional Coders, Nancy provides coding certification courses, outsourced coding, chart auditing, consultative services and seminars in CPT and ICD-9 coding, evaluation and management coding and documentation, and compliance planning. Nancy frequently speaks on coding, compliance, and reimbursement issues to audiences from the provider community specializing in primary care and surgical specialties. She is a fellow of the American College of Medical Practice Executives. She is on the MGMA-ACMPE Section Steering Committee and is a past president of MA/RI MGMA. She is the founding president of the Rhode Island chapter, AAPC.

David N. Gans, MSHA, FACMPE, is vice president of innovation and research practice management resources at MGMA-ACMPE.

Sarah J. Holt, PhD, FACMPE, is the administrator of several healthcare organizations in Cape Girardeau, Missouri, providing practice management for Cape Girardeau Surgical Clinic, Inc., & Breast Care Center and for Cape Medical Billing Corp., a medical practice billing company. Additionally, she is the administrator of Cape Girardeau Doctors' Park, which offers a full range of medical services on an 80-acre complex of 35 medical buildings. Holt received a PhD in policy analysis with a healthcare emphasis from St. Louis University, a master's in counseling from Southeast Missouri State University, and an undergraduate degree in education. She has done extensive research on how medical office insurance staff members make decisions relating to insurance reimbursement and how complexity influences organizations. She teaches health policy and healthcare reimbursement at the graduate level at Southeast Missouri State University and speaks on healthcare management topics to audiences of physicians, management, and staff.

Sara M. Larch, MSHA, FACMPE, is a specialist leader in the healthcare practice Deloitte Consulting LLP. She has more than 30 years of healthcare-industry experience in large physician groups in academic medical centers and multihospital systems. She has c-suite experience as COO of a 900-physician faculty practice plan and as vice president of a five-hospital integrated delivery system, leading their newly formed employed physician group. Working in those groups, she designed physician governance and created new physician employment models, led teams that reduced denial rates from 32 percent to 12 percent, increased the net collection rate by 34 percent, and centralized self-pay collections from 22 entities into one. She is currently focused on the model of the employed physician within large healthcare organizations. Larch is past board chair of the Medical Group Management Association (MGMA) and past president of the Academic Practice Assembly and Association of Managers of Gynecology and Obstetrics. She is coauthor of the book The Physician Billing Process: 12 Potholes to Avoid in the Road to Getting Paid (MGMA, 2009). In 2012 Larch received MGMA's Harry J. Harwick Lifetime Acheivement Award.

Daniel D. Mefford, CPA, MBA, FACMPE, has more than 23 years of experience in physician practice management. As a senior consultant with the Practice Resource Management Group, he works with medical practices to improve productivity, reduce costs, and align compensation systems to meet their strategic goals. He has held executive leadership roles in small and large group practices and has provided consultative services to virtually all specialties. He has a particular interest in group practice integration and operational efficiency. Additionally, he specializes in developing ancillary revenue streams from such sources as diagnostic laboratory, imaging, and surgery centers. His extensive financial and practice management background allows him to balance patient care priorities with the realities of administrative efficiency and financial profitability.

Michael O'Connell, MHA, FACMPE, FACHE, is vice president of clinical and support services for Marymount Hospital, a Cleveland Clinic hospital, in Garfield Heights, Ohio. He is responsible for hundreds of employees and numerous departments at three campuses, as well as corporate compliance, environment of care, safety, and a $45 million surgery construction and renovation project. In 2005, he coauthored "Human Resources Management in Group Practice," which appeared in *Physician Practice Management: Essential Operational and Financial Knowledge* (published by Jones and Bartlett), now in its second edition. In 2006, he authored *Human Resource Management* (MGMA). O'Connell has contributed to healthcare publications including MGMA Connexion and was nominated for the 2009 MGMA Article of the Year. He has a master's of health administration from Saint Louis University in Saint Louis, Mo., and a bachelor's of science degree from University of Illinois in Urbana, Ill. He is also certified in healthcare management and a medical practice executive and is a fellow in the American College of Medical Practice Executives and American College of Healthcare Executives.

Rhonda W. Sides, CPA/ABV/CFF/CGMA, CVA, is principal for healthcare services and forensic/valuation services for Crosslin & Associates in Nashville, Tenn. Rhonda has over 20 years of experience in medical practice management, cost accounting, and healthcare consulting for physician practices. She served as an adjunct MBA professor for three years at the Massey School of Belmont University in Nashville, where she taught healthcare cost accounting. Rhonda lectures nationally for various healthcare and financial organizations on combining the practicality of accounting with the needs of medical practice management. She has coauthored two books, *Valuation of a Medical Practice* and *Accounting Handbook for Medical Practices,* both published by John Wiley & Sons. To learn more about Rhonda's services, contact her at rhonda.sides@crosslinpc. com or visit www.crosslinpc.com.

Lee Ann Webster, MA, CPA, FACMPE, has extensive experience with medical practices both as a practice administrator and as an independent accountant. Since 1997, she has served as practice administrator for Pathology Associates of Alabama, P.C., in Birmingham. She previously worked in national and local CPA firms, where she performed accounting, auditing, and tax services for clients in a variety of industries, including a significant amount of work for physicians and physician practices. Lee Ann is a fellow in the American College of Medical Practice Executives (ACMPE) and a certified public accountant in the state of Alabama. She is a past president of the Pathology Management Assembly of the Medical Group Management Association (MGMA) and a past chair of the ACMPE Professional Papers Committee. Lee Ann is a summa cum laude graduate of William Jewell College in Liberty, Missouri, and earned her master of arts in accounting from the University of Alabama.

Deborah Walker Keegan, PhD, FACMPE, is a nationally recognized consultant, keynote speaker, and author. Known for her dynamic, educational, and high-energy presentation style, her seminars and books are rich with "real-life" case material that are relevant and practical for today's healthcare environment. With more than 25 years of experience as a medical practice executive and healthcare consultant, she assists clients in resolving a wide range of challenges, including practice operations, revenue cycle assessment, physician–hospital integration, physician compensation plan redesign, and strategic planning and organizational evaluation. Dr. Keegan is president of Medical Practice Dimensions, Inc., and a principal with Woodcock & Walker Consulting. She earned her PhD from The Peter F. Drucker Graduate School of Management and her MBA from UCLA. With rich experience in consulting, education, and industry research, Dr. Keegan brings knowledge, expertise, and solutions to healthcare organizations. To contact Dr. Keegan or learn more about her services, go to www.deborahwalkerkeegan.com.

Robert F. White, MBA, has more than 25 years of healthcare leadership experience working with a wide variety of subspecialties. Robert worked at Massachusetts General Hospital for 15 years in the anesthesia and oral surgery departments. Serving in both financial and administrative roles, he learned budgeting and financial operations from a unique perspective. Robert has also managed retina surgery and OB/GYN practices and served as director of financial reporting for Anesthesia Healthcare Partners, a private anesthesia management company in Georgia. He is currently a practice administrator for Women's Care Florida — Winter Park OB/GYN. He earned his undergraduate degree in management and public policy and administration from Suffolk University and his MBA from the University of New Hampshire Whittemore School of Business and Economics. Robert is married with three children and lives in Orlando, Florida.

Contents

PART I
FUNDAMENTALS OF FINANCIAL MANAGEMENT

PART II
USING FINANCIAL MANAGEMENT INFORMATION
TO MANAGE OPERATIONS

PART I

Fundamentals of
Financial Management

CHAPTER 1

Introduction to Financial Management

By David N. Gans, MSHA, FACMPE, and Marilee E. Aust

After completing this chapter, you will be able to:

- Describe the purposes and uses of this text.

- Summarize the organization and content of this text.

- Define the role and function of the financial manager of a medical group and its principal activities.

- Sketch some typical profiles of financial managers in medical groups.

- Specify the ways that financial managers can develop effective competencies to carry out their responsibilities.

- Explain how financial managers can train others to understand the various functions of accounting and finance.

PURPOSES AND USES OF THIS TEXT

During the last several decades, the popularity of medical group practice has experienced dramatic challenges — from start-ups and mergers and acquisitions to disintegration and, now, reintegration. This occurrence evolved from the long-standing belief that ambulatory medical service delivery can be carried out most efficiently through the group practice. In today's environment of increasing healthcare services costs, the effective management of high-quality and low-cost medical services demands that all members of medical groups become familiar with the basics of sound financial management principles, techniques, and practices.

Since its inception, MGMA-ACMPE has been involved in the development, publication, and distribution of professional books and publications that deal with effective financial management of medical groups of all sizes.

Even though a great deal of assistance is available to financial managers from other organizations, there is a need for an organized source that covers all the fundamental aspects of a medical group's financial management. The objective of this text is to provide a resource or a vade mecum for the financial manager. A *vade mecum* is a handbook for ready reference; the words are derived from Latin and mean "come with me." The authors and editors encourage you, the reader, to come and explore the systems of financial management as they relate to healthcare. This resource will be especially useful to health professionals because it applies financial theories and concepts to the ambulatory healthcare setting. The publication provides myriad examples and leads the reader through specific multistep processes to achieve maximum effectiveness.

In addition, this text can serve as a valuable resource for physicians. The authors believe that a financially literate medical practitioner is a more effective and efficient provider of medical services. With greater financial knowledge, the physician can perform vital clinical tasks in the most efficient and least costly manner possible while maintaining high-quality care delivery.

BACKGROUND AND PROFILES OF MEDICAL GROUP FINANCIAL MANAGERS

Managing the financial affairs of a medical group requires a solid foundation and understanding of accounting, finance, and business in general. An understanding of third-party reimbursement procedures, contract negotiations (the modus operandi of insurance processing), governmental and regulatory laws and rules, and the patient-physician relationship are some of the financial manager's other more important knowledge areas.

For individuals with little formal education in accounting and finance, this text should prove to be a valuable tool. For financial managers that have had some or a great deal of previous accounting and finance experience, this text can serve as a collection of useful and relevant references about the basic aspects of the financial management function of a medical group practice.

THE ROLE AND ACTIVITIES OF FINANCIAL MANAGERS IN MEDICAL GROUPS

The responsibility for the financial management function within medical groups is usually vested in one individual. That person may be called by many different titles depending on the size of the medical group or the customs and preferences of the group's upper management and/or owners. Often, these staffers are called financial or accounting managers. In other groups, they may carry job titles such as the following:

- Chief executive officer
- Chief financial officer
- Controller
- Practice administrator
- Office manager
- Business office manager
- MSO administrator/director

In small groups, financial management may be only part of the many functions for which the practice administrator/business office manager is responsible. As the group expands, the financial areas will tend to separate from the general phases of practice management and become the responsibility of another individual who may be designated as the finance or accounting manager. The financial manager may also have staff members who will be assigned a segment of the total financial management area and who report to the practice administrator or the chief executive officer, depending on the organizational structure.

The following job descriptions illustrate some of the possible ways in which a group practice's overall financial management may be organized. They are provided merely as examples of possible arrangements. Each group must decide on its own title, manner, and breakdown of financial responsibilities depending on the mission, preferences, and capabilities of individuals.

Chief Executive Officer (CEO)

Responsibilities: This is the highest nonphysician executive position in the organization, typically found in the larger, more sophisticated medical practices, or in an integrated system (e.g., physician hospital organization, management services organization).

Duties:

- Develops and monitors organizational policy in conjunction with other management personnel and the governing body of the organization.
- Responsible for the overall operation of the organization, including patient care and contract relations, as well as activities that relate to the future growth of the organization such as strategic planning and marketing.

- Oversees a team of senior management personnel who have direct responsibility for these functional areas.
- Serves as a liaison between the organization and its constituents such as staff members, business partners, and individuals in the community.
- Also serves as the liaison between the organization and the governing body of the organization.
- May hold a designation as a fellow in the American College of Medical Practice Executives (FACMPE).

Reports to: Board of directors

Chief Financial Officer (CFO)

Responsibilities: The organization's senior financial position, typically found in larger, more sophisticated medical practices. The CFO develops financial policies and oversees their implementation.

Duties:

- Monitors a variety of financial activities, including budgeting, analysis of the organization's financial performance, accounting, billing, payer contracting, collections, and the preparation of tax returns.
- Prepares or oversees the preparation of annual reports and long-term projections to ensure that the organization's financial obligations are met.
- Obtains funds for capital development.
- May hold a designation as a Certified Public Accountant (CPA).

Reports to: Senior administrative officer or the governing body of the organization

Controller

Responsibilities: The second-in-charge financial officer in the organization.

- Assists the CFO with the organization's financial responsibilities.
- Develops and oversees activities relating to implementing and maintaining the integrity of the organization's financial reporting system, including implementing internal accounting procedures, analyzing finances, and developing internal auditing procedures.
- Assists with or oversees the budgeting process.
- Assists with the preparation of financial reports and tax returns.

Reports to: CFO or senior administrative officer

Practice Administrator

Responsibilities: This is a top nonphysician administrative position; however, the practice administrator often has less overall authority than a CEO and reports to a governing body often comprised of physician owners.

Maintains broad responsibilities for all administrative functions, including operations, marketing finance, managed care and third-party contracting, physician compensation and reimbursement, human resources, medical and business information systems, and planning and development.

Reports to: Governing body of the organization

Office Manager

Responsibilities: Typically found in a practice that does not have a practice administrator position. Manages the nonmedical activities of a larger medical practice with a more limited scope than that of a practice administrator. May initiate or lead strategic development activities. The focus of this position usually rests on the daily operations of the organization. May oversee some financial activities, such as billing and collections.

Reports to: Physician management

Business Office Manager

Responsibilities: Directs and coordinates all business office activities in an organization; typically found in practices that have a CEO, practice administrator, or CFO. Monitors the medical billing system. Oversees responsibility areas such as third-party reimbursements, physician billing, collections, contract administration, and management reporting. May assist with the preparation of financial reports, tax returns, and payroll.

Reports to: Senior administrative officer or top financial position in the organization

MSO Administrator/Director

Responsibilities: Oversees all activities of a hospital, health system, or investor-owned management services organization (MSO) that provides practice management services and other business functions to physicians' practices. Develops and monitors organization policy in conjunction with other management personnel and any governing body of the organization. Responsible for the overall operation of the MSO, including daily operations of multiple practice sites and contract relations, as well as activities that relate to the future growth of the organization, such as strategic planning and marketing MSO services to physician clients. Oversees a team of senior management personnel who have direct responsibility for these functional areas. Serves as a liaison between various organization levels and external entities, from the physicians to the equity partner(s) in the MSO and any governing body.

Provides or oversees the provision of consulting services to newly integrated practices.

Reports to: Senior administrative officer within a hospital or health system or to the governing body of the MSO

As you can observe from the diversity of the above job descriptions, the financial management function is carried out in a variety of organizational arrangements and structures. The important point is that these activities are performed by individuals who need to know the crucial elements of financial management and must complete the necessary tasks with a high level of competence.

WAYS TO DEVELOP FINANCIAL MANAGEMENT COMPETENCIES

Managers with financial responsibility usually do not have a uniform background but gravitate to the position from many previous roles within and outside of the healthcare environment. Thus, many individuals who do not possess a financial background have a great need for knowledge, starting with the fundamentals of accounting and finance. These persons should find this text to be a great resource in orienting them to the areas where they need to develop competencies.

Beyond the basics, there is a growing necessity for experienced managers to stay informed about new developments in healthcare management. At this writing, the most current pressing educational needs of financial managers include the following:

- Healthcare reform
- Continuous quality improvement
- Cost accounting for pricing and managing the practice
- Government payment regulations
- Capital budgeting and acquisitions
- Benchmarking
- Physician profiling
- Outcomes-based research
- Fraud and compliance
- Accountability perspectives

Aspects of these subjects will be covered in later chapters of this text. Since we will deal with the fundamentals of all subjects from the perspective of financial managers, in-depth treatments will be left to other sources.

Individuals who have become proficient as financial managers in medical groups have discovered various ways to gain more knowledge about the financial setting and about the changing state of the art of healthcare. They include:

- Attending short-term professional education courses.

- Joining and becoming active in professional associations and societies, such as MGMA-ACMPE's American College of Medical Practice Executives (ACMPE).

- Exploring the offerings of a local community college, particularly if it has courses in the fundamentals of accounting and finance. Also, examining self-study texts and materials that cover the basics in detail.

- Reading healthcare and medical group periodicals to gain familiarity with the "industry" and learning about the latest developments in financial management.

- Networking with other financial managers to obtain information and assistance when needed.

- Requesting assistance from the accounting firm that services the medical group.

- Hiring and working closely with a healthcare financial management consultant who will assist in the establishment of new or the revision of old systems.

- Becoming an Internet browser by exploring healthcare subjects and references and/or participating in e-mail discussion groups (e.g., http://community.mgma.com/Home or http://www.egroups.com).

HOW TO MULTIPLY THE KNOWLEDGE OF FINANCIAL MANAGERS

Financial managers must take advantage of every opportunity to convey the financial message to all members of the medical group, especially physicians. When occasions arise to discuss any financial report or information, the financial manager must be ready to explain the content and meaning of the report. In addition, the financial manager should periodically hold in-house meetings or training sessions for nonfinancial principals of the group. These could include a review of the latest set of financial statements and operating statistics.

The head of the financial management function must encourage his or her staff members to grow and develop in their positions. Efforts to promote financial and healthcare expertise among staff members might include the following:

- Preparing and maintaining current detailed policy and procedure manuals for all members, which explain the accounting and information processing systems of the group. To encourage use, present them in a user-friendly format, such as flow charts.

- Developing an on-the-job program for staff personnel by careful appraisal of each staffer's present strengths and needs. Tailor individualized programs with outside course work, self-study readings, job rotation, and experience to develop broader ranges of competencies.

- Conducting short in-house training sessions about new and important developments for the members of the financial staff, if the staff size is large enough.

- Encouraging all staff members to "show and tell" other staff persons the nature of their jobs and encouraging everyone to have a basic understanding of everyone else's financial functions.

ORGANIZATION AND CONTENT OF THIS TEXT

This third edition includes the following:

- Significant updating of previously existing material.

- Expansion of other material deemed to be critical and most important for financials in the future.

- Addition of a new component — accountability and the healthcare industry's efforts to address the important issues surrounding this important concept.

Part I of this book, Fundamentals of Financial Management, will cover the basics of accounting and financial matters that form the foundation of the financial manager's position in medical practices. Part II, Using Financial Management Information to Manage Operations, will show how core financial data and other supplementary information can be used to assist in the overall management of the medical practice. Both sections provide information about emerging forces and developments that will dominate the healthcare scene in the years ahead.

Chapter 2 discusses the key elements that form the basis for managing the operations of a medical practice. Starting with a review of the major organization structures that comprise a practice, it goes on to describe the main functions of a financial management operating system. The accounting and finance functions are overviewed together with the system of internal control. Significant key indicators to measuring a medical group's financial performance are also included.

Chapter 3 covers the process of accounting and the composition of the accounting system. Our treatment will be basic, touching on the essence of the process and explaining the fundamental concepts and techniques used to record, summarize, and report a medical practice's financial affairs. The contents and structure of the basic financial statements are present along with a summary of the basic assumptions underlying them.

Chapter 4 explains the nature of a financial information system and the important categories of information that medical group practices design and include in their systems. The new *Chart of Accounts for Health Care Organizations (COAHCO)* developed by MGMA-ACMPE is described and shown to be the central organizer of information in practice records. Key factors and key steps necessary in selecting information-system components and vendors are summarized for practice use.

Chapter 5 focuses on the major vehicles used to convey financial operating results and the practice's financial status — that is, the income statement and the balance sheet. Other major types of operating reports and their desired characteristics are cited, as well. The key indicators, which supply important measures for appraising the financial success of medical groups, are also listed and explained. These indicators are regularly distributed by MGMA-ACMPE.

Chapter 6 delves into the basic rules of measuring and reporting costs and expenses in operating reports and the logic of the chart of accounts' classification bases. The subject of cost accounting is introduced by defining the cost concepts and applications that are used and by explaining how costs behave in relation to varying activity levels. Responsibility accounting — an orientation of the accounts to arrange accounting information to assist planning and controlling operations — is presented together with an explanation of how the new 2011 *MGMA Chart of Accounts* can accommodate this form of accounting.

Chapter 7 explains how a physician practice can estimate its cost of doing business down to the individual procedure level while taking into account not only the direct costs of a procedure but also the indirect overhead costs of the practice. Instructions and examples for each step in the process are provided, including illustrations of formulas and calculations that can be tailored to a specific practice. Also included is discussion of how management may use the resulting data to make better-informed decisions for their practices.

Chapter 8 deals with measuring and managing cash flows, an important asset of medical groups. The objectives of cash management and how to accomplish this end are covered in a practical way. This section includes sample cash reports and cash budgets, as well as a discussion regarding internal control over cash. Illustrating the development and interpretation of the third basic financial statement — the cash flow statement — is included. How to forecast and budget future cash flows is shown along with the possible problems and consequences of faulty cash management practices. Also included is the use of short-term investments in the cash management process.

Chapter 9 addresses the nature of accounts receivable arising from patient care, as well as the accounting practices and techniques to manage the collection of these amounts due. Strategies for improving cash flows from receivables are identified and illustrated. The medical group's financial position is significantly affected by each of the revenue cycle key functions. This chapter helps analyze the group's charge and collection trends and turn that information into actionable improvements. It also looks at the medical group's use of vendors and other ways to optimize collection performance and keep the accounts receivable at best-practice rates.

Chapter 10 begins Part II, and it highlights the impact of managed care on financial management. The introduction of the major stakeholders in the managed care systems and definitions of basic concepts that differentiate managed care from FFS segue into an outline of the continuum of managed care contracting. This includes a discussion of various risk arrangements and how to control cost. After a contract is negotiated, the question of how to manage the contract becomes most important. The chapter provides information on how to negotiate and how to ensure that the practice understands the financial implications of a contract that will help to build a good skill set for the financial management of managed care contracts.

Chapter 11 focuses on one of the most important activities for medical practices: planning and budgeting for operations. The preliminary phases of using the objective-setting process and the development of strategies are highlighted as essential steps before budgeting. The composition of budgets used in medical practices is delineated and described together with the functioning of a flexible budgeting system. A section dealing with budgeting physician compensation contains practical approaches for considering this important factor in the overall budgeting scheme. Analyzing simple cost-volume-profit structures of medical groups is shown as a way to determine break-even points, and the relationships of these variables are useful in assessing their impact on group profits as they change.

Chapter 12 spotlights the sensitive areas of operating a medical practice and how financial analysis can provide a means to uncover weaknesses and areas for improvement. Starting with an exposition of evaluating the performance of profit and cost centers, we move to an updated version of MGMA-ACMPE's efforts to provide financial and nonfinancial information about successful medical groups with which to compare the performance of your group. This new service also involves relaying comparison data from MGMA-ACMPE's annual Cost Survey. Provider profiling and the type of data comprising these profiles are covered. MGMA-ACMPE's software package, DataDive, is explained and described. Specific focus is placed on how medical group operations might be examined to improve productivity, implement cost reductions, and increase the group's income potential. In addition, sources of assistance that financial managers can turn to are identified.

Chapter 13 explains and illustrates MGMA-ACMPE's approach to benchmarking, as well as the major current tools for managing operations — benchmarking and total quality management. With quality being the center of attention for delivering medical services, extensive ideas are included on defining quality and its applications in healthcare. Couched in a total quality management (TQM) framework, the chapter provides an explanation of the concept of quality and the meaning of total quality in the context of healthcare today. How a TQM effort can be established in a medical group is then covered.

Chapter 14 evaluates short- and long-term investment alternatives. The types of short-range decisions and the relevant costs and benefits applying to these alternative choices are explained. This chapter also emphasizes long-range investment decisions, starting with a review of the time value of money concepts and ending with how these variables are employed in the process of determining appropriate capital investment opportunities. The basic approach to capital budgeting is also covered.

Chapter 15 approaches the financing aspects of medical practices. The authors explain the reasons why medical practices need capital and articulate how these factors relate to the specific financial needs of different kinds of medical groups. Also, relationships are identified between the capital funding sources and the strategic directions of the practice. The various sources of capital are described so that financial managers can select the most appropriate types to fit their purposes. Steps for seeking a capital partner are highlighted, as well as a summarization of the elements of a business plan.

Chapter 16 calls for the financial manager to take the lead in organizing and integrating the activities of the practice, both financially and otherwise, to focus on accountability. The chapter begins by defining and describing the elements of accountability. A general model is set forth to show how individuals and group relationships interrelate and how each can be held accountable for the activities undertaken. Specific applications are developed, illustrating how accountability perspectives can add dimension to all group members' work and lead to better problem identification and results improvement. Broader aspects of accountability issues in the healthcare industry are highlighted, with emphasis on the fraud and abuse efforts now being made to ameliorate these problems, including developing a compliance program. Finally, potential theft and fraud occasions within a group practice are identified, with measures cited to minimize their occurrence.

Chapter 17 sets the stage for the "new financial management" required in an era of healthcare reform. The chapter discusses the new skills and data metrics needed to ensure a medical practice's financial health in the midst of payment, structure, and delivery system reform. Changes in both expenditure management and revenue cycle management are described so that a medical practice can position itself for success in value-based purchasing and healthcare commoditization. New payment models are detailed, including fixed payment arrangements, and the impact of these models on financial management and operations are explored. Emerging models of payer, hospital, and physician alignment are described with a discussion of each of these stakeholder perspectives on financial integration for the future.

To the Point

- This text is useful to the person just entering a position in the financial management of a medical group practice or to the experienced individual who desires a refresher on the various areas of financial management. Further, physicians will find that this volume contains a complete compendium of all financial matters that affect a medical group practice.

- The medical group financial manager requires a background with a solid foundation and understanding of accounting and finance and of business in general. The responsibility for the financial management function within medical groups is usually vested with one individual. That person is called by many different titles, such as CFO, controller, practice administrator, office manager, or business office manager.

- Beyond the basic fundamentals of accounting and finance, there is a growing necessity for all financial managers, experienced or not, to stay informed about new developments in healthcare management. Some areas are healthcare reform, continuous quality improvement, cost accounting for pricing and managing the practice, and government payment regulations.

- There are many ways that financial managers can continue their personal development in all subject areas vital to their position, such as attending short-term continuing education courses and joining and becoming active in professional associations, such as the American College of Medical Practice Executives (ACMPE).

- Financial managers should take every opportunity to convey financial information to all members of the medical group, especially physicians, and to make sure that everybody understands it. The financial manager must also take steps to consciously promote his or her medical staff's continuing development.

CHAPTER 2

Key Elements in Financial Management

Edited by Pawan Arya, MD, MBA-HCM, MCMC, CMPE, CPC, CPC-H

After completing this chapter, you will be able to:

- Identify the typical organizational structures, including the different legal forms, used in the management of medical groups.

- List the major functions comprising the financial management operating systems of a medical group, and summarize the usual evolution of a financial information system.

- Describe the major accounting and financial functions performed in a medical group office.

- Specify and describe the types of financial information needed to manage a medical group practice.

- Explain the elements of a system of internal control and how internal control relates to the operation of a medical group practice.

- Identify the significant indicators used to measure performance of a medical group practice.

The first consideration facing a medical group is to decide what form of organization to adopt to operate its practice. We will explain the primary management structures and legal forms that most groups adopt. Then, we'll describe the financial management operating systems, especially those related to the accounting and finance functions, which are so essential to information collection and dissemination. The need for financial information that drives the development of accounting systems is summarized next. Internal control considerations, incorporated into the systems, are also explained. Once a medical group has started operating, key performance indicators should be used to monitor operating activities. All these issues are covered in this chapter.

LEGAL TYPES OF ORGANIZATIONS

Choosing a legal structure for a medical group depends upon a variety of factors, such as:

- The types of organizations permitted by state law
- The nature of the organization's mission
- The identity of "owners" in a proprietary organization
- The perceived needs and goals of the organization
- The income tax laws, regulations, and application
- Retirement/pension/profit-sharing planning requirements

Some structures occur by default, while others result from executing a plan developed after receiving the opinions of lawyers and accountants. Some organizational structures are driven by legal requirements, while in others, tax ramifications are the driving force. In still others, organizational structure evolves through the influence of personalities in the group despite the organization's legal structure. The article, "Choosing Your Medical Practice Entity"[1] from the online *Physicians' News Digest* provides useful information on organizational structures.

The types of legal structures permissible for group practices vary from state to state. Typical types of organizations are:

- Sole proprietorships with employed and or contracted physicians
- Sole proprietorships that share facilities and some expenses

- General partnerships and limited liability partnerships
- Limited liability companies
- Business corporations
- Professional corporations (PC) and personal service corporations (PSC)
- Not-for-profit corporations
- Cooperatives

The owners have different rights and responsibilities in relation to one another and to third parties in each of these legal structures. These types are described below in some detail.

Sole Proprietorships

As the name suggests, a single physician owns all the assets of the practice and has complete autonomy and authority to make decisions. Most sole proprietors operate under an assumed name popularly called a DBA or "doing business as." The name will need to be registered with the city after making sure that it is not already registered by any other business. There is no legal limitation on the size of the business that is operated as a sole proprietorship or the number of professionals the proprietor may employ. Even though the practice might become quite large with many employed and or contract physicians, the control and reporting requirements are kept quite simple, and the sole proprietor is the ultimate and final authority. The employee physicians of such sole proprietors are salaried and receive a form W2 at the end of the year. The contracted physicians receive a form 1099 for tax filing.

The individual physicians employed or contracted by the sole proprietor are responsible for their own claims of medical liability; however, the sole proprietor may also be involved because of the practice ownership and is required to have malpractice insurance for the business entity. AllBusiness.com[2] lists the following advantages and disadvantages of sole proprietorship.

Advantages of sole proprietorship:

1. It's the simplest form of business entity to set up. The legal cost is minimal, and formal legal and business requirements are few.
2. It's the easiest form of legal entity to terminate or liquidate.
3. Taxes are paid by the sole proprietor under his or her social security number, and there are no taxes payable on the business.
4. The sole proprietor has complete autonomy, is free to follow his or her vision and has complete authority for running the organization. He or she may employ any number of physicians as employees or contractors to provide services.
5. The sole proprietor retains all the profits, and if he or she so chooses, may multiply revenue streams by diversifying the scope of services provided without having to seek someone else's consent to do so.

Disadvantages of sole proprietorship:

1. The sole proprietor is responsible for all administrative tasks and decision making and has the ultimate responsibility for compliance with all federal, state, and local laws, such as state and federal labor laws, Occupational Safety and Health Administration (OSHA), and HIPAA privacy and security statutes, to name a few.

2. As a small group with fewer resources, hiring good talent is difficult. It is hard to provide good benefits such as health insurance and paid time off.

3. Because of their small size, sole proprietorships have limited ability to negotiate contracts with vendors for goods and services and pay more compared to bigger groups.

4. Sole proprietorships have no negotiating ability with payers, and therefore, the reimbursement for services is smaller compared to larger groups.

5. The liability to the creditors is complete.

6. Exposure to risk is complete in terms of liabilities for bill payments.

Space-Sharing Sole Proprietors or Groups

The pressure of the economy and the need to keep overhead costs low encourages some physicians to share space, staffing, and utilities. In other cases, a physician or a group may simply sublet some space to a physician from another specialty. This helps defray some of the overhead cost. All such arrangements are governed by terms of contract and should be in writing, clearly stating the cost of renting and the scope of services.

While subletting space, the most important thing to consider is the fair market value. If the space is being sublet to a physician who will depend solely on the referrals of the landlord physician, the rent charged should be equivalent to the rent if the physician had an independent office not based on the referrals made to the physician, otherwise this will run afoul of the anti-kickback statute (Stark Rule).

The physician should consider many things before subletting the space to another physician or subletting from another group.[3] These include:

■ Procure and review the original lease document to determine whether subleasing or sharing space is allowed.

■ Decide what space in your office you want to lease without creating hardship to you, and during what periods of the day or week.

■ Publicize your need for a subtenant through professional networking, medical society publications, or various Web sites. Sometimes it helps to hire an agent for a finder's fee.

■ Find a physician or other healthcare professional who benefits your patient population.

■ Have a written sublease agreement that lasts at least a year, includes the services to be provided, and a noncompete clause, which ensures that the renting provider does not provide the same services as you.

- Set rent payment terms and charge fair market rent.
- Specify how the contract can be terminated if necessary.
- Check a potential subtenant's references.
- Inform patients referred to a subtenant of the nature of the relationship.

Things to consider when renting space from another physician or group:

- Look for an office through professional networking, medical society publications, or various Web sites, or you may wish to engage an agent.
- Find a space that will be available during the hours you need.
- Pick a location that will allow you to expand the patient population you can serve.
- Assess whether your practice will fit with the one already in the space.
- Sign a written agreement that lasts at least a year.
- Ask what additional technology or administrative services will be provided.
- Ensure the contract can be terminated easily if necessary.
- Check a potential sub-landlord's references.
- Review the original lease document to make sure that the lease is unfettered, that the tenant group has no restriction on subletting the space, and that you will be allowed to post your signs.
- Check the terms of the lease, making sure the remaining term meets your needs and expectations.
- Call the building landlord to ensure that the physician subleasing the space to you is up to date on his or her payments.

Another variation of space sharing exists where a realtor develops a medical space and rents turnkey spaces to the physicians. In such cases, since the landlord does not benefit from the referrals, there is no impact from the anti-kickback statute.

Partnerships

There are two types of partnerships:[4] general partnerships and limited partnerships (LPs). The partnerships are governed by the terms of agreement in the form of responsibilities, share of equity and revenue, and scope of goods and services provided by each. In a general partnership, each partner can incur obligations on behalf of the partnership, and each assumes unlimited liability for the partnership's debts. For example, if there is any unpaid bill or the partnership goes into bankruptcy, the creditors can go after both or any of the partners that may have assets.

LPs are an attractive alternative to general partnerships. In an LP, generally one partner is responsible for managing the affairs of the partnership and is therefore also responsible for any liability that the partnership may incur. The other partners with no management role are called limited partners. The role of limited partners is limited to contributing initial investment in exchange of a firm's profits. Limiting the risk to the general partner makes this an attractive alternative to the general partnership. In fact, a limited partner's role usually involves nothing more than making an initial capital investment in exchange for a share of the firm's profits. The liability of the limited partners cannot exceed the share of contributions made by the limited partner while the managing partner has an unlimited liability.

The limited partnership offers two main advantages: (1) it gives freedom to the managing partner, specifically the freedom to run the practice without any interference from other partners; and (2) it protects the limited partners from liability beyond their share of equity in the practice. If the practice is not going in the right direction, the other partners may choose to be more involved, but that would remove limited status and make them equally vulnerable to any liability.

In general partnerships, all partners are jointly and severally liable for all actions of each partner. A limited partnership, however, provides some protection of reduced liability to limited partners. A limited partner's liability is reduced to the capital that he or she has invested and to the partnership's assets. Unlike general partners, limited partners are not permitted to participate in the management of the organization. A limited partnership is not commonly used as the legal structure for a group practice, but it is often used as an investment vehicle to acquire land, buildings, or equipment for the practice.

Corporations

Corporations are artificial entities that are created by state statute and that are treated much like individuals under the law, having legally enforceable rights, the ability to acquire debt and to pay out profits, the ability to hold and transfer property, the ability to enter into contracts, the requirement to pay taxes, and the ability to sue and be sued.

The rights and responsibilities of a corporation are independent and distinct from the people who own or invest in them. A corporation simply provides a way for individuals to run a business and to share in profits and losses.

Types of Corporations

The corporations can be one of several types depending on the functions they perform and the articles of incorporation. A medical group corporation is generally one of two types: (1) a private business corporation or (2) a not-for-profit corporation, such as a community health center. Other types of corporations, such as municipal and quasi-public, are not normally seen in medical practices.

Private corporations: Private corporations are in business to make money for the shareholders, whereas nonprofit corporations are generally designed to benefit the general public. Any profit generated by such nonprofit companies is not distributed as dividends but is utilized to provide more services and improve the quality of services. Municipal corporations are typically cities and towns that help the state to function at the local level. Quasi-public corporations would be considered private, but their business serves the public's needs, such as offering utilities or telephone service.

A private corporation can be one of the two types. One is the public corporation, which has a large number of investors, called shareholders. These corporations trade their shares on a security exchange. Another type of private corporation is one that is closely held, and has relatively few shareholders, often all members of the same family with little or no outside market share. In such cases, the family members run the business together. Such corporations are generally used as instruments for raising funds (generally as bonds) and limiting liability of the individuals.

In a corporation, any liability arising out of a claim is the responsibility of the business entity, and the shareholders are immune to such claims. In some cases, however, the courts may pierce the "veil" of a corporation and hold the shareholders, officers, or board of directors personally responsible for the corporation's liability. This occurs generally when the corporation is a "sham," engages in fraud and or other unlawful acts, or is used solely for the personal benefit of its shareholders, directors, or other officers. Courts traditionally require fraud, illegality, or misrepresentation before they will pierce the corporate veil.[5]

Courts may pierce the corporate veil in taxation or bankruptcy cases, in addition to cases involving plaintiffs with contract or tort claims. Federal law in this area is usually similar to state law. The instrumentality and alter-ego doctrines used by courts are practically indistinguishable. Courts following the instrumentality doctrine concentrate on finding three factors: (1) The people behind the corporation dominate the corporation's finances and business practices so much so that the corporate entity has no separate will or existence; (2) the control has resulted in a fraud or a wrong, dishonest, or unjust act; and (3) the control and harm directly caused the plaintiff's injury or unjust loss.

However, so long as the officers of the corporation conduct the corporation's business per the bylaws and statutes of the state, they are protected from any liability claims. Such actions include:

- Scrupulously treating the assets of the corporation as assets owned by the corporation, and the corporate assets are not undercapitalized.
- Taking corporate actions through resolutions of the board of directors and its committees or pursuant to a delegation of authority from the board of directors and not treating the corporation as a personal business entity.
- Executing all corporate contracts and undertaking all corporate commitments in the name of the corporation.

In a business corporation, a shareholder owns property, which is represented by shares of stock. Specific rights ascribed to shareholders include:

- The right to vote for the election of directors.
- The right to a distribution of dividends from the corporation.

  ▪   The right to assets remaining upon liquidation of the corporation after payment of the corporation's debts.

The directors are elected by shareholders, and acting together, they have an overall responsibility for managing the corporation and its affairs. Typically, shareholders are entitled to one vote for each share they own. The board of directors may delegate some, all, or none of their management authority to particular officers, directors, or committees of the board of directors or to management.

Professional corporations: For medical practices, a professional corporation (PC) is a well-known choice. A PC allows the licensed professionals to practice as a corporation. When professionals gained the right to incorporate in the early 1970s, this form offered many tax benefits. However, over years of amendments to the tax codes, the professional corporations have lost their tax benefits. Earlier, the PCs also offered the advantage of saving into the retirement funds, which could be borrowed right back and invested in the business. However, several tax-saving plans are now available, and the PC does not offer much additional benefit.

In terms of liability, the PC does not offer any additional benefit. The purpose of allowing the professionals to incorporate was to provide them with tax benefits and not shield them from personal liability.

Except for certain brief periods in specifically limited circumstances, shares of stock in professional corporations cannot be transferred to an unlicensed individual. One instance might be when stock in the corporation is transferred to a shareholder's heirs upon his or her death, subject to the requirement that the stock be redeemed by the corporation or transferred to a licensed professional within a specific period of time.

Personal service corporations: Most professional corporations qualify as personal service corporations (PSCs) for federal tax purposes, provided that they also qualify under state law. To qualify as a PSC under Internal Revenue Service (IRS) rules, a professional corporation must be organized under state law and then pass two federal tests: the function test and the ownership test. The function test requires that substantially all (95 percent) of the business activities of the professional corporation involve services within specific occupations in the fields of health, law, engineering, accounting, actuarial science, consulting, or performing arts. The ownership test requires that substantially all the professional corporation's outstanding stock be held directly or indirectly by qualified people: (1) employees who are currently performing professional services for the corporation, (2) retired employees who did so prior to their retirement, or (3) their heirs or estates. If a professional corporation organized under state law does not qualify as a PSC, then it is treated as a general partnership for federal tax purposes.

PSCs are taxed like regular C corporations, but with a flat corporate tax rate of 35 percent rather than a graduated rate depending on the level of income earned. The PSC files a corporate tax return and also issues form K-1 to all shareholders/employees to show their individual shares of the corporation's profit or loss. Any income that is retained in the PSC is subject to the corporate tax rate, while any salaries paid to employees are considered tax-deductible business expenses. Like most small corporations, however, PSCs are likely to pay out all business income to shareholders in the form of salaries, bonuses, and fringe benefits, thus reducing corporate taxable income to zero.[6] Of course, the shareholders/employees still must pay personal income taxes on the income they receive.

Not-for-profit corporations or foundations: A not-for-profit organization is a group organized for purposes other than generating profit and in which no part of the organization's income is distributed to its members, directors, or officers. Nonprofit corporations are often termed "nonstock corporations." They can take the form of a corporation; an individual enterprise (e.g., individual charitable contributions); unincorporated association, or partnership, foundation (distinguished by its endowment by a founder, it takes the form of a trusteeship); or condominium (joint ownership of common areas by owners of adjacent individual units incorporated under state condominium acts). Nonprofit organizations must be designated as nonprofit when created and may only pursue purposes permitted by statutes for nonprofit organizations. Nonprofit organizations include churches, public schools, public charities, public clinics and hospitals, political organizations, legal aid societies, volunteer services organizations, labor unions, professional associations, research institutes, museums, and some governmental agencies.

Nonprofit entities are organized under state law. For nonprofit corporations, some states have adopted the Revised Model Nonprofit Corporation Act (1986). For nonprofit associations, a few states have adopted the Uniform Unincorporated Nonprofit Association Act (see Colorado §§ 7-30-101 to 7-30-119). Some states exempt nonprofit organizations from state tax and state employment programs, such as unemployment compensation contribution. Some states give nonprofit organizations immunity from tort liability (see Massachusetts law giving immunity to a narrow group of nonprofit organizations), and other states limit tort liability by enacting a damage cap. State law also governs solicitation privileges and accreditation requirements, such as licenses and permits. Each state defines nonprofit differently. Some states make distinctions between organizations not operated for profit without charitable goals (like a sports or professional association) and charitable associations in order to determine what legal privileges the respective organizations will be given.

For federal tax purposes, an organization is exempt from taxation if it is organized and operated exclusively for religious, charitable, scientific, public safety, literary, and educational purposes, as well as for the purpose of preventing cruelty to children or animals, and/or developing national or international sports. Social security tax is also currently optional, although 80 percent of the organizations elect to participate.

Not all states allow not-for-profit corporations to employ licensed professionals or to deliver services through licensed professionals. The states that do permit not-for-profit corporations to engage in this type of activity treat these organizations as a form of professional corporation.

This type of organization, sometimes called a foundation, is the only kind that qualifies for exemption from federal income tax. While currently there are over 30 types of not-for-profit organizations classified as exempt from federal taxes, the most preferred type is the 501 (c)(3) charitable designation. To qualify as a tax-exempt organization, consult the Internal Revenue Code (www.irs. gov/taxpros/article/0,,id=98137,00.html). Generally, the community health centers fall under this category. In order to qualify, a community health center would be required to demonstrate, among other requirements, a charitable purpose (which may include the delivery of medical services on a free or part-pay basis) or an educational or research purpose. In addition, the not-for-profit corporation must also show that "no part of its net earnings inure to the benefit of any private shareholder or individual."[7] This provision requires that employee salaries be limited to reasonable amounts for services actually rendered. Usually, this is achieved by a governing board, instead of the officers planning and approving salaries and benefit packages.

Limited liability companies: A rather new form of legal entity — a limited liability company (LLC) — has emerged, and all states have adopted LLC statutes. The enabling acts, which authorize the formation and operation of the new entity, combine the best attributes of corporations and partnerships into a single entity. LLCs are formed by filing articles of organization with a state corporate commission like a corporation. Owners are referred to as "members" and, unlike S corporations, there is no limit on the maximum number of members an LLC may have. An S corporation (subchapter S corporation) is a firm that has elected to be taxed as a partnership under the subchapter S provision of the Internal Revenue Code. Of course, the attractive element of the LLC is that there is no personal liability for contract or tort liabilities.

There is a great deal of flexibility as far as management options go, such as a corporate form of management with officers and directors or a partnership form of management with a single class of members. Furthermore, members may customize their operating agreement, such as adoption of a partnership model with disproportionate distributions of cash or property and special allocations of nontaxable income and loss. It is equally possible to adopt a corporate model with common and/or preferred classes of membership interests.

From the tax standpoint, LLCs are considered partnerships for federal and state tax purposes. This enables the income/loss results to pass through to individual members, thereby eliminating the double taxation effects of the corporate form of organization. Other tax advantages realized from the LLC form make it more desirable than S corporations and limited partnerships.

ORGANIZATIONAL STRUCTURES

The pressures of regulation, environment, medical technology, and incentives have been the driving forces behind the formation of physician medical groups. Since their inception, these groups have shown a capability to combine separate, but functionally interrelated, delivery components into a unified whole. The cohesiveness makes possible a defined system for delivering efficient, effective healthcare.

Several important advantages are associated with forming medical groups. These include:

1. Achieving economies of scale by optimizing the use of resources such as space, staffing, and utilities and spreading the cost of operations to a larger patient base.

2. Diversifying the scope of services to multiple specialties. This helps capture greater market share, ensures a minimum referral base for the specialists, and diversifies revenue streams.

3. Engaging in ancillary services, such as in-house laboratory and imaging services. In addition, the larger groups may be able to sustain ambulatory surgical centers.

4. Providing better access to care because groups with multiple streams of services can cater to multiple patient needs.

5. Implementing new technologies by developing better operational and management structures and better quality control and resource utilization.

6. Ensuring compliance with federal and state laws such as OSHA, labor laws, HIPAA privacy, and security laws, as larger groups are better equipped to do this.

7. Contracting with vendors for better pricing of goods and services because of their strength in numbers and market share.

8. Negotiating better reimbursement rates with payers, compared to smaller groups.

9. Marketing more effectively because bigger budgets and larger patient databases enable larger groups to market their services to a wider patient population, resulting in higher growth in revenue.

When investigating the kind of organization, the physicians must decide which legal entity will best meet their needs, lifestyle, and career goals. Commonly observed physician organizational structures are as follows:

1. Solo-physician practice
2. Group practice
   a. Single specialty
   b. Multispecialty
3. Hospital-owned physician practice
4. Staff-model health maintenance organization
5. Independent contractor
6. Locum tenens physician
7. Community health center

8. Medical cooperative
9. Accountable care organization

Solo-Physician Practice

A solo-physician practice, as the name suggests, is a single-physician practice. This differs from the business entity sole proprietorship, which may have more than one physician but only one physician owns the stock and other physicians may be employees or provide contracted services. A sole practitioner as the owner has all the responsibility and liability of the sole proprietorship. One has a small setup with the responsibility of managing the operations and meeting all regulatory needs. Solo physicians experience mostly the same advantages or disadvantages of a sole proprietorship. A solo physician may be a primary care physician or a specialist. This form of practice is slowly on the decline because of the pressures from the healthcare environment, insurance carriers, and runaway overhead costs of running the practice.

Group Practice

Group practices can be a single-specialty or a multispecialty practice. A single-specialty practice comprises two or more physicians providing a specific type of care, which may be primary care or a specialty. The advantages of single-specialty group practices are lower overhead costs because of economies of scale, increased financial security, and controlled lifestyle. As the names suggest, a single-specialty group practice offers a single type of service, whereas multispecialty practices offer services in multiple specialties.

Legally, the group practice may have any of the legal business entity forms, such a sole proprietorship, general partnership, limited liability partnership (LLP), LLC, PC, professional limited liability corporation (PLLC), or a business corporation. The responsibilities and liabilities of each partner will depend on the nature of the business entity, and the compensation will depend on the article of organization (in case of partnership) or article of incorporation (in case of a corporation).

The single-specialty groups have the advantage of focusing on what they do best and achieving an economy of scale better based on the need for similar resources. Because of nonconflict of interest with primary care or with other specialist groups, they are also able to optimize referrals. Single specialties may also have some leverage with insurance carrier fee negotiation because of the greater market share. However, since the single-specialty groups depend on outside referrals, they are at risk, especially in the current environment where medical groups are consolidating to form big groups and hospitals are largely acquiring solo physicians and medical groups, thereby shrinking the referral base.

Multispecialty group practices offer various types of medical care in one organization. Such groups may be situated in one or multiple locations, depending on the size and the types of services they offer. If the groups are large enough, they may add some ancillary services, such as laboratory, imaging, and physical therapy services. The overhead cost will generally depend on the size of the practice and the nature of services provided. The calls, compensation, and benefits will depend on the size of the group. The major advantage of multispecialty groups is that they generate enough internal referrals and are relatively immune to external forces of integration. However, this may also put them at a disadvantage because of the difficulty in getting referrals from outside physicians. Physician autonomy declines as the size of group increases.

Hospital-Owned Physician Practice

Because of declining reimbursements, hospitals are under pressure to find new streams of revenue and augment referrals. This has led to fierce competition for referrals for outpatient procedures and for filling hospital beds. In order to maintain a steady supply of referrals, hospitals have recently been buying private practices very aggressively by offering financial stability, better compensation benefits, and a better lifestyle. Since hospitals have larger negotiating power, they are able to get better rates with insurance carriers and pass on the benefits to the physicians while maintaining a loyal referral base.

Staff-Model Health Maintenance Organization

A staff-model health maintenance organization (HMO) is similar to large multispecialty group practices. The ownership of such organizations may belong to physicians or insurers. The physician-owned HMOs are things of the past. However, insurance-owned physician group models still exist in some parts of the country. In this model, the insurance owns the integrated healthcare delivery system that owns the hospitals and health centers. All physicians are employees of the HMO. Kaiser Permanente[8] is one such example. However, this model may reemerge because of the Patient Protection and Affordable Care Act passed on March 23, 2010.

Independent Contractor

Independent contractor physicians are generally contracted with a physician or a group to provide specific services. There has to be a contract between the physician group and a contracted physician regarding the term of contract, the scope of services, and the compensation formula. The contracted physician generally has no decision-making ability with the group and limited autonomy since he or she must perform as per the terms of the contract.

The group that contracts with the contracted physician or group should also have a business associate agreement in place because of access to patient information. Also, if there is an expectation of referrals for ancillary services, the law looks at these arrangements very closely. The compensation cannot be based on the number of referrals generated by the physician contractor. For example, a contracted physician may not be compensated based on the number of procedures the physician will perform at the ambulatory surgical center owned by the physician group. This will run afoul of the anti-kickback statute.

Locum Tenens Physician

A locum tenens is an alternative to more permanent employment. Locum tenens offers physicians the opportunity to work in a practice or an area for a short period of time, from a few weeks up to a year. Not infrequently, the pay rate is higher than for the permanent position. Such physicians operate on per diem terms and may work on their own or through larger organizations. A locum tenens arrangement is common in anesthesiology. Coverage is generally needed to cover the absence of the regular anesthesiologist in smaller ambulatory surgical centers.

Community Health Center (CHC)

CHCs are not-for-profit organizations that receive funding from a variety of sources to provide family-oriented primary and preventive healthcare, outreach services, and dental care to uninsured, underinsured, and special populations in medically underserved areas. Known as "safety net providers," CHCs exist in areas where economic, geographic, or cultural barriers limit access to primary healthcare for substantial portions of the population. A large number of patients served by CHCs live below the poverty level, and without this safety net, the vast majority of these people would not receive even basic healthcare or dental services.

Initially conceived and funded under the Public Health Service Act, CHCs continue to receive Section 330 grants from the U.S. Department of Health and Human Services (HHS), Bureau of Primary Health Care (BPHC). Additional support is received through funding from state and local government grants and contracts, as well as through patients and third-party payers, such as state Medicaid programs, Medicare, commercial insurance, and managed-care organizations.

Medical Cooperative

Medical cooperatives are consumer run, nonprofit organizations. Generally the cooperatives are integrated healthcare delivery systems and have the authority to contract reimbursement rates with the insurance carriers to provide healthcare delivery in a demographic area. The American Recovery and Reinvestment Act of 2009 encourages the formation of such medical cooperatives.[9]

Accountable Care Organization

The Patient Protection and Affordable Care Act[10] requires the Centers for Medicare & Medicaid Services (CMS) to develop and establish within CMS an instrument to research, develop, test, and expand innovative payment and delivery arrangements. One such innovation is an accountable care organization (ACO). ACOs will be responsible for containing the cost and improving the quality of care received by patients and will receive a share from the savings the organization will earn for the Medicare program. The HHS secretary developed a national, voluntary pilot program encouraging hospitals, doctors, and post-acute providers to improve patient care and achieve savings through bundled payments. A new demonstration program for chronically ill Medicare beneficiaries will test payment incentives and service delivery systems using physician and nurse practitioner-directed home-based primary care teams.

MEDICAL GROUP GOVERNANCE

Governing a small medical group is similar in many instances to operating a small business; the only difference is that physicians generally fill two roles: They are the owners and also the primary providers of services. The complexity of governance increases with the number of physicians, the diversity of services provided, the number of locations, and the overall size of the group. As the size grows, the hierarchical structures become more complicated. As the number of physicians in the group increases, a need arises for governing bodies, medical directors, and group practice administrators. With more growth, the role of the financial manager emerges, and responsibility for the financial management of the group's affairs becomes vested in one individual: the physician executive, the practice administrator, or a chief financial officer (CFO).

As groups get bigger, professional administrators may take over almost every management task and influence major policies and decisions through their knowledge of healthcare-industry practices, insurance and reimbursement complexities, and legal issues. As the group continues to grow, it becomes necessary for physicians to leave administrative complexities to a full-time, nonphysician administrator. However, the physicians continue to provide leadership, and the group functions based on the physician leaders' mission and long-terms goals. The governance is remarkably different in medical groups that assume the business entity-type of corporation, particularly a C corporation.

The governing body is very important in ensuring appropriate control over day-to-day activities and long-term planning. The adopted structure affects the processes of managing the organization. In ambulatory care organizations, for example, the legal structure of the practice can be important from both the practice and operating points of view. The legal entity is often related to important practice considerations, such as liability for personal injury, retirement plans, and taxation.

When groups are formed independently of other institutions, it is necessary to have the appropriate legal documentation for that structure, such as a partnership agreement, articles of incorporation, and bylaws. This documentation clarifies the role of the governing body, shareholders, directors, and managers. The duties and responsibilities of the governing body must be carefully and comprehensively specified, and procedures for the election, meeting, and documentation of the governing body or partners' major policy decisions must be ensured. In addition, the governing body should hold regular meetings, review the bylaws and other governing documents periodically, establish working committees to facilitate various responsibilities (such as physician compensation), prescribe roles for the chairperson of the governing body, and decide on the election and removal of the chairperson.

In a partnership, an executive committee may be elected to fulfill the role of a governing body, while in corporations, the shareholders or an elected board of directors may constitute the governing body. Also, the board of directors may decide to delegate the major governance responsibilities to an executive committee made up of board members.

Ultimate responsibility for defining and monitoring the successful fulfillment of the practice's goals and objectives rests with the governing body, regardless of the form it may assume. The responsibility should be related to patient care services, community relations, short- and long-term planning, outreach services, financial success, and other appropriate objectives set by the group.

Even though the governing body has the final responsibility for all operations, it frequently delegates operating tasks to a physician executive and or a nonphysician executive. The physician executive is generally responsible for establishing practice protocols, clinical policies, and procedures, as well as supervising the quality of care, appointing the medical staff, selecting and approving medical staff officers, and developing or modifying the rules and regulations of the medical staff. The nonphysician executive is responsible for the administration and operations of the group. In smaller groups, the governing body lays down the policies and procedures, while an administrator is responsible for running the day-to-day operations of the group. Physicians are generally independent in following their own clinical judgment for patient care without any hindrance or guidance.

In the area of financial management, the governing body oversees the success of the practice in terms of financial viability, profitability, or the equivalent for a not-for-profit practice and other indicators of financial stability. In a successful organization, the governing body should set financial goals for the practice and monitor the practice's progress in achieving them.

Good communication is the centerpiece of a strong and positive culture in any organization. Both formal and informal communication systems exist. Communication between the various levels of hierarchy generally presents policies and procedures, changes, and updates. These are in writing, in the form of memos or policy papers. Informational messages may be in the form of e-mails or posted on bulletin boards.

MAJOR ACCOUNTING AND FINANCE FUNCTIONS

Successful management of any medical group practice requires the establishment of a sound financial management system. A practice's financial viability depends on an accurate accounts receivable (A/R) and accounts payable system, payer and vendor contracting, accounting/bookkeeping, managing cash flow, data analysis, benchmarking, financial reporting, strategy planning, and investing. In addition, a practice needs to set up bank accounts that meet the needs of the practice and choose the type of accounting system the practice will adopt between cash accounting and accrual accounting.

Banking

The practice's first step is to set up business accounts in a bank. The bank branch should be close so that making deposits takes minimal time. The bank will require articles of organization for a partnership and articles of incorporation for a corporation. Sole proprietors will just need a copy of their "doing business as" (DBA) registration certificate from the city. The bank will go through the application process before the account is finally set up. Banks offer multiple types of accounts. The group should perform due diligence to see what types of accounts meet their financial needs and the fee charged for the accounts. If not set up properly, the bank fee could run into hundreds of dollars each month.

An ideal bank account should have unlimited deposit and check-writing capability without incurring bank fees and should also pay some interest on the revolving balance that remains with the bank. In addition, the bank should provide credits for the revolving balance to offset the cost of supplies, such as checks and deposit slips. No single bank can accomplish all this. Therefore, one may have to open at least a couple interlinked accounts to achieve this goal. For example, a money market account normally allows unlimited deposits. For writing checks, one will need a checking account, which normally provides limited check-writing ability. Therefore, a group should develop a smart payment system and utilize credit cards for payment where possible. This will reduce the need to write checks.

Credit Cards

The medical practice will need to set up business credit cards in order to pay some vendors and also for sundry purchases for everyday needs directly from stores. Various types of cards are available these days; some offer miles that can be used for executives' travel and others provide cash back. Some credit cards have annual fees, while others do not charge any fee. The group should look at its needs and determine the right card for them. The process is relatively simple in small groups and gets complicated as the business gets bigger.

Remote Deposits

These days, most banks offer remote deposits for checks, which allow you to avoid writing deposit slips and making trips to the bank, and help get money into the bank faster.

Electronic Deposits

Most major insurance carriers offer electronic deposits, and some carriers have made this mandatory. Medicare allows paper checks only under some exceptions. This is to the medical practice's advantage since it considerably shortens the revenue cycle and also saves the time required to make deposits.

Credit Card Merchant Services

Depending on the group's size, it will need to set up merchant service accounts in order to accept credit card payments. This helps with the timely collection of copays and deductibles. Setting up merchant accounts requires some negotiating ability, since the rates vary from one merchant to the other, and there is always room for negotiation.

Accounting Software

Several software brands are available that cater to the different needs of diverse users. Accountants require the data to be sent to them as backup files that they can open on their end and work on. Therefore, the medical practice should consult with its accountants on the products they use for compatibility. Common brands[11] in the market are listed below in no particular order of preference:

- Sage Peachtree Accounting
- QuickBooks Pro
- Bookkeeper
- AccountEdge

Bookkeeping

Bookkeeping is an important part of accounting. Basically, it means recording the payments received for services rendered, paying bills, and reconciling receipts and payments to the bank accounts. In solo practices, this function may be performed by the doctor or a family member. For a small group, normally the office manager performs this function. As the group gets bigger, more specialized employees assume the role. Very large groups and corporations have a chief financial officer to oversee the functions of a large accounting department. A new startup will need bookkeeping operations that include the following setup:

Vendor center: A new startup bookkeeping operation will need a vendor center. Vendor names, addresses, and contact information must be correctly recorded since this will be used to write checks and make payments. Each vendor will need to be linked to the type of expense from the accounts list.

Chart of accounts: Each payment needs to be linked to the nature of the expense. A chart of accounts is the listing of accounts into various categories of expense. The list below provides a sample of what the chart of accounts may look like, though it is not exhaustive. Appropriate allocation of expenses to the chart of accounts is important for running management reports. This will show how much is being spent on each product or service purchased. Your accountant or the bookkeeper will set up the chart of accounts if you do not have a background in bookkeeping.

- Cleaning
- Dues and subscriptions

- ▨ Insurance
  - – Health insurance
  - – Liability insurance
  - – Property insurance
- ▨ Maintenance
- ▨ Payroll expense
  - – Salary and wages
  - – Medicare tax
  - – Social Security tax
  - – Federal Unemployment Tax (FUTA)
  - – State unemployment tax
- ▨ Phones
- ▨ Professional fees
  - – Accountants
  - – Lawyers
- ▨ Rent
  - – Base rent
  - – Operational expense
  - – School county tax
- ▨ Supplies
  - – Medical supplies
  - – Office supplies

Accounts payable: Payment of bills is popularly known as accounts payable. The person responsible reviews the invoices for accuracy and matches these with packaging slips (for goods purchased) or proposals for services to ensure the accuracy of payments. Care should be taken to avoid duplicate payments because of duplicate invoicing. The checks should clearly list the vendor's business account number and the invoice number so that proper credit may be applied. Depending on the practice's needs and utilization, payments to most vendors can be made online to save on the cost of supplies and postage. Some payments can also be made with credit cards.

Payroll: Payroll is a type of accounts payable where the employer pays employees' wages after withholding the taxes. Solo physicians or small groups may do their own payroll, but then they are also responsible for payroll taxes, and that could be a hassle. These days, a number of banks offer payroll services at a nominal cost. This takes a lot of responsibility away from smaller groups.

- ▨ Employee deductions:
  - – FICA (Federal Insurance Contribution Act) tax, which includes Social Security (6.2 percent) and Medicare tax (1.45 percent). The taxable income for the Social Security tax for year 2012 was $110,000. There is no such cap for Medicare contributions. The employer contribution totals 7.65 percent. The employee contributes the same amount.
  - – Federal and state income taxes, depending on the deductions claimed on form W-4.

- The law requires certain minimum disability insurance for each W-2 employee. The disability insurance carrier requires the employer to fill out a worksheet that will determine the percentage of disability benefit that will be taxable. The employer will make payroll deductions from employees based on this worksheet.
- The other deductions may include health insurance, disability insurance, 401K contributions, and so on.

■ Employer liabilities:

Employers have certain payroll liabilities, too. These are in the form of taxes and contributions. Some of the major ones are as follows:

- FICA taxes (as noted above)
- Federal and state unemployment tax
- Other miscellaneous taxes that may be imposed by states from time to time, such as the commuter tax for New York City and certain nearby areas.

Cash receipts: Recording the cash receipt is a bookkeeping function. However, a lot goes into providing services and getting the money in the bank. This includes charge entry for services, claims transmission, payments receipt, payments posting, working on A/R, and transferring claims. One example is the preauthorization of services before they are provided to avoid claim denials. The entire process is known as revenue cycle management, and it is the function of the billing department. The billing department may comprise one person (sometimes even the physician himself or herself) or a large department consisting of many employees, each performing a specialized function.

MAJOR DRIVERS OF FINANCIAL INFORMATION

A financial report is only as good as the information entered into the books. A financial report should answer the following questions:[12]

1. How much profit is the practice making?
2. How many assets and liabilities does the practice have?
3. How well is the practice making use of the capital investment?
4. What is the cash flow for a given period of the revenue cycle?
5. Did the practice reinvest any profits?
6. Does the practice have adequate funds for future growth?

The management of a medical practice requires current and relevant financial information. The information is needed for the following reasons:

■ Estimating profit (or loss) from the practice operations
■ Determining income distribution to the partners
■ Cost reporting, benchmarking, and cost control
■ Filing income tax returns
■ Providing information for creditors in case the practice needs to raise capital

- ■ Collecting information for financial planning and budgeting
- ■ Assessing and managing risk
- ■ Informing decision making for short-term and long-term goals

Estimate of Profit and Loss

An estimate of profit and loss is necessary for a number of reasons. Most importantly, the information tells the owners about the health of the practice, whether the revenue is going up or down, and if the cost of doing business is increasing or decreasing. Such information at the end of the year will show the overall performance for the year and the profit or loss for the practice. Employers will use this report to determine whether the staff will get raises and year-end bonuses. Contributions to the profit-sharing plans will also be determined based on the profit generated for the year, since these are at the discretion of the employer, as opposed to 401K plans where some contributions may be mandatory under safe harbor plans.

Income Distribution to the Partners

The information provided by profit and loss statements each month will determine the net profit that can be distributed. The actual distribution will, however, be determined based on the partnership agreement if it is a partnership. In the case of corporations, the profit generated by the corporation will be distributed based on the articles of incorporation. The practice may retain some income to maintain cash flow. Some groups distribute a uniform amount each month based on historical data and then reconcile quarterly or even annually as dictated by the necessity. Various MGMA-ACMPE publications provide information on physician salaries and compensation agreements. The administrators and financial officers should take full advantage of these resources.

Cost Reporting, Benchmarking, and Cost Control

The accounting system gathers information on the vendor payments and the nature of the cost. When recorded accurately, the reports will provide information on the nature of the expenses for each month. For example, it will provide information on the percentage of cost resulting from the payroll, rent, medical and office supplies, cleaning and biohazard waste disposal, and other sundry expenses. This helps create internal benchmarks to see how the cost varies from month to month and from year to year. The data can also be used to compare with industry standards to see how the practice measures up against other similar practices in the area. MGMA-ACMPE reports provide a wealth of information that helps practices point to the areas that require more effective monitoring to control cost. For example, if the salaries and wages as a percentage of practice expense are higher compared to other similar practices, the employers would know that better operational efficiencies are needed to control the payroll expense.

Information for Tax Filing

All for-profit organizations are required to file annual tax returns. In addition, the partners are required to file tax estimates quarterly and make advance tax payments. An accurate estimate of income, profit, and loss requires appropriate entry of payments and receipts. Such expenses and income can be recorded in two ways:

Cash basis: Under cash basis, revenue is recognized when the payment is received. Similarly, the expense is recorded when the bill is actually paid.

Accrual basis: Under accrual basis, revenue is recognized when the service is provided to the patient (regardless of when cash is collected), and expenses are recognized when the invoice is generated by the vendors (regardless of when the cash is paid).

The following example will clearly illustrate the difference between cash and accrual accounting: For the services provided in January 2012, if the payments are received in February, the income will be recorded for February in cash accounting, whereas in accrual accounting, the revenue is recorded when the services were provided, that is, for January. Similarly, in accrual accounting, an expense is recorded when the supply is ordered even though the invoice may be paid in 30 to 90 days, depending on the payment terms. In cash accounting, however, the expense is recognized when payment is actually made.

There are pros and cons of each accounting system. For medical practices, recording income before the cash is actually received could be misleading because of payment uncertainty. This also advances the tax liability. Compared to other businesses, physicians are not allowed to write off uncollected fees as bad debts, and therefore, recording revenue ahead of payments could have serious tax consequences. To avoid problems with the IRS, most medical practices adopt the cash accounting method.

Accrual accounting offers some benefit if the information is needed for the creditors. This system inflates the revenues. In addition, accrual accounting could be useful if the practice accurately records A/R after discounting based on each individual insurance fee schedule and all accounts payable when the liability is incurred, including the payroll. This form is then used for management reports because the reports clearly indicate the cash expectations and liabilities. These two bases of accounting will be explained in greater detail in chapter 3.

Information Required by Creditors

The creditors, such as banks, that advance large capital for practice growth, expansion, and diversification needs require the practice to provide financial information to ensure the group's credit worthiness. Even the vendors that supply large ticket items, and even if the payments will be made each month, would like to know if the group has enough cash flow for making timely payments. For example, for a large oncology group, the bill for drugs could run into millions of dollars each month. A payment default of even one to two months could set the vendor back by millions of dollars, and the practice may file for bankruptcy before the vendor even becomes aware.

The information generally required by creditors includes profit and loss statements, cash flow statements, balance sheets, latest A/R reports, and income tax returns from the previous year. The extent of the information needed will depend on the amount of the loan being requested. In most cases, where the loan amount is large, the creditors will want the owners' personal guarantee, and the owners will be required to provide personal financial information. Creditors are also known to have the owners sign off on a lien on the practice's A/R just in case the practice defaults on payments.

Assessing and Managing Risk

The major concern of any business is its ability to maintain its profitability, and this, too, is the case with medical practices. Like the famous line "Show me the money!" from the movie *Jerry Maguire,* the financial statements show exactly where the money is and help evaluate and manage the financial risk. A major concern for administrators is to maintain cash flow so they can pay the liabilities in a timely manner. One may have substantial cash at the end of the month but not necessarily when the bills are due or when it is time to do the payroll. Cash flow statements show when and how much money will be available. This helps answer questions such as, "How much money did I spend on supplies last month? Do I have the ability to pay on the due date? Is there any expectation of large cash outflow as with malpractice insurance?" Financial statements help answer all these questions, which are important aspects of financial risk analysis, and manage it by catering for cash as needed.

Information for Financial Planning and Budgeting

When recorded accurately, the financial reports provide a wealth of information in terms of the medical practice's financial activities, which can be utilized to plan for the future. For example, the report will help create a budget for the upcoming year, help allocate resources for each activity, and prepare for future activities. Large profits may motivate the practice owners to set aside some funds for improvements, diversification, addition of new services, and investment in technology, or even save for future growth and avoid borrowing.

For solo practitioners and small groups, the process of financial planning is relatively simple unless the physician has goals for major expansion and diversification. For larger groups, a complex system of planning exists. For example, a group operating in multiple locations will need to evaluate the productivity of each center, see what center is more profitable, and take corrective action for the location that is incurring a loss. The practice may want to close an office if it sees no potential for income or fails to turn it around to generate profits.

Similarly, a multispecialty group would like to see what specialty is generating more profits and may want to focus greater effort on expanding the services that contribute more to revenue. Likewise, the group may want to integrate or add services that provide upstream referrals for services that generate more profit.

The planning process may include the following steps:

- Begin with a formal statement of short-term and long-term goals;
- Develop budgets for the next year, which include a cost budget, revenue budget, and then master budget;
- Allocate resources based on the budgets;
- Establish strategic planning based on practice decisions; and
- Initiate decision making.

Most small groups have limited financial planning; however, as the activities become more complex and group size increases, planning and control systems become more formalized. This evolution is also important in view of capitated contracts offered by many HMOs. Knowing average per patient costs will help in negotiating contracts with such payers. This helps mitigate the risk of entering into loss-making contracts.

Medical group leaders may have short-term and long-term goals, and accordingly, they may have short-term and long-term plans. MGMA-ACMPE's *In Practice Blog*[13] provides a concise explanation of short-term and long-term planning.

Short-term planning: Short-term plans generally involve small changes in how things are done and are not capital intensive. For example, using dictation software will eliminate the cost of transcriptions and reduce overall cost. Another example may be using an auto-attendant for the phone system that will eliminate the need for a switchboard secretary.

Long-term planning: Long-term plans generally revolve around growth (capacity expansion) and diversification. While the growth is geared toward capacity expansion for the same services in the same location or expanding the same service into a new market, diversification involves adding new services. Since any such activity will involve the need for additional resources, the practice must analyze the cost of doing so, compare this to the expected returns, estimate return on investment (ROI), and determine the opportunity cost.

The cost associated with providing services has two components: the variable cost and the fixed cost. Small changes in volume may only impact the variable cost, such as the cost of supplies, and fixed cost may remain the same. Small growth without increasing the fixed cost helps improve utilization of capacity and resources. However, the increase in growth over a certain point may result in the need for capacity expansion, and that leads to increases in fixed cost. This may include an increase in staffing, renting additional space, buying new equipment, and so on.

In many medical practices, a wide range of activity can occur before some of the fixed costs move up to a higher level. Such an increase in cost is referred to as step-fixed cost. For example, a practice may have the capacity to see 30 patients per day, and the number increases to 40 patients a day due to an intensive marketing program. This may only increase the variable cost, and the practice utilizes the spare capacity to optimize the use of its resources. However, because of the addition of a new physician, the patient visits per day go up to 60. This will require additional staffing and equipment. The cost increase for procuring these resources is called a step-fixed cost. This cost will again remain constant within a certain range before there is another increase in step-fixed cost. Chapter 11 presents more details on these types of decisions.

Decision Making

Decision making is the final step in financial management. Having reviewed the finances, strategic plans, the expected ROI, and opportunity cost, the practice leaders make decisions, which may be short-range or long-range decisions, and these coincide with short-term plans and long-term plans. For a small group, the process is simple, and the physicians make decisions based on short-term and long-term goals. The process is more complex in larger groups or corporations where different committees may be involved.

Short-range decisions: Short-range decisions generally do not require extensive resources and can be achieved within normal budget and cash flow. For example, the practice decides to add a patient portal to the EHR. The cost of doing so is limited and is achievable within the normal cash flow. Or the practice decides to replace a couple old computers or hire an additional employee for managing A/R.

Long-range decisions: Long-range decisions revolve around a practice's mission, vision, and long-term goals. These are made after extensive planning and cost and benefit analysis. Such decisions may involve capacity expansion and diversification. Major renovations or moving to a new location may be part of these decisions to expand or diversify. Chapter 14 will cover more details on long-range decisions.

INTERNAL CONTROL

Effective management of a medical group requires effective management of its resources. And since all resources come at a cost, effective financial management is the key to the overall management of the medical group. The goal of financial management is to ensure increases in shareholder value by increasing profits, which means proper management of resources, A/R, and accounts payable. Monitoring of these activities comes through adequate internal controls.

Monitoring of financial activities is needed to:

- Ensure proper utilization of resources and promote efficiency
- Reduce the risk of asset loss through theft or pilferage
- Ensure the reliability of financial reporting
- Ensure compliance with laws and regulations

In 1992, in response to the needs of its senior executives, the Committee of Sponsoring Organizations of the Treadway Commission developed the *Internal Control—Integrated Framework*[14] for effective ways to better control their enterprises and to help ensure that organizational objectives related to operations, reporting, and compliance are achieved. This document, most widely used as an internal control framework by businesses in the United States and numerous countries around the world, provides principles-based guidance for designing and implementing effective internal controls. The internal control framework may be adapted for medical group management.

What Is an Internal Control?

Internal control is a process, implemented by an organization's governing body, management, and other personnel to provide reasonable assurance that objectives are achieved in the following areas:

- Effectiveness and efficiency of operations
- Reliability of financial reporting
- Compliance with applicable laws and regulations

The first area addresses a medical group's basic objectives, which include delivery of quality healthcare services, keeping the overhead cost low, safeguarding resources, and maintaining profitability. The second area relates to maintaining accuracy of financial records that will provide reliable financial reports, which will be used by the group leaders for making important short-term and long-term decisions. The third area deals with complying with federal, state, and local regulations to which the group is subject. Accurate reports are necessary to comply with several regulations. For example, form 5500 needs to be submitted by the group if there is a 401K plan in place, and some reports are required for workers' compensation insurance and for disability, and payroll taxes need to be paid in a timely manner.

The *Internal Control—Integrated Framework* report describes internal control as consisting of five interrelated components derived from the way management operates a business. The extensiveness of implementing various components will depend on the size of the organization. As the organization gets bigger, the processes and components become more formal, but each organization can adapt these to their organizational needs.

1. **Control environment:** Establishing appropriate internal control mechanisms is part of a practice's efforts to reach high levels of accountability and professional ethics. The people and their attributes, such as integrity, ethical values, and competence, as well as the environment in which they operate are at the heart of any organization's success. This, along with the operating style of the group's leaders, their philosophy, the way they assign responsibility and delegate authority, and how they communicate the organization's mission and goals provide the building blocks for the control environment. Building strong core values creates a positive control environment in the organization.

2. **Risk assessment:** Medical groups face multiple threats from internal and external forces. From a financial standpoint, this could be the loss of data due to failure to back up, failure to preauthorize procedures leading to claim denials, loss of capitated contracts, a reduction in the fee schedule for services by the insurance carrier, or even the risk of an employee stealing the cash collected from the patients. Such incidents could impact cash flow and the ability to pay bills. Through internal controls, the management takes steps to mitigate this risk and keep these within acceptable levels.

3. **Control activities:** Control policies and procedures must be established and executed to reasonably ensure that actions to address the risks in achieving the entity's objectives are effectively carried out. In a medical organization, these activities include approvals, authorizations, verifications, reconciliations, reviews of operating performance, and security of assets. Even though the scope of control activities will depend on the size or the organization, even small groups must have some control activities.

4. **Information and communication:** Surrounding these control activities are information and communication systems that enable the entity's people to capture and exchange the information needed to conduct, manage, and control its operations. Pertinent information must be identified, captured, and communicated in a form and timeframe that enables people to carry out their responsibilities. Information systems produce reports containing operational, financial, and compliance-related information that make it possible to run and control the business. They deal not only with internally generated data, but also with information about the external events, activities, and conditions necessary to informed decision making and external reporting. Effective communication also must occur in a broader sense, flowing down, across, and up the organization. All personnel must receive a clear message from top management that control responsibilities must be taken seriously. They must understand their roles in the internal control system, as well as how individual activities relate to the work of others. They must have a means of communicating significant information upstream.

5. **Monitoring:** Internal control systems must be monitored periodically. This is a process that assesses the quality of the system's performance and ongoing activities over a period of time. Monitoring is necessary to ensure that the internal controls remain dynamic and prevent any system failure. The monitoring may be done during the normal course of operations or through special evaluations or audits or a combination of both.

There exists a synergy and linkage among these five components of internal control, forming an integrated system that reacts dynamically to changing conditions. The internal control system is intertwined with the entity's operating activities and is most effective when controls are built into the entity's infrastructure, philosophy, and operations and is part of the essence of the enterprise, such as "this is how we do business." Such "built-in" controls in a medical group support quality of care and cost containment, and enable quick response to changing conditions.

What Internal Control Can Do

Internal control, therefore, can help a medical group achieve its performance and profitability targets and prevent loss of resources. It can help ensure reliable financial reporting and help the group comply with laws and regulations, avoiding damage to its reputation and other consequences. Thus, it can assist a group in getting where it wants to go and avoiding pitfalls and surprises along the way. Specific internal control procedures will be mentioned in later chapters when recordkeeping and various financial processes are covered.

What Internal Control Cannot Do

However tight the internal controls might be, they cannot determine the outcome of strategy plans and management decisions. If the decision is bad or the strategy is flawed, the outcome may not be as expected. At best, one can achieve optimal results with good internal controls even though the overall outcome will not be as expected.

SIGNIFICANT INDICATORS OF FINANCIAL PERFORMANCE

Determining the financial success of a medical practice on a continuing basis requires the preparation and dissemination of key financial reports. These financial reports are significant indicators that track progress toward the practice's goals and objectives. Any substantial changes to these reports without any foreknowledge of an event indicate a problem that may need immediate attention. The most common reports include revenue reports, collections and cash balances, operating statements, balance sheets, cost reports, A/R reports, special reports, and MGMA-ACMPE reports.

Revenue Reports

Daily, weekly, and/or monthly reports showing gross charges for the services rendered and payments received for services provided earlier are key indicators of operational activity. The breakdown of charges by physician, location (if the group has multiple locations), specialty, and types of insurance carrier provides the management with an overall picture of the practice's operations and identifies areas of strength and weakness. If the group follows budgets, comparing these actual performance reports with the budgeted amounts is useful and may necessitate mid-year corrections to the budget.

Collections and Cash Balance

A cash receipts report reflecting the types and sources of collections for each day is a valuable tool for managing cash. The report should also indicate the cash balance(s) available in the bank repository(ies). Sound cash management procedures call for a continuous forecasting of cash receipts and payments for the next several months. Thus, collection reports should be integrated with the cash forecasts to ascertain whether actual receipts and payments are tracking closely with predicted trends. Maintaining sufficient cash to pay for the recurring expenditures should be a dominant focus of a manager's daily activities.

Operating Statements

The operating statements, or income statements as they are commonly called, are financial statements that show the operating results of a particular period. The reports show earnings, expenses, and revenue for the period. Such operating reports will generally be run monthly, quarterly, and annually or as frequently as the medical group needs to keep track of its operations.

Balance Sheets

A statement of a company's assets, liabilities, and stockholder equity at a given period of time, such as the end of a quarter or year, is known as a balance sheet. A balance sheet is a record of what a company has and how it has come to receive it. A balance sheet is divided in two main sections, one that records assets and one that records liabilities and stockholder equity. The assets should generally equal the liabilities and stockholder equity because the latter are how the company paid for its assets. Examples of items recorded as assets include A/R, property, equipment, and so on. Examples of liabilities include accounts payable and long-term bonds.

Cost Reports

A vital aspect of running a successful practice is to deliver the highest quality medical services for the least possible cost. An important tool for assisting group management in reaching this objective is the collection of various cost reports that are meaningfully arranged to provide a picture of costs incurred throughout all phases of the practice operations.

The management would like to know how the resources of the group are being spent. Cost reporting is simple for small single-specialty groups and may not be any more than that derived from the profit and loss report. For larger groups, however, and especially those with multiple offices, it gets more complicated. Such reports will provide the following information:

- Direct cost attached to each procedure, specialty, location, and physician.
- Indirect cost that cannot be directly assigned to any particular group, activity, procedure, physician, or location. For example, the administrative cost to manage the entire group and the cost of billing are difficult to allocate to a single procedure, specialty, physician, or location.
- Cost comparison to the budgeted amounts or to the internal or external benchmarks.

Accounts Receivable Reports

Keeping track of A/R is like having a physician's finger on a patient's pulse. It provides vital information on the health of the medical practice. A monthly aging report shows exactly how much balance is due from each responsible party. The two important measures of A/R activity are days in A/R and A/R in each bucket of 0–30 days, 31–60 days, 61–90 days, 91–120 days, and more than 120 days. A/R days in receivable is calculated by dividing the total amount in A/R by the average daily charge. For example, if the average charges per day are $1,500, and the total amount in A/R is $150,000, then the practice has 100 days in A/R; that is, the practice has 100 days worth of charges in A/R.

The industry standard is to measure in 30-day increments as follows (note the percentage of accounts that might be expected to fall into each bucket based on median benchmarks for internal medicine from the MGMA-ACMPE):[15]

- 0–30 days: 65.47 percent
- 31–60 days: 13.45 percent
- 61–90 days: 6.13 percent
- 91–120 days: 11.49 percent

Special Reports

Special reports may be needed by the management to address certain issues, plan growth strategies, and benchmark outcomes. For example, a referring physician report comparison will show the referral pattern by each referring physician. Comparing the numbers to those in earlier periods will determine whether the referrals from particular physicians have declined. If so, the physicians may want to approach the doctor to see how the group could best serve that referring physician's needs. Similarly, a patient demographic report by zip code could indicate where most patients are coming from, and based on this, the group may like to open another office in an area where there is no patient base. Also, the practice may want to run a report by referral sources after an ad campaign to determine the effectiveness of its marketing effort.

MGMA-ACMPR Reports

Each year, MGMA-ACMPE publishes survey reports based on data collected from member medical groups' financial data. Some of these survey reports are discussed briefly. Additional information may be found at the MGMA-ACMPE Web site.

DataDive Cost Survey Module: The Cost Survey presents summary statistics of medical group practice revenues, expenses, and staffing information for each year. MGMA-ACMPE has conducted this survey for over 50 years. The MGMA-ACMPE 2011 DataDive Cost Survey Module presents data from more than 1,950 medical groups representing more than 43,000 providers — the largest provider population of any cost survey in the United States. The survey report for 2011,

Cost Survey: 2011 Interactive Report Based on 2010 Data, is currently being offered by MGMA-ACMPE. For more information, visit www.mgma.com/store/Surveys-and-Benchmarking/Cost-Survey-2011-Interactive-Report-Based-on-2010-Data-CD-Site.

This resource can be used for:

- ▨ Comparing cost data by category to identify possible improvement areas in a practice
- ▨ Determining how payer mix can affect a practice's bottom line
- ▨ Reviewing staffing costs compared to total revenue and other variables
- ▨ Using cost reduction to improve profitability — even in a sluggish economy

Procedural Profile Module of DataDive: DataDive is an online application that allows medical practices to analyze and compare physicians' procedural behavior with practices in the same specialty and region.

This resource can be used for:

- ▨ Recognizing significantly different coding patterns for individual providers:
  - – Compare your physicians' behavior with behavior in similar practices performing in the top quartile by work RVUs or collections
  - – Provide data to support physician education or behavior modification when deemed appropriate
  - – Infer the diversity of your patient mix compared to your peers (e.g., illness, age, complexity)
  - – Provide insight into potential new service lines
- ▨ Comparing your data internally will help you:
  - – Evaluate expense allocation and staffing ratios based on types of procedures performed, giving you the ability to correlate and allocate expenses appropriately
  - – Determine the complexity of your patients and the mix of procedures and how those impact patient access, scheduling, and resource allocation
- ▨ Data in this module include:
  - – Top procedures for your specialty, categorized by region and populations
  - – Top procedures by CPT chapters: surgery, medicine, E&M, anesthesia, laboratory, and radiology
  - – Coding profiles by level of compensation or level of production

Physician Compensation and Production Survey: MGMA-ACMPE's annual *Physician Compensation and Production Survey Interactive Report*, based on 2011 data from 59,375 providers in 2,846 groups, spotlights the critical relationship between compensation and productivity for providers.

The information can be used for:

- Evaluating physician and nonphysician provider performance through peer comparison
- Analyzing pay-level factors to assess physician compensation systems and set realistic compensation and production targets
- Estimating the potential impact of adding physicians
- Determining fair market value and assessing compensation methods for compliance
- Tracking provider compensation trends in specialties

Management Compensation Survey: The *Management Compensation Survey Report*, an annual census of medical group practice members, is a comprehensive guide to management compensation data. The survey report summarizes compensation, retirement benefit package, selected fringe benefits, and annual days off information for key administrative positions that range from entry-level managers to senior management and physician executives. Based on this survey data, organizations can compare compensation packages against those of other practices and structure competitive salaries and benefits.

Patient Satisfaction Comparison Survey (PSCS): Conducting patient satisfaction surveys in a medical practice can lend exceptional insight into how to improve quality, care, and referral rates. When performed thoughtfully and with adequate follow-up, the results of these surveys can immediately affect the way a medical practice does business. Satisfied patients are essential to a practice's continued success, no matter what the practice size, specialty, or location. The PSCS enables a medical practice to compare their practice with other service participants in terms of patient satisfaction. PSCS informs practices about the patients' views on:

- Waiting time
- Provider's personal manner
- Length of time spent with the provider
- Provider's technical skills
- Other key parts of the practice system

This tool also utilizes patient demographics such as age, gender, and education, as well as information about major medical conditions that the patient previously had or has now. MGMA-ACMPE partnered with the Response Division of HCIA, Inc., to provide the PSCS service.

Management Services Organization Benchmarking Survey: MGMA-ACMPE and Medimetrix Consulting jointly conducted the first comprehensive survey of management services organizations' (MSOs) financial and operational indicators. This survey report will help MSOs evaluate performance and compare selected operational and financial results against the emerging industry standards. A growing segment in healthcare integration, MSOs can assess how corporate performance is influenced by product portfolio, provider and corporate staffing levels, managed-care penetration, information system capabilities, and other demographic and operational circumstances.

To the Point

- Physicians generally fill two roles in medical groups: owners or principal stockholders and primary operators and deliverers of healthcare.

- Practice groups adopt various arrangements of organizational structure depending on their size, as well as the objectives and personalities of the individuals involved. Usually, there will be a governing body, such as a board of directors or an executive committee. The operations may be delegated to a physician executive/medical director who is responsible for the clinical and administrative affairs of the group. As the group grows larger, these two functions are divided, and separate individuals occupy each position. Eventually, the administrative function may be segregated into several areas, one of which will be headed by a financial manager.

- The selection of the legal structure depends on a variety of factors. The usual types of organizations are proprietorships, partnerships, corporations, limited liability companies, and not-for-profit organizations.

- Financial management operating systems assist in the management of the practice's financial viability. There are various subsystems, including a financial information system, that deal with financial planning and control.

- Most financial information systems evolve from a simple cash-basis system into a sophisticated computerized system. Enhancements are added to the system to provide information about production, productivity, costs, and bases for income apportionment.

- The major accounting and finance functions are cash collections and payments, A/R, accounts payable, payroll, and general accounting.

▪ There are five different needs for financial information that medical groups possess, many of which cannot be met by conventional financial statements:

1. Information required by law, such as income tax returns
2. Information required by contract, such as creditor agreements
3. Information for physicians' income distribution
4. Information for financial planning and control
5. Information for decision making, both in short-range and long-range orientations

▪ Internal control is a process that assists in keeping a medical group's activities on course toward its profitability and other goals, and in minimizing surprises along the way. Internal controls promote efficiency, reduce the risk of asset losses, and help ensure the reliability of financial statements and compliance with laws and regulations.

▪ Significant performance indicators are financial reports or statistics that denote whether or not progress is being made toward the practice goals and objectives. They are watched closely and frequently on a daily basis by the group's administrator and financial manager.

▪ MGMA-ACMPE publishes annual survey reports summarizing important medical group financial and clinical data for each year. These survey reports are:

– *DataDive Cost Survey Module*

– *Procedural Profile Module of DataDive*

– *Physician Compensation and Production Survey Report*

– *Management Compensation Survey Report*

– *Patient Satisfaction Comparison Survey*

– *Management Services Organization Benchmarking Survey*

REFERENCES

1. Hursh, D. 2008. "Choosing Your Medical Practice Entity." *Physicians' New Digest*. Retrieved from www.physiciansnews.com/business/908hursh.html. Accessed February 4, 2012.

2. AllBusiness.com. 2007. "Advantages and Disadvantages of Sole Proprietorship." Retrieved from www.nytimes.com/allbusiness/AB4113314_primary.html. Accessed February 4, 2012.

3. Eliot, V. S. 2010. "Sharing Your Space: Things to Consider When Looking for an Office Mate." Retrieved from www.ama-assn.org/amednews/2010/02/01/bisa0201.htm. Accessed February 5, 2012.

4. Laurence, Beth. n.d. "Learn about Business Ownership Structures." Retrieved from www.nolo.com/legal-encyclopedia/learn-about-business-ownership-structures-29785.html. Accessed February 5, 2012.

5. Free Dictionary by Farlex. n.d. "Piercing the Corporate Veil." Retrieved from legal-dictionary.thefreedictionary.com/Piercing+the+Corporate+Veil. Accessed February 8, 2012.

6. "Professional Corporations." n.d. *Reference for Business, Encyclopedia of Business, 2nd Edition*. Retrieved from www.referenceforbusiness.com/small/Op-Qu/Professional-Corporations.html. Accessed February 8, 2012.

7. Internal Revenue Service. 2005, October 17. "Notice of Proposed Rulemaking Standards for Recognition of Tax-Exempt Status if Private Benefit Exists or if an Applicable Tax-Exempt Organization Has Engaged in Excess Benefit Transaction(s)." *Internal Revenue Bulletin, 25*, 42. Accessed February 9, 2012.

8. Kaiser Permanente. 2012. "About Kaiser Permanente." Retrieved from http://xnet.kp.org/newscenter/aboutkp/index.html. Accessed February 11, 2012.

9. Davis, K. 2009. "Cooperative Health Care: The Way Forward." *The Commonwealth Fund*, June 22. Retrieved from www.commonwealthfund.org/Blog/Health-Cooperatives-The-Way-Forward.aspx. Accessed February 12, 2012.

10. DPCC. n.d. "Responsible Reform for Middle Class: Patient Protection and Affordable Care Act." Retrieved from http://dpc.senate.gov/healthreformbill/healthbill04.pdf. Accessed February 12, 2012.

11. TopTenReviews. 2012. "Accounting Software Reviews." Retrieved from http://accounting-software-review.toptenreviews.com. Accessed February 18, 2012.

12. Tracy, J.A., n.d. "The Purpose of Financial Reporting." *Dummies.com*. Retrieved from www.dummies.com/how-to/content/the-purpose-of-financial-reporting.html. Accessed February 18, 2012.

13. Medical Group Management Association. 2009. "Financial Decision-making Tips for a Profitable Medical Practice." *In Practice Blog*, November. Retrieved from www.mgma.com/blog/Financial-decision-making-tips-for-a-profitable-medical-practice. Accessed February 18, 2012.

14. Committee of Sponsoring Organizations. 1992. "Internal Control-Integrated Framework." Published by AIPCA. Retrieved from www.cosco.org/ic.htm. Accessed February 19, 2012.

15. Physicians Practice. 2008. "Days in A/R." *Physicians Practice.com*, June. Retrieved from www.physicianspractice.com/display/article/1462168/1627515. Accessed February 19, 2012.

CHAPTER 3

The Accounting Process and Accounting Systems

Edited by Daniel D. Mefford, CPA, MBA, FACMPE

After completing this chapter, you will be able to:

- Differentiate between the fields of accounting — financial and management.

- Explain the basic accounting process, including the analysis of transactions and identification of important accounting principles.

- Contrast the two bases of accounting and when each may best serve medical groups.

- Describe the general contents and structure of the basic financial statements.

- Summarize basic assumptions underlying financial statements and their qualitative characteristics.

- Recount the major data flows, information processes, and accounting subsystems used by a typical medical group.

- Define the role of the independent auditor and the purpose of audit reports and other accountants' reports.

The core discipline for supplying relevant and useful financial management information is accounting. This chapter presents a description of the accounting process and the two bases of accounting typically employed by medical practices. The content and structure of financial statements for conveying meaningful information about operations will be explained and illustrated. Important underlying assumptions and the generally accepted bases used in the accounting process will be summarized. The principal accounting subsystems, which capture and disseminate important information flows, will be described. Finally, the role of auditing and the purposes of various reports rendered as a result of this process will be covered.

ACCOUNTING — THE CHIEF DISCIPLINE OF FINANCIAL MANAGEMENT

Financial information to manage medical group operations comes from the accounting data and the accounting information system established to record and summarize all transactions affecting the practice. The information provided by accounting is useful for making informed judgments and decisions. Thus, accounting information is composed principally of economic data about business transactions, expressed in terms of money.

Accounting provides a conceptual framework for gathering economic data and the language for communicating these data to an organization's management and to individuals and institutions outside of that entity. As a result of accelerated economic growth and technological advances, a number of specialized fields in accounting have evolved. The two most important ones are financial accounting and management accounting.

Financial Accounting and Management Accounting

Financial accounting is concerned with the measurement and recording of transactions for a business entity and the periodic preparation of various reports from such records. These reports contain useful information about the organization's financial affairs. The basis upon which information is recorded and the manner in which it is reported is governed by a set of underlying concepts, assumptions, and standards, called generally accepted accounting principles (GAAP). The use of these principles assures the consistency and comparability of financial statements issued by enterprises.

The conventional financial statements emanating from financial accounting are the following:

- The operating statement or income statement
- The balance sheet or statement of financial position
- The cash flow statement, which shows sources and uses of cash for a period of time, such as a month, quarter, or year, and the resulting change in cash balance

Examples of all these statements will be presented later in this chapter.

Management accounting is concerned with the internal accounting information necessary for the planning and control of an entity's business and for making decisions. Management accounting employs both historical and estimated data in reports assembled for internal use. It overlaps financial accounting to the extent that management uses the financial statements or reports in directing operations and in planning future operations. However, management accounting goes beyond by providing additional information and reports for management that may not be in accordance with generally accepted accounting principles. The criterion for the adoption of management accounting principles is their usefulness to management. Examples of management accounting disciplines are budgeting and cost accounting. Management accounting reports usually contain more detailed information and do not have to follow the legal and GAAP requirements that apply to externally oriented financial statements. Both types of accounting — financial and management — are used in medical practices. While we have distinguished these two fields in this description, our treatment will be merged and will be referred to under the general reference of accounting.

BASIC ACCOUNTING PROCESS

Accounting Measurements

Cash basis accounting is used for many small businesses and, as stated previously, is the basis used by most medical practices. However, accounting rule-making bodies, which influence and develop accounting standards for application by businesses and professions, have concluded that GAAP requires the use of accrual basis accounting in audited financial statements bearing the unqualified opinion of a certified public accountant (CPA). However, for most purposes, particularly for internal financial reporting to managers and owners, medical practices do not normally need audited financial statements. Let's examine each of these bases more fully.

Cash Basis Accounting

Most medical groups use the cash basis of accounting for internal uses as well as for tax and, if needed, for external reporting. Recent MGMA-ACMPE surveys (see Exhibit 3.1) show that approximately 75 percent of all medical groups use

EXHIBIT 3.1 ■ Frequencies for Medical Group Variables

Internal accounting method	Count	Percent
Cash or modified cash	830	71.55%
Accrual	330	28.45%
Total	1,160	100.00%

Tax reporting accounting method	Count	Percent
Cash	866	74.91%
Accrual	290	25.09%
Total	1,156	100.00%

this basis for tax reporting and about 72 percent for internal reporting. This widespread use appears to have two reasons:

1. Preparation of an accrual set of financial statements involves substantial additional costs and expertise. Many practices may need to employ outside accountants and CPAs to convert cash-basis financial statements to accrual formats.

2. The cash basis is simple and easy to understand. With few exceptions, such as recording depreciation on long-lived assets, the accounting records, the checkbook, and the financial statements are consistent.

When the cash basis of accounting is followed, revenues are recognized (recorded in the records) when cash is collected, and expenses are recognized when cash is paid. Thus, cash-basis financial statements exclude accounts receivable (A/R), accounts payable, accrued expenses, deferred costs, and referred revenues related to operations. If a "pure" cash basis is used, all expenditures, including those for long-lived assets, supplies, and liability insurance premiums, are expensed when cash outlays are made to procure them. The balance sheet prepared on a "pure" cash basis would have only two items: (1) cash as the asset and (2) the owner's equity (ownership interest in the practice). However, as a practical matter, the "pure" cash-basis method is usually modified to record long-lived assets as well as payables and receivables relating to the borrowing and investing of cash. Thus, most groups that are not on the accrual accounting basis will follow a modified cash or income tax basis of accounting.

Accrual Basis Accounting

There is a movement by medical groups to adopt accrual basis measurements to evaluate financial performance in group practices. Accrual accounting provides a more accurate measurement of efforts expended to generate revenue if revenue is recorded when patient services are rendered rather than when payment is received for them. Such is the requirement of accrual accounting as the basis for revenue recognition — that is, to record revenue when services are performed or when purchased products are delivered. Similarly, measurement accuracy is enhanced under the rule of accrual accounting for expense recognition; that is, expenses are recorded when resources (assets) have been used up or consumed in the generation of patient revenue, regardless of when cash was expended to acquire those resources. Thus, under accrual accounting, cash receipts and cash payments do not govern the time period when revenue and expenses are recorded in the group's accounts. The delivery of patient services and the using up of resources are the determining points for revenue and expense recognition in accrual accounting.

As we have intimated, cash-basis accounting usually results in a mismatching of revenues and expenses among one or more accounting periods. No such mismatching occurs when accrual accounting is followed since revenues recognized for a period are matched with the best estimates of expenses consumed in producing that revenue. Groups that employ cash-basis measurements will find that monthly comparisons of operating results will be distorted. Thus, to have better reporting upon which to evaluate the performance of group practitioners, accrual measurements are being adopted for internal reporting purposes, while the cash basis is continued for income tax reporting.

Accrual Basis Transactions

A business transaction is the occurrence of an event or of a condition that must be reflected in the records of the business, for example, the payment of a $75 utility bill, the purchase of supplies for $380 on credit, or the acquisition of equipment for $50,000. These transactions are recorded in terms of money, which is the common denominator to achieve a uniform unit of measurement.

Resources owned and used by a business enterprise or professional practice are called assets. The rights or claims to these resources by the business or practice are referred to as liabilities or owners' equities.

The rights of creditors are represented by the obligations or debts of the business or practice and are called liabilities. The rights of owners are owners' equity. An expansion of the first equation to recognize the two types of equities would be:

$$\text{Assets} = \text{Liabilities} + \text{Owners' Equity}$$

This second equation is known as the basic accounting equation. It might also be restated as:

$$\text{Assets} - \text{Liabilities} = \text{Owners' Equity}$$

All business transactions, from the simplest to the most complex, can be stated in terms of the changes that occur in the three elements of the basic accounting equation. To determine the precise effect on the equation from a transaction, the event must be analyzed carefully with the objective of ascertaining which elements have been increased or decreased by that transaction. A fundamental truism, which forms the crux of the accounting recording process, is that all transactions are recorded so that the monetary total of the elements comprising the equation remain in balance after the amounts for each transaction have been reflected in the accounts.

An example of this process would be the initial investment in a medical practice. If the investment of $200,000 was obtained by borrowing $150,000 from a bank and using $50,000 of personal savings, the accounting records for the practice would record the transaction as follows:

$$\text{Assets} = \text{Liabilities} + \text{Owners' Equity}$$
$$\text{Cash} = \text{Notes Payable} + \text{Capital}$$
$$\text{increase} \quad \text{increase} \quad \text{increase}$$
$$\$200{,}000 = \$150{,}000 + \$50{,}000$$

Each transaction would be recorded in this fashion, with entries made to maintain the monetary balance of the three elements. That is, every entry(ies) on one side of the equality is offset by an entry(ies) of equal amount on the same or other side. Thus, the system of accounting is referred to as a double entry system. Note that all three major categories have many subcategories, such as cash, notes payable, and capital.

This method of recording transactions is presented with a much fuller treatment in the series of exhibits in Appendix 1–12 on pages 574–585, which show the various transactions completed by a newly formed medical group, The Denell Group, PC.

Examples of Transactions

Appendices 1, 2, 3, 7, 8, and 9 provide detailed examples of typical transactions. The accrual basis of accounting, used in Appendices 1, 2 and 3, provides a much more complete picture of the activities transpiring for the first three months of operation than the modified cash basis used in Appendices 7, 8, and 9. Note the construction of the transactions information, that is, the basic accounting equation:

$$\text{Assets} = \text{Liabilities} + \text{Stockholder's Equity}$$

Stockholder's Equity is broken down into Capital + Retained Earnings (a culmination of all prior revenue and expenses).

All transactions are recorded according to the double entry accounting rules to maintain the equality of the basic equation. This can be verified by equating the balances at the end of each month. With the exception of the note payable involved with the equipment purchase (transaction 2 in month 1), the only transactions entered into under the modified cash basis are those involving either the receipt or payment of cash. Under the accrual basis, many transactions each month show the recognition of revenue when it has been earned (services delivered), and the recognition of expenses when they have been consumed in generating revenue, regardless of when cash movements were involved.

BASIC FINANCIAL STATEMENTS

Earlier, the three basic financial statements — income statement, balance sheet, and the statement of cash flow — were described. The examples of transactions in Appendices 1–12 include these three statements developed from the transactional information for both the accrual and the modified cash basis. Appendices 4, 5 and 6 show the accrual basis and Appendices 10, 11, and 12 present the modified cash basis. The major points to consider about each of these statements are:

Income Statement

Income statements present the revenues for the period matched by the expenses incurred to produce those revenues. In comparing Appendices 5 (accrual basis) and 11 (modified cash basis), the following comments are relevant:

- ■ More revenue is reflected under the accrual basis than under the modified cash basis because of the difference in the timing of revenue recognition.

- ■ Similarly, the expenses under accrual accounting are greater than those under modified cash accounting, again due to the difference in expense recognition rules.

- ■ There is a dramatic difference in Income before Physician Salaries. Under accrual accounting, there is a net income amount each month, whereas under modified cash accounting, there are losses during the first two months and for the three months to date.

- ■ Physician salaries under accrual accounting seem to be based on Income before Physician Salaries, but under modified cash accounting, there is no apparent correlation between these two elements.

- ■ Note that these discrepancies in revenue and expense are due only to a difference in timing of the recognition of those financial statement elements.

Balance Sheet

The balance sheet presents a listing of all assets (resources) owned and used in the practice, all liabilities (debts or obligations) owed to outsiders and stockholders' equity, which represents the ownership interests in the practice. This statement embodies the basic accounting equation in its arrangement of Assets = Liabilities + Stockholders' Equity. Some interesting comparisons can be drawn by comparing the accrual balance sheets (Appendix) with the modified cash-basis balance sheets (Appendix):

- ■ At the end of each accounting period, the accrual assets include A/R, supplies, and prepaid insurance while the liabilities include accounts payable and interest payable. It should be noted that these accounts are excluded from the modified cash-basis counterparts. The inclusion of these elements shows the broader picture presentation in accrual based balance sheets. Both types of statements have the same elements of stockholders' equity: capital stock and retained earnings (but with differing amounts).

■ Note the decline in total assets under the modified cash assets, largely because there is no recognition of A/R (which is increasing under the accrual basis due to increasing patient revenues).

■ The accrual balance sheet provides a more accurate and complete portrayal of what actually happened during the first three months of the practice.

Cash Flow Statement

The cash flow statement presents a picture of the cash flows experienced by an organization during a time period. The statement reflects this information through a classification of three kinds of cash flow:

1. Cash provided (used) by operations
2. Cash provided (used) by investing
3. Cash provided (used) by financing

Both cash inflows and cash outflows are included in each of these three categories. Appendices 6 and 12 show the cash flow statement under the two bases of accounting. Note that they are the same since cash movements are identical under each of these bases. Some relevant comments about the Denell Group cash flow statement in Appendix 12 are:

■ Cash is being used by operations (as opposed to cash being provided by operations, which is the more desirable result) during all three months, largely because the physicians are withdrawing cash (as salaries), and cash received is less than cash paid for various expenses except physician salaries. Since the cash balance in the practice is declining, and if no new infusions of cash are made by the owners, cash will have to be obtained through borrowing or through additional investment by the physician owners.

■ The only other cash flows occurring during the three-month period are the initial investment of $100,000 in the practice, the purchase of equipment for $125,000, the borrowing via a note payable of $100,000, and the payment of $5,000 on the note.

IMPORTANT GENERALLY ACCEPTED ACCOUNTING PRINCIPLES UNDERLYING ACCRUAL BASIS ACCOUNTING

Accrual accounting is based on the set of standards called GAAP. Accounting principles have been developed by individuals and professional groups to help make accounting data more useful in an ever-changing society. Based on reason, observation, and experimentation, the principles represent guides for the achievement of desired results. As the complexity of business operations increases, these principles are continually reexamined and revised to keep pace with the changing environment. The criterion for determining an accounting principle is its acceptance by the users of financial statements.

Responsibility for the development of accounting principles has rested primarily with practicing accountants and accounting educators, working both independently and under the sponsorship of various accounting organizations. These principles are also influenced by business practices and customs, ideas and beliefs of stock exchanges, and other business groups. Presently, the dominant body in the development of GAAP is the Financial Accounting Standards Board (FASB). Created in 1973, it is an independent board comprised of CPAs, business executives, financial analysts, and educators. As problems in financial reporting arise, the FASB conducts extensive research to identify the principle issues involved and the possible solutions. After due deliberation, new standards are formulated and issued. These are then adopted by the financial and business community and become part of the continuing body of GAAP.

Some of the important GAAP guidelines used in practice for all businesses, including medical practices, are:

1. Assets and liabilities should be recorded at their initial cost, which is the value of the consideration given. Known as the historical cost principle, it forms a basic rule for recording acquisitions of assets and liabilities. Cost is used because it is a reliable measurement and can be objectively determined much easier than other valuation methods, such as market values.

2. Revenue from the sale of goods and services should be recognized when the practice has delivered the goods and performed the service and is entitled to collect from the patient. This rule is called the revenue recognition principle. As stated previously, the receipt of cash for these items is only of secondary importance. However, if there is a great deal of uncertainty of cash being collected, then revenue recognition should be delayed until cash is collected. The general rule, though, under accrual accounting is to record revenue when services are performed. If some of the revenues are not expected to be collected — that is, a small portion of the total recognized for the period — then an estimate of the uncollectible amount can be made, which then reduces the reported revenue and adjusts the receivable balance at the end of that period.

3. Recognition of expenses (the asset or cost that is used in providing a service) depends on the nature of the expense.

4. For those costs directly related to specific revenue, such as eyeglasses in the optical department, costs should be carried as an asset (inventory) until revenue is recognized for the sale of the glasses. Then the cost of the glasses is treated as an expense (cost of goods sold).

5. For long-lived assets, there is no direct relationship between the cost of the asset and revenue generated by the asset. For example, there is no direct relationship between the purchase price of X-ray equipment and

revenues from the service for a particular patient. For expense recognition in these cases, a systematic and rational plan of allocating a portion of the cost of the asset to specific time periods over its useful life must be established. This process is called depreciation (for tangible long-lived assets) or amortization (for other long-lived assets, such as prepaid insurance or goodwill).

6. Costs that do not have a direct relationship to particular revenue or that do not relate to long-lived assets should be considered expenses during the period that they have been incurred. These costs usually relate to the passage of time. Some examples are interest expense and practice promotion expenses. In applying all of the above expense recognition rules, an underlying objective is to use the matching principle as much as possible — that is, matching as many appropriate expenses expiring that produced the level of revenue recorded for that accounting period.

ASSUMPTIONS UNDERLYING AND QUALITATIVE CHARACTERISTICS OF FINANCIAL STATEMENTS

The financial statement form and content are influenced by the business environment in which a practice operates. They follow a set of basic assumptions that are the foundation blocks in the development of GAAP, assumptions relating to the entity, going-concern, accounting period, objectivity, and monetary unit.

Entity

The entity assumption refers to separating the activity of a business enterprise from the personal affairs of the owners. Accounting information should pertain only to the economic activities of the individual business and should be separate from the personal financial affairs of the owners. Accordingly, entities as specific areas of interest defined by the owners or managers establish boundaries for elements to be included in the financial statements. A medical practice operates and is reported as a separate financial unit, independent of the persons owning, managing, or working for it. Further, one entity may be the legal organization owning and operating the practice (i.e., the professional corporation or the partnership), another may be a part of the practice for which responsibility has been defined (i.e., each specialty or department), and yet another possibility is a combination of legal entities to represent the larger economic entity (consolidation of the practice corporation and the realty corporation). Financial statements may be prepared for each type of entity. Possible types of entities will have slightly different presentations of the financials statements. Corporations present their earned equity in the form of retained earnings, while partnerships and limited liability companies may present their respective owners' equity as "partners' equity" or "net worth." The latter and S corporations may be more likely to pay parts of their physician compensation in the form of dividends than a C corporation, where such dividends may face double taxation.

Going-concern

By this assumption, it is assumed that a practice will have an indefinite life, at least into the foreseeable future, unless there is information indicating the contrary. Thus, we can ignore liquidation values of assets and most temporary fluctuations in market values. However, assuming a long life for a practice poses problems to evaluating performance over a short time period (month, quarter, year). According to the matching principle, revenue and expenses must be matched with applicable time periods to measure net income. To do so, we must introduce systematic estimates into the accounting process, such as depreciation expenses that represent an estimate of asset-cost allocation to periods that benefit from the use of that asset.

Accounting Period

Since the going-concern assumption establishes that entities have an indefinite life, it is necessary to define an arbitrary time constraint on businesses to take periodic reckonings on how well they are doing and to determine their financial status. In the long run, a business's success or failure is best measured when it liquidates because under liquidation, a discrete monetary value for the whole enterprise is reached. Since we cannot wait indefinitely for such information, we divide a business's existence into artificial time periods — months, quarters, or years — and report results for these time periods. To accomplish this, we must make certain estimates and judgments about revenues and expenses to reflect their status for a given time period.

Objectivity

Business activity involves an exchange of goods or services at a specified price agreed upon by the parties in the exchange. The normal accounting procedure is to record these transactions at their cost, which is measured by the value of the resources given up in the exchange. The measurement of these exchanges must be objective and verifiable, such as an invoice, a memorandum, or a contract. Therefore, the support for all transactions must be based on documentation that contains objective data that describe the nature of the exchange.

Monetary Unit

The monetary unit is considered the common denominator by which economic activity is conducted and measured. In the United States, accounting systems measure and report the results of transactions and events in U.S. dollars that represent the value of the resources exchanged at the time of their acquisition. Financial statements of businesses in other countries would be expressed in the currency unit of that country. Further, the assumption is made that the monetary unit of measure is unchanging in terms of its purchasing power — an assumption that is unrealistic in the real world. The accounting profession has not yet determined a feasible way to adjust accounting data for price-level changes.

Other foundation blocks in the overall conceptual framework of accounting are the qualitative characteristics of financial statements. They relate to the need to make accounting measurements useful to decision makers. The most important of these are relevance, reliability, full disclosure, conservatism, consistency, and comparability.

Relevance

To be relevant, accounting information must be capable of making a difference in a decision. But the needs of various users of financial statements differ. For example, lenders are interested in the practice's ability to repay its loan. Owners and managers are interested in the practice's ability to provide quality care and generate an adequate income stream to its owners. Although general-purpose financial statements may meet creditors' needs, these statements may have to be supplemented with internal reports and nonfinancial data to meet the needs of owners and managers. Relevancy also involves the timely distribution of the proper type of information to various users.

Reliability

Reliability is the quality of information that gives assurance that it is reasonably free of error and bias and that users can depend on it to truly represent the economic conditions or events in question. To be reliable, accounting information must be capable of eliciting a high degree of consensus among independent measurers who use the same measurement methods.

Full Disclosure

The financial statements must present a complete picture of the practice's financial position, operations, and cash flows. Since the financial statements are considered general-purpose presentations, they are intended to fulfill the needs of all external users who do not have access to the practice's internal records. Thus, financial statements should include all information that would influence the decisions of these users.

Conservatism

Conservatism is an accounting guideline used to present overstatements of periodic earnings and financial position. Thus, a conservative practice in accrual accounting is to postpone the recognition of revenue until the collection of cash is relatively certain or is in hand. But the recognition rule for losses is less rigid; losses are recorded at the first sign that they may occur. There is nothing in the conservative convention urging accountants to deliberately understate assets or earnings. Rather, the rule means, when in doubt, choose the solution that will be least likely to overstate assets and earnings. In medical practice, widespread use of cash-basis accounting is predicated on conservatism.

Consistency

Consistency occurs when an accounting entity applies the same accounting treatment from period to period to similar accounting events. This practice ensures comparability of accounting data among the various periods. Consistency does not mean that the business cannot switch from one acceptable method of accounting to another. When it can be demonstrated that another method is preferable to the current one, then it is permissible to adopt the new one. The impact of any change in accounting methods must be disclosed in the financial statements.

Comparability

Because many accounting measurements are influenced by the assumption that organizations will have long lives, it is necessary to be sure that information prepared for short periods of time is comparable. The accrual basis of accounting and acceptable procedures have evolved to provide comparable results of operations and financial position over short time periods when fluctuations may distort comparisons if a cash basis of accounting were followed.

GUIDELINES FOR USE OF CASH AND ACCRUAL ACCOUNTING IN MEDICAL PRACTICES

Medical practices can use any accounting methods they choose for planning, control, evaluation of financial performance, and decision making. Most of the information needed to meet external reporting requirements can be drawn from the accounting records. But for internal financial reports related to planning and control, it may be necessary to supplement the general accounting data with other nonfinancial and budgeted data.

To place internal financial reporting in the proper perspective, the following comments are relevant:

- Internal reporting is not governed by GAAP. Conformity with GAAP is an external reporting requirement only. Internally, the dictum is "Is the information relevant and useful?"
- While it may be mandated to issue periodic financial statements to external users, internal reporting is optional. Many practices do no internal reporting beyond the general-purpose financial statements used for taxes or creditors.
- Internal reporting embraces nonfinancial information, such as the number of patients served, number of hours worked, and number of procedures undertaken. The format of these reports usually focuses on parts of the practice, such as specialty areas or departments, as well as on the practice as a whole.
- The frequency of internal reports can vary — daily, weekly, or monthly — depending on specific needs — for example, a daily cash report. External financial statements are usually prepared at least annually and more often as needed.

- The emphasis of internal reports should be on showing whether the group is accomplishing its goals, objectives, and plans. External reporting is an historic account of the past financial activities of the practice.

Concerns with the Use of Accrual Accounting

The accounting and financial reporting system should present the clearest and most complete picture of the group's financial performance. This result is best achieved through the use of accrual based accounting. Administrators of medical groups frequently voice three major concerns with its use: (1) measuring income for tax purposes, (2) measuring income for distribution to physicians, and (3) measuring the financial position of the group for buy-in or buy-out by physicians.

Measuring income for tax purposes: Group administrators fear that the use of accrual accounting in the books and in the financial statements will require its use for income tax purposes. This is not necessarily true. Accounting policies for tax reporting may differ from those for financial reporting. The IRS requires only that a taxpayer's records clearly show the amounts used in the tax return. The general accounting system can be developed such that accrual, cash, or modified cash basis information can be derived from one set of records to satisfy tax, external, and internal reporting needs.

The increasing proportion of a medical practice's revenue being realized in the prepaid or capitated form has brought an interesting twist to the choice of cash or accrual basis for tax reporting. Since the timing of cash receipts for prepaid contracts moves to a time period prior to the rendering of patient services and paying expenses, using the cash basis for tax reporting results in paying taxes before services are rendered and many related expenses are paid. This effect is the opposite of what occurs in a fee-for-service environment, when services are provided before payments for them are received and taxes are then paid thereafter. Thus, with a practice's total revenue now comprising a larger prepaid component, it would seem that the accrual basis would be the preferred tax-reporting basis to defer tax payments until after services are rendered and cash for them is received.

Measuring income for distribution to physicians: The amount of cash to be distributed to a group of physicians depends on a distribution formula and the amount of cash available. In many group practices, the statement of revenue and expenses (based on the cash basis) is used as the measure of income available for distribution. It is understandable to physicians, and if cash must be retained for equipment purchases or debt repayment, this purpose can be easily explained. The accrual based income statement is intended to report physician performance and not to measure the amount of cash available for distribution to physicians or for any other cash distributions. Whether accounted for on the cash or accrual basis, income before distributions to physicians on the income statement may be more than, equal to, or less than the amount of cash available for any specific purpose. Thus, it may be difficult to explain to physicians why income is high but cash available for distribution is low. The cash flow statement, the third basic financial statement (which is the same under either cash or accrual), is intended to explain all sources and uses of cash. Determining the amount of cash available for physician distribution should be a part of the cash management system, which involves more considerations than merely the income statement.

Measuring the financial position for buy-in or buy-out by physicians: The negotiation and determination of the provisions of buy-in or buy-out agreements relating to medical practices must embrace more aspects than the financial statements. For example, these agreements must consider tax situations, the ability of physicians to make the required investment, and the formula for income distribution. The agreement should include whatever all parties involved want it to. The omission or inclusion of patient receivables in the formal financial statements, for example, should have no impact on what is designated in the buy-in or buy-out agreement.

Optimal Conditions for the Use of the Cash Basis

As stated previously, about 75 percent of all medical groups use the cash basis of accounting. Since the tax laws permit the delay of reporting patient revenue until it is collected in cash, these advantages have dictated the use of the cash basis for tax reporting. Because accounting records must reflect what is in the tax return, relatively few medical groups have formally introduced a second set of accounting measurements directed specifically at performance evaluation and decision making. Even though tax compliance is necessary, it should not preclude the practice from adding other measurements to the accounting system to provide information for management, as long as the benefits exceed the costs.

Despite the above comments, the cash basis of accounting is most appropriate for both tax filings and management information purposes when the following conditions are present:

- The operation's level is stable with minimum seasonal variations during the year.
- Patient receivables are collected evenly throughout the year, and the age of these receivables does not materially change.
- Long-lived assets are leased rather than purchased, and the rent is paid monthly.
- Supply inventories are replenished as used.
- Large expenses, such as professional liability insurance premiums, are paid monthly rather than annually.
- Total revenue is derived mostly from fee-for-service.

When these conditions are not present and comparisons of operating results for short time periods (e.g., monthly) are important, practices may find advantages in adopting accrual accounting for internal reporting or adding some accrual techniques to cash-basis measurements. The accrual techniques may be recorded formally in the accounting records or may be developed through informal analysis techniques of the cash-basis records. For example, many practices maintain their records on the accrual basis during the year but prepare a set of adjusting entries at the end of the year to reflect the cash-basis for tax reporting. At the beginning of the next year, the adjustments to reflect the cash basis are reversed, and the practice continues on the accrual basis. This way, the practice is able to meet the monthly needs for performance measurement and also meet the tax needs at the end of the year. There is a clear trail of tax measurements in the records to satisfy the tax requirements.

COMPONENTS OF ACCOUNTING AND FINANCIAL MANAGEMENT SYSTEMS: DATA FLOWS AND PROCESSES WITHIN SYSTEMS

The informational needs for financial management were summarized earlier in this chapter. These needs might be visualized as six different forms of data flows:

1. Determining revenue
2. Determining expenses
3. Providing external reports
4. Determining physician income distribution and productivity
5. Managing the practice — short-range
6. Managing the practice — long-range

Each of these flows is presented in Exhibit 3.2.

Determining Revenue

Crucial elements in achieving a successful practice are the processing of information about patient services and billing and collecting for those services. The basic steps to capture the necessary data involve the following procedures:

- Registering patients, which includes documenting their medical history, current symptoms, and treatments/procedures provided
- Processing charges and fees for services rendered
- Billing insurers and patients for services performed
- Processing the collection of cash payments
- Recording the charges and collections to patient accounts
- Following up on delinquent accounts and adjusting balances for uncollectible amounts

Determining Expenses

The companion "matching" element to revenues is determining the proper amount of expenses. The steps involved in this process are:

- Securing authorization to incur various costs, such as payroll, supplies, outside referral fees, and other services, needed to operate the practice

EXHIBIT 3.2 ■ Data Flows within an Accounting System of a Medical Group

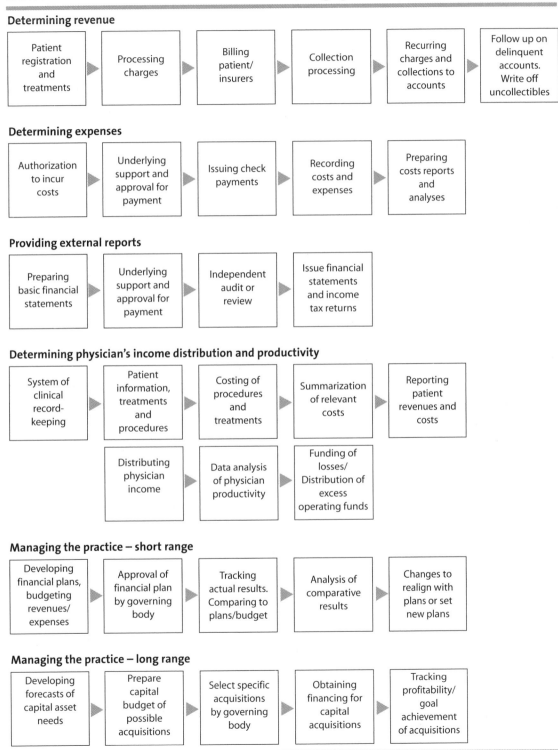

- Compiling the necessary underlying documentation and support for expenditures made and approving these items for payment
- Issuing check payments on a timely basis
- Recording costs and expenses in the appropriate accounting records
- Summarizing recorded expense data in various forms for use in preparing internal financial reports

Providing External Reports

After all revenues and expenses have been properly reflected in the accounting system, these data can be used in reporting the financial results to third parties who require this information. To satisfy these needs, the following procedures are necessary:

- Preparing the basic financial statements, including the balance sheet, statement of income, and the statement of cash flows
- Preparing the income tax return(s)
- Having the financial statements and income tax return(s) reviewed or audited by an independent party, such as a CPA firm
- Issuing and distributing the reviewed/audited set of financial statements and income tax return(s)

Determining Physician Income Distribution and Productivity

A major objective of accounting and financial management systems is to provide meaningful information about the method(s) followed to distribute income to the physician owners. Another objective is to make the physicians aware of relevant data concerning their productivity. The steps to accomplish these objectives include:

- Establishing and maintaining an adequate and current system of clinical recordkeeping, including correct use of CPT-4 and ICD-9 coding
- Compiling, classifying, and recording various information about treatments and procedures rendered to patients
- Determining the costs of treatments and procedures and recording them in the appropriate accounting records
- Summarizing relevant costs of patient care by various groupings, such as by types of service and physician
- Preparing reports showing patient revenue and costs by physician
- Distributing income to physicians based on a previously agreed-upon formula
- Analyzing data and reports on physician productivity and making appropriate changes in the modus operandi of the practice
- Determining amounts of additional funding needed to cover losses or amounts of excess operating funds for distribution to physicians or shareholders

Managing the Practice — Short-Range

As medical groups adopt more formal approaches to practice management, financial planning processes become core components of short-range practice management. The involved actions and data flows are:

- Developing a detailed financial plan (the budget) for the following year, including a forecast of revenues and expenses
- Obtaining the approval of the financial plan by the governing body of the medical group
- Tracking actual financial results and comparing them with the financial plan and budgeted amounts
- Analyzing the comparative results, which are arranged by the appropriate areas of responsibility and segments of the practice
- Achieving effective changes to operations that are indicated by the analysis or revising the plan to accommodate a changed environment

Managing the Practice — Long-Range

Further sophisticated management approaches deal with long-range factors. They usually include:

- Developing forecasts and projections of future capacity needs, which entail more capital assets and larger facility accommodations
- Preparing a capital budget showing the financial benefits and costs of possible capital acquisitions
- Deciding, by the governing body of the group, on the specific long-range capital acquisitions
- Obtaining the necessary financing to acquire the assets needed to enlarge the group's capacity for service
- Tracking the actual results of profit and goal attainment forecasted by each capital acquisition

Exhibit 3.3 furnishes a visual overview of the accounting subsystems of a medical practice and shows how these subsystems provide data for the purposes behind the various data flows.

ACCOUNTING SUBSYSTEMS

Earlier in chapter 3, we introduced the notion of transactions. Financial transactions are important in recording a historical chronology of events that reflects an impact on the accounting model that is used for recording and reporting financial information. Exhibit 3.3 shows how transactions flow into and through various accounting subsystems and how financial information is classified and summarized to produce the financial statements and other reports.

EXHIBIT 3.3 ■ Accounting Subsystems

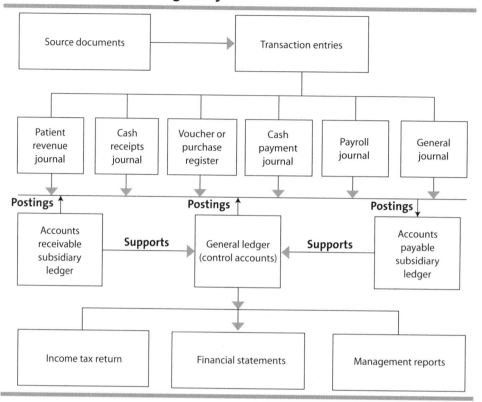

As transactions occur, documentation, such as patient charge tickets, purchase orders, cash receipts, bank deposit slips, canceled checks, and other business memoranda, is accumulated. These source documents form the basis for entering transactions into the accounting records. Usually there is a separate book of entry for each type of transaction, and these various journals are shown in the horizontal "repository" boxes of transaction entries. These journals are the first part of a series of accounting subsystems used for the recording, summarizing, and reporting of specialized financial information. They are:

- **Patient revenue journal** — records all patient charges for services rendered, both by the medical group and by referral sources.

- **Cash receipts journal** — records all cash received from patients, reimbursement agencies, and other sources.

- **Voucher or purchases register** — records all purchases of supplies, services, and capital acquisitions after the proper documentation is assembled, such as the purchase order, receiving ticket, and vendor invoice, and the transaction has been approved by a person in authority. A voucher is used to assemble all the underlying support for a transaction and requires an independent verification of these evidences along with authoritative approval.

- ■ **Cash payments journal** — records all checks issued as payments for approved vouchers evidencing completed transactions.

- ■ **Payroll journal** — records the amounts of all salaries and wages paid to all employees of the group as well as all required and elective deductions from the gross payroll. An individual payroll record must be maintained for each employee.

- ■ **General journal** — records all other transactions that are not entered into one of the specialized journals.

After transactions have been recorded in one of the journals, the accounting data are posted to accounts in the general ledger and, where appropriate, in one of the subsidiary ledgers, such as A/R or accounts payable. The general ledger contains accounts for all elements that appear on the financial statements — the balance sheet and the statement of income. These accounts serve as the mechanism to increase or decrease each element's balance depending on the transactions entered. The recommended MGMA-ACMPE *Chart of Accounts* to be used for this purpose will be covered in detail in chapter 4. The subsidiary ledgers serve as detailed records for each customer (A/R) or for each vendor from which goods or services have been purchased (accounts payable). Thus, transactions affecting patients' charges and receipts are entered twice — once in the A/R control account in the general ledger and again in the specific customer's account in the subsidiary A/R ledger. The same dual entry would occur when other subsidiary ledgers are used.

Once accounting data have been summarized in the various ledgers, they can be used for any kind of reporting, both external and internal to the group. The data, after final adjustments, would be organized into the required format following generally accepted principles of reporting the basic set of financial statements. Similarly, the account data can be taken and placed into the proper categories for income tax return preparation. Also, the account data can be organized in many different ways to report management accounting information to the governing body of the medical group, the physician owners, and other managers of the group's practice.

In the later chapters, these accounting recording subsystems will be related with broader aspects of the financial management system and its components.

Payroll Administration

Aside from physician salaries, a practice's largest expense item is usually staff salaries, associated payroll taxes, and fringe benefits. Most financial managers may not get involved intimately with the preparation of the payroll or the payroll tax returns. Rather, many groups rely on an outside payroll service organization to write payroll checks, to keep detailed employee records related to payroll data, to file federal and state tax returns, and to provide employees with relevant documentation as needed. In cases where an outside service is used, the financial manager should have a general knowledge about payroll matters so that the service can be properly supervised. Also, the financial manager should be able to answer questions from staff members about payroll without contacting the outside service.

Some of the related payroll areas that financial managers should gain familiarity with include the following:

- Federal wage and hour requirements, including:
  - Exempt and nonexempt employees
  - Minimum wage requirements
  - Overtime pay
  - Employer records
  - Workers with disabilities
  - Termination
  - Leaves of absence
- Discrimination, including:
  - Federal legislation (Civil Rights Acts) regarding prohibited actions, sexual harassment, and employer obligations
  - Age discrimination
  - Disabilities
  - Affirmative action
- National Labor Relations Board provisions about prohibited practices and penalties
- Payroll requirements, including:
  - Federal and state income tax
  - Federal insurance contribution act (FICA)
  - Deposit of payroll taxes
  - Unemployment taxes
  - Federal and state tax returns
- Workers' compensation regulations and requirements
- Practice-specific deductions relating to benefits, such as:
  - Health insurance
  - 401K plans
- Postemployment issues, including:
  - Covenants not to compete
  - Wrongful discharge
  - Insurance contribution, such as COBRA

Financial managers should obtain copies of relevant payroll-related laws and regulations and may want to subscribe to a payroll information service to gain access to an ongoing stream of updated information. If an outside service is used, they may be asked to supply the above-listed information or it may be provided by the external CPA or accounting service firm that handles the filing of the income tax returns and/or conducts an annual financial statement review or audit. If the financial manager is an experienced accountant or possesses a payroll background, the group may establish its own internal payroll system.

Processing and Control of Accounts Payable

Accounts payable are amounts owed to vendors and suppliers for goods and services acquired by a medical group on a credit basis and for which the suppliers have not yet been paid. Usually these claims are unsecured and are frequently referred to as open accounts. The terms of these payable transactions normally require payment within 30 to 60 days after receipt of the goods or services.

The control of accounts payable involves maintaining a detailed record of individual accounts payable by vendor and using a tickler file or memory jogger showing dates that the obligations should be paid. The terms of these transactions usually stipulate the taking of cash discounts, such as 2/10, net/30. (That is, if the invoice is paid within 10 days from the date of the invoice, the payer can take a 2 percent discount from the amount due; if the discount is not taken, then the total amount due is to be paid by 30 days from the date of the invoice.) Missing or not taking cash discounts can be costly, thus, the system should ensure that all cash discounts are taken as offered.

Other controls of accounts payable entail assuring that amounts due to vendors are authorized, authentic, and supported by underlying documentation, such as purchase orders and receiving reports, as well as invoices showing the complete details of the transaction. Before a payment is made on any account payable, the check signer should check the supporting evidence to ensure that unauthorized or erroneous disbursements are not being made. A few other hints on effective management of accounts payable include the following:

- Ask suppliers to bill the medical group for all purchases on a set series of dates each month to prevent payments from bunching up and to ease the demands on cash outflows.
- Find out if vendors will grant a larger discount for paying cash at the time of purchase rather than being billed at a later date. Sometimes, discounts up to 5 percent are possible.

AUDITING AND AUDIT REPORTS

Nature and Purpose of an Audit

Accounting is a process of collecting, summarizing, and communicating financial information about economic events and their results as they relate to business entities. There are various groups besides the owners who have an interest in the economic affairs of these entities. For public corporations, these groups might be investors, creditors, financial analysts, governmental officials, employees, and others concerned with the operations of the business. For medical practices, these external parties might be creditors, suppliers, third-party reimbursement entities, and other governmental agencies.

Among these parties, there is a need for assurance that the financial statements prepared and distributed by management contain information that is fairly presented in accordance with GAAP. The purpose of auditing is to provide an independent process that ensures that this outcome occurs and that the statements can be relied upon to depict what they purport to represent. There are four key aspects of the auditing process that help to add to the credibility of the financial statements:

1. Auditing is a systematic process based on logic and reasoning. It is planned and conducted in a methodical, not haphazard, manner.

2. The auditor obtains and evaluates evidence. Evidence is collected throughout the audit as the auditor makes decisions about the financial information presented by management's financial statements.

3. The evidence compiled by the auditor is used to ascertain the degree of correspondence between the assertions (elements on the financial statements prepared by management) and established criteria (GAAP).

4. Finally, the auditor communicates the results of the audit to interested parties, such as stockholders, creditors, and so on. The communication is called the auditor's report.

Independent auditors (usually CPAs) conduct audits and render an opinion in their audit reports about the fairness of the presentation of financial statements issued by management. This process is called attestation, and an audit is sometimes referred to as an attest engagement.

The Audit Report

Audit examinations are carried out following a prescribed set of standards that measure the quality of the auditor's performance as well as the objectives to be attained by the use of certain procedures. These auditing standards rarely change, and if they do, it's only because of the official decree of the Auditing Standards Board, a professional body of CPAs who constantly monitor the effectiveness of existing standards and developments. Generally accepted auditing standards (GAAS) are important for several reasons:

■ To define the broad objectives of every independent audit

■ To provide a gauge for judging an auditor's performance

■ To set recognized standards of the profession through the business and legal world

There are 10 generally accepted auditing standards, which are divided into three broad categories: (1) general standards, (2) standards of field work, and (3) standards of reporting. These standards, as developed by the Auditing Standards Board and approved by the members of the American Institute of Certified Public Accountants (the professional organization of CPAs), are listed in Exhibit 3.4. Financial managers should be aware of these standards when they assess their practice's auditing services — both internal and external.

Auditors' reports are addressed to the governing body of the organization requesting the audit. An introductory paragraph identifies the responsibilities

EXHIBIT 3.4 ■ Generally Accepted Auditing Standards

General standards

1. The examination is to be performed by a person or persons having adequate training and proficiency as an auditor.
2. In all matters relating to the assignment, independence in mental attitude is to be maintained by the auditor(s).
3. Due professional care is to be exercised in the performance of the examination and the preparation of the report.

Standards of field work

1. The work is to be adequately planned, and assistants, if any, are to be properly supervised.
2. A sufficient understanding of the internal control structure is to be obtained to plan the audit and to determine the nature, timing, and extent of tests to be performed.
3. Sufficient competent evidential matter is to be obtained through inspection, observation, inquiries, and confirmations to afford a reasonable basis for an opinion regarding the financial statements under examination.

Standards of reporting

1. The report shall state whether the financial statements are presented in accordance with generally accepted accounting principles.
2. The report shall identify those circumstances in which such principles have not been consistently observed in the current period in relation to the preceding period.
3. Informative disclosures in the financial statements are to be regarded as reasonably adequate unless otherwise stated in the report.
4. The report shall either contain an expression of opinion regarding the financial statements, taken as a whole, or an assertion to the effect that an opinion cannot be expressed. When an overall opinion cannot be expressed, the reasons therefore should be stated. In all cases where an auditor's name is associated with financial statements, the report should contain a clear-cut indication of the character of the auditor's work and the degree of responsibility, if any, the auditor is taking.

of both the client (XYZ Company) and the auditor regarding the financial statements. The second paragraph contains the auditor's description of the scope of the examination and is called the scope paragraph. In the third paragraph, the auditor renders an opinion about the fairness of the presentation of the financial statements in what is usually referred to as the opinion paragraph. The report is signed by a partner of the CPA firm involved. The date printed on the report is the actual date the audit field work was completed. This indicates the point at which the auditor was in a position to render an opinion.

An unqualified audit opinion, illustrated in Exhibit 3.5, means that the auditor believes that the financial statements are presented fairly, that they conform with GAAP, that they are applied consistently each year, and that the statements include all necessary disclosures. It means that the statements fairly present the financial position, results of operations, and cash flows.

Auditors can render three other types of opinions:

1. A qualified opinion in which the auditor expresses certain reservations in the report regarding the scope of the audit and/or the financial statements. When the auditor's reservations are more serious, one of the two other following types of opinions are rendered.

2. A disclaimer of opinion in which auditors state that they cannot give an opinion because of scope limitations (e.g., the auditor has been precluded from completing certain significant audit procedures) or some other reason (e.g., the auditor is not independent).

3. An adverse opinion in which the auditors state that the financial statements do not present fairly the financial position of the company, the results of its operations, and the cash flows. In this case, it is claimed that the client is making a serious departure from GAAP.

EXHIBIT 3.5 ■ Standard Auditor's Report, Example of an Unqualified Audit Opinion

We have audited the accompanying balance sheet of XYZ Company as of December 31, 2XXX, and the related statements of income, retained earnings, and cash flows for the year then ended. These financial statements are the responsibility of the company's management. Our responsibility is to express an opinion on these financial statements based on our audit.

We conducted our audit based on generally accepted auditing standards. Those standards require that we plan and perform the audit to obtain reasonable assurance about whether the financial statements are free of material misstatement. An audit includes examining, on a test basis, evidence supporting the amounts and disclosures in the financial statements. An audit also includes assessing the accounting principles used and significant estimates made by management as well as evaluating the overall financial statement presentation. We believe that our audit provides a reasonable basis for our opinion.

In our opinion, the financial statements above present fairly, in all material respects, the financial position of XYZ Company as of December 31, 2XXX, and the results of its operations and its cash flow for the year ended in conformity with generally accepted accounting principles.

(Signature)

Types of Audits

The independent examination of an organization's financial statements is called a financial statement audit. The audit report provided in this setting gives assurance to external users that the financial statements are prepared in accordance with established criteria (GAAP). There are other types of audit activities that can be performed, which provide benefits to the organization.

One other type of audit, an operational audit, is performed to determine the extent to which some aspect of an organization's operating activities is functioning effectively and efficiently. In these audits, auditors observe and test various areas of one or more of a firm's activities, such as the production process of a manufacturing company. Operational audits would assess the performance of the production process, identify opportunities for improving the process, and develop recommendations for upgrading company activities. Unlike a financial statement audit, the reports and analyses generated by an operational audit would not circulate externally but would be used by management only.

A third type of audit, a compliance audit, is conducted to determine the extent to which an organization and/or its personnel are performing their duties in a manner consistent with organizational policies and procedures. For example, a common organizational policy relates to the adherence to internal control procedures. Such a compliance audit would be conducted to identify deviations from these procedures. Another type of compliance audit would deal with an organization's compliance with federal laws, regulations, contracts, and grants. For example, an audit might be performed to investigate whether funds received from various sources were used for the specified purpose(s). In medical practice, there might be a compliance audit to tell whether the accounting procedures for billing patients were in compliance with Medicare and Medicaid regulations. There can also be tax compliance audits performed by IRS and state tax agents.

Types of Auditors

There are three types of auditors generally involved in the various audit examinations. These are the independent (external), internal, and government auditors.

Independent (external) auditors: The audits of financial statements are performed by independent accountants, usually CPAs. Also, the fact that CPAs are independent — that is, they do not hold an ownership interest or have management involvement in the clients they audit — lends the utmost credibility to their attestations.

Internal auditors: Unlike independent auditors, internal auditors are employed by a single organization and only perform services for that firm. Internal auditors conduct operational and compliance audits for their employer. Essentially, their role is to determine the following:

- ◼ Whether the organization and its employees are complying with established policies and procedures

- The efficiency and effectiveness of some aspect of the organization's operational activities

As employees, they lack the degree of independence of external auditors. However, they usually report to the governing body or to some committee of the board of directors. As medical groups grow in size and scope of operations, it is likely that more groups, especially those that are part of large integrated systems, will employ internal auditors to conduct compliance types of audits and reviews.

Government auditors: These auditors conduct audits under the auspices of various governmental agencies such as the General Accounting Office and the IRS. They usually perform compliance audits to evaluate whether federal laws and regulations are being complied with.

Compilation and Reviews of Unaudited Financial Statements

There are two other types of services besides financial statement audits that independent external auditors perform — a compilation or a review of unaudited financial statements. In either case, the work performed is not an audit and should not be construed as equivalent to an independent audit.

In a compilation, the accountant merely assembles (or assists the entity in assembling) financial statements. No assurance is provided in a compilation engagement; thus, the accountant cannot issue an opinion or provide any other form of assurance regarding the compiled financial statements.

In a review, the auditor is trying to provide limited assurance about the fairness of the company's financial statements. Two procedures performed by the accountant in a review engagement beyond those normally required in a compilation are inquiries of client personnel and analytical procedures. Inquiries relate to the client's use of accounting principles, practices and procedures, and actions taken by meetings of stockholders and the board of directors that may affect the financial statements. Analytical procedures will normally consist of comparing components of the financial statements with components of comparable prior periods and with budgets and forecasts. The report on reviewed financial statements does express a limited (or negative) assurance statement that "we are not aware of any material modifications that should be made . . . for them to be in conformity with GAAP."

To the Point

- Financial accounting deals with measuring and recording transactions for businesses and preparing periodic financial statements in accordance with GAAP. Management accounting is concerned with internal accounting information needs to assist managers in planning and controlling the business operations.

- Cash basis accounting involves recognizing revenues only when cash has been received and recognizing expenses only when cash has been paid for them. Accrual basis accounting provides for a more accurate measurement of net income by recognizing revenue when services have been rendered and expenses when resources have been used up or consumed in the generation of patient revenues, regardless of when cash was received or expended. Most medical groups use a modified cash basis, which involves recording long-lived assets as well as payables and receivables relating to the borrowing and investing of cash.

- The fundamental foundation of financial accounting and the core concept used in recording transactions affecting medical group operations is the basic accounting equation of Assets = Liabilities + Owners' Equity.

- The three basic financial statements are the balance sheet, the income statement, and the statement of cash flows. The balance sheet presents a listing of all assets, liabilities, and owners' equity elements. The income statement shows the revenues and expenses recognized in an accounting period with the net balance of those two elements being referred to as net income or net loss. The statement of cash flows presents a picture of cash flows experienced by a medical group for a designated time period. The cash flows are classified as cash provided (used) by operations, investing, and financing.

- Accrual accounting is based on the set of standards called generally accepted accounting principles (GAAP). Some important GAAP guidelines include the historical cost principle, which requires that assets and liabilities be recorded at their initial cost; the revenue recognition principle, which specifies that revenue from the sale of services and goods should be recognized when the practice has performed the services or delivered the goods and is entitled to collect from the patient; and the matching principal, which is applied to expense recognition rules whereby the appropriate expenses used and expiring production levels of revenue are matched with those revenues to determine the net income for an account period.

▪ A set of basic assumptions form the foundation of GAAP and include the following: the assumptions of entity, going-concern, accounting period, objectivity, monetary unit, relevance, reliability, full disclosure, conservatism, consistency, and comparability.

▪ The informational needs for financial management can be visualized as six different forms of data flows and processes:

1. Determining revenue
2. Determining expenses
3. Providing external reports
4. Determining physician income distribution and productivity
5. Managing the practice — short-range
6. Managing the practice — long-range

▪ An audit is a systematic process performed by an independent professional accountant that results in a report that provides assurance that the financial statements prepared by an organization's management contain information that is fairly presented in accordance with GAAP. Usually, audits are performed by CPAs who have a specified educational background, have relevant experience, and have passed a rigorous examination to obtain a license to practice and perform audit engagements.

▪ The three types of audits are financial audits, operational audits, and compliance audits. The three kinds of auditors are independent external auditors (CPAs), internal auditors, and government auditors.

CHAPTER 4

Choosing Financial Information Systems for Medical Group Practices

Edited by Nancy M. Enos, FACMPE, CPMA, CPC, CPC-I, CEMC

After completing this chapter, you will be able to:

- Explain what a financial information system (FIS) is.

- Identify the most important types of FIS for medical group practices.

- Become familiar with the new MGMA-ACMPE Chart of Accounts for Healthcare Organizations.

- Understand the relationship between FIS, practice management systems, and EHR.

- Initiate and conduct a thorough selection process for choosing a financial management system.

Modern information systems (IS) involve far more technology than ever before in the history of medical practices. While IS for medical groups will continue to face the challenges of merging clinical with financial data, this chapter will focus on the financial portion of IS. Clinical components will be mentioned as they impact other financial data needs. An IS will be defined, and IS categories will be introduced. A description of the MGMA-ACMPE *Chart of Accounts for Healthcare Organizations* will lead into practices' need for accounting from an IS viewpoint. Later, other practice and patient management issues will be explored. In the remaining section, the financial manager will learn how to select IS components.

Most of the chapter's organization is based on specific IS categories. Information applicable to many different IS categories, such as the advantages and challenges of outsourcing and customization of specific functions, are mentioned throughout the text. The increasing number of "SaaS," or Software as a Service, options will also be discussed.

For the purposes of this chapter, EHR are considered part of a practice management system. Currently, many practices have access to this increasingly important IS function, and the numbers continue to grow quickly. The importance of EHR will grow as the overall need for computerized information continues to include more and more facets of healthcare delivery services.

Government legislation is driving changes in healthcare today under the American Recovery and Reinvestment Act of 2009 (ARRA). The provisions of HIPAA are expanded under the HITECH Act. Incentives, such as meaningful use of EHR, raised the bar for use of computerized EHR systems. Because the patient record contains information that can be potentially linked to many other clinical and financial records, it is mentioned first in the following introduction of the selected practice management functions. Interoperability is a major factor in the selection of an IS, and a good understanding of the relationship between systems and workflow is essential.

WHAT IS AN INFORMATION SYSTEM (IS)?

An IS provides financial managers with financial information to track their organizations' activities and offers support for decision-making processes. Modern IS now involves far more technology than ever before in the history of medical practices. It minimizes paperwork, decreases labor-intensive processes, curbs costs, enhances workflow, and improves quality of care. In short, an IS increases the physicians' and staff's overall effectiveness. One of the fastest growing areas of healthcare technology is the Internet. Healthcare systems are using it for clinical care, most notably in remote rural areas.

Rules of meaningful use and accountable care organizations are based on standards of performance tied to federal funds and performance metrics, and that opens the door to increases in analytic work. Under federal mandate, information must flow through custodial walls, which is where cloud computing provides the pathway for information sharing and access from multiple access points.

What is Meaningful Use?

A provision of healthcare reform, meaningful use is a measure intended to drive the adoption of EHR for practices that were slow to move away from their paper charts. The incentive payment will provide funds for eligible professionals (EPs) who "meaningfully use" an EHR system to qualify for government incentives. The goal of meaningful use under ARRA is to accelerate the adoption of EHRs among providers. This requires two major steps:

1. Adopting and using a "certified" EHR.
2. Using that certified EHR in a certain manner. For Stage I of meaningful use, EPs are required to report that they are documenting certain types of information.

The goal of the U.S. government is clear: to improve patient care quality and reduce costs through EHRs. To accomplish this, they have outlined an incentive program, which has three main stages that build on each other. The first stage is finalized, the second and third are still pending, and the dates have been in flux.

- Stage I: Requires that EPs record specific quality measures in the EHR
- Stage II: Requires that EPs transmit information between provider groups
- Stage III: Requires that EPs focus on using the quality measures to improve their standard of care

What is the HITECH Act?

HIPAA was introduced in August 1996. The privacy, security, and administrative simplification provisions have been implemented over the past decade. When President Obama signed the ARRA, the act included important changes for privacy. The Health Information Technology for Economic and Clinical Health Act (HITECH) provisions of ARRA in Title XIII include changes to the original HIPAA provisions.

The key changes from HIPAA to privacy under the HITECH Act are:

1. Enforcement
2. Notification of breach
3. EHR access
4. Business associates and business associate agreements
5. Requirements for marketing communications, restrictions, and accounting

Information is power. Quality organizations and accountable care organizations (ACOs) are changing the way doctors practice medicine. With the best technology tools and complete information, medical group practice leaders will be able to successfully negotiate profitable contracts with third-party payers. For the most part, no one individual software program alone can offer all the necessary information. Practices will need a system of components capable of working together to analyze the data in order to make informed decisions. One of the challenges financial managers will continue to face is the ever-increasing need to integrate financial data with clinical data. Current pressures to benchmark one group's data against other clinics will increase with growing competition in the healthcare market.

What Is Cloud-based Software as a Service?

The latest trend is the cloud-based SaaS EHR and practice management system. The system is designed to address a wide range of specialties within physician practices, inpatient clinics and hospitals, federally qualified health centers, and medical billing services. They also offer physician referral tracking networks, online patient portal applications, built-in dashboards to monitor meaningful use, key indicators and clinical workflow, and revenue cycle management applications.

In addition to core charting, e-prescribing, and lab test tracking, EHRs offer a number of powerful modules that connect various systems. These include clinical decision support alerts that prompt physicians to perform examinations or tests based on symptoms or diagnoses entered into the system. The systems also offer continuity of care documentation that supports information sharing across the continuum of care. Patient information, such as a library of patient education documents and care instructions, are often built in.

FINANCIAL MANAGEMENT SYSTEMS

When planning for the implementation of a financial information system (FIS), managers need to know who will access the system and what existing systems will interface with the FIS. While the lack of adequate funding is a major obstacle to IS implementation, it is possible to take an incremental approach to an IS project. With proper planning and budgeting, even the smallest groups can afford to automate some of their mission-critical functions over time. Consideration of cost savings through outsourcing some financial functions, such as payroll, should be fully evaluated before incorporating these functions into a new IS purchase. Several other accounting functions lend themselves to outsourcing. Small groups can use an outside payroll service supplied by either a bank or an automated payroll service firm. The associated expense of outsourcing this function is offset by the gains in internal productivity and increased efficiency by the accounting staff. Another benefit of outsourcing is risk mitigation. By having a system of checks and balances, the reconciliation process between the payroll vendor and the practice can detect and prevent any potential theft or embezzlement.

The first step in selecting an appropriate IS is to carefully research the information an entity needs to effectively manage the practice today and in the future. This must include a determination of what types of data entry and report writing will be needed. Some systems do not require manual data input but will interface with existing systems. IS also significantly differs from one vendor to the next by their built-in report-writing capabilities. When identifying IS needs, it is important to consider future expansion or growth of the practice and to recognize and plan for the tremendous amount of time and effort required to complete the data entry and to learn the new system.

IS CATEGORIES

Many different IS categories exist. A group will not need to invest in all components within each category but should choose several across the spectrum in order to gain a variety of timely indicators to successfully and strategically manage a practice. In addition, not all components need to be purchased simultaneously. A system may be built based upon the practice's need for automation while some of the less-critical functions may not need to be automated at all. In this book, the major categories of IS are organized in these four areas: (1) financial management (including contract management), (2) practice management, (3) patient management, and (4) decision-support systems.

Financial Management

The financial IS category includes general and cost accounting, patient accounting systems (including claims systems), and contract management. All operate in a symbiotic relationship; that is, what affects one system can impact all other systems. The core accounting component that provides a financial reporting framework is the chart of accounts.

Chart of Accounts for Healthcare Organizations

The concept behind a chart of accounts (COA) is to visually organize the host of financial report categories. Although each entity has its own unique chart of accounts, there is a common thread of core structure throughout all COA. Specifically, all transactions are classified as asset, liability, equity, revenue, or expense account categories. This organization of information allows for standardization of financial and tax compliance reporting through the healthcare field, which is vital for any type of comparison, such as determining total provider expenses per full-time equivalency (FTE).

Since 1979, MGMA-ACMPE has made available a COA for medical group practice. MGMA-ACMPE periodically updates the chart to provide an industry standard that reflects the many changes within healthcare delivery systems. In subsequent years, the name of the publication changed, and the tool was updated in 1985, 1996, and 1999 to reflect changing account and record-keeping needs of medical groups.

The new and revised (January 2011) MGMA-ACMPE *Chart of Accounts* gives the healthcare accounting structure needed to provide accurate and detailed reports for management decision making (see Exhibit 4.1).[1]

General Accounting

As mentioned in chapter 2, a generic accounting system includes cash collections and payments, A/R, accounts payable, payroll, and the general ledger. Because cost accounting depends on the specific environment of a practice, financial managers should insist on flexible, user-friendly, and easy-to-customize software components when choosing or upgrading an FIS.

Cost Accounting

Due to ever-increasing competition in the health services delivery markets, medical group practices need specific cost accounting information to help them identify the profitability of their activities. In this context, financial managers seek cost information regarding discrete changes, such as the addition of new services, the purchase of satellite offices, additional staff, expanded information systems, and so on. Cost accounting is also an indispensible tool to evaluate variances in the cost effectiveness of services or providers.[2] A detailed discussion on how to develop, use, and analyze a practice's cost accounting data is in chapter 6.

Administrators should strive to automate as many cost accounting processes as possible. They can either develop their own system or purchase one of the commercially available products. Group practices may not have the internal resources to develop their own system and should instead invest in an off-the-shelf product. Vendors will offer (for a fee) to customize their product to better address a group's needs. Independent of a medical group's choice, it behooves the practice administrators to ask upfront what questions the cost accounting software is supposed to answer. This should include decisions on how much detailed information is needed and how the information should be organized to encourage the intended end-users to incorporate the data into their decision-making processes.

EXHIBIT 4.1 ■ Healthcare Accounting Structure

Account Numbers	Account Labels
1000	Assets
1100	Cash
1200	Short-Term Investments
1300	Accounts Receivable
1400	Inventories
1500	Prepaid Expenses and Other Current Assets
1600	Investments — Long-Term Receivables
1700	Property, Furniture, Fixtures, and Equipment
1800	Accumulated Depreciation — Property, Furniture, etc.
1900	Intangible and Other Noncurrent Assets
2000	Liabilities
2100	Current Liabilities — Payables
2200	Current Liabilities — Payroll
2300	Current Liabilities — Other
2400	Long-Term Liabilities
3000	Owners' Equity Accounts
3100	Partners' Equity (General Partnership)
3200	Stockholders' Equity (Corporation)
3300	Net Assets (Not-for-Profit Organization)
3400	Partners' Equity/Stockholders' Equity (Limited-Liability Partnership/Corporation)
4000	Operating Revenue
4100	Gross Charges (Accrual and Modified Cash)
4200	Adjustments to Fee-for-Service Charges (Accrual and Modified Cash)
4300	Cash Received (Cash and Modified Cash)
4400	Bad Debt Recovery (Accrual, Cash, and Modified Cash)
4500	Patient and Payer Refunds (Accrual, Cash, and Modified Cash)
4600	Third-Party Settlements (Accrual, Cash, and Modified Cash)
5000	Operating Expenses — Support Staff
5100	Salaries — Support Staff
5200	Bonuses — Support Staff
5300	Support Staff Benefits
5400	Temporary Staff Expenses
6000	General and Administrative Expenses
6100	Building and Occupancy Expenses
6200	Furniture, Fixtures, and Equipment
6300	Administrative Supplies and Services
6400	Employee-Related Expenses
6500	Vehicles and Travel
6600	Promotion and Marketing

(Exhibit 4.1 continues on the next page)

EXHIBIT 4.1 ▪ **Healthcare Accounting Structure** *(continued)*

Account Numbers	Account Labels
6700	Insurance
6800	Information Technology
6900	Bad Debt Expense
7000	Clinical and Ancillary Services
7100	Clinical Furniture, Fixtures, and Equipment
7200	Clinical Supplies and Services
7300	Radiology Expenses
7400	Laboratory Expenses
7500	Ambulatory Surgery Expenses
7600	Other Ancillary Services Expenses
7700	Research Expenses
7800	Purchased Professional and Medical Services
7900	Cost of Goods Sold
8000	Physician and Nonphysician-Related Expenses
8100	Physician Compensation
8200	Physician Benefits
8300	Nonphysician Provider Compensation
8400	Nonphysician Provider Benefits
8500	Residents, Fellows, and Postdocs Compensation
8600	Residents, Fellows, and Postdocs Benefits
8700	Distributions to Nonphysician Owners
9000	Nonoperating Revenue and Expenses and Provision for Conversion to Cash Basis Accounting
9100	Nonmedical Revenue
9200	Nonoperating Expenses
9300	Current Income Tax
9400	Deferred Income Tax
9500	Business Taxes
9600	Business Assessments
9900	Provision for Cash Basis Conversion

PRACTICE MANAGEMENT SYSTEMS

This generic term refers to a multitude of functions: patient accounting includes both accounting (posting transactions, managing A/R and collections, monitoring bad debt, and billing consolidation by payer) and electronic claims processing (including the ability to handle fee-for-service [FFS] and capitation billing and payments, copayments, and deductibles). Appointment scheduling and reporting are also important functions of a practice management system.

Obviously, patient accounting is a critical component to overall practice management. The efficiency and effectiveness of patient accounting can "make or break" an organization's financial health. Because of the high volume of submitted claims, automation of these functions may take priority over some of the other operations management subsystems.

This subsystem should be able to track and report lag time from date of service to date of billing. If there is a significant amount of lag time, perhaps the physicians and/or mid-levels are not completing their paperwork in a timely manner. The use of a fully integrated practice management system with EHR can automate the coding process and eliminate the need for manual coding and charge entry. The system should track missing charges, checking scheduled services against billed services. An organization should also have the capability to track and report the A/R aging, which is the lag time from date of billing to date of payment, by payer. When analyzing the data, a practice should note which payers are easier to work with on claims processing and pay faster than others. Are the slowest payers providing a low percentage of the overall revenue? If so, perhaps those contracts should not be renewed. Overall, is the age of the A/R increasing or decreasing? It is important to track these various indicators over time to stay on top of potential problems rather than wait until a financial crisis develops.

Claims Systems Features

Managed care has definitely complicated claims processing. Historically, claims were processed manually by a staff person who only needed to know if the patient was current with his/her insurance, what services were covered, whether or not the deductible was met, and the amount of the co-insurance. Now it is nearly impossible for an entire staff to efficiently and effectively process, let alone adjudicate, the volume of claims with the various payers and numerous contract restrictions. Thankfully, technology has allowed medical groups to automate this arduous process. Because of the different designs of such claims systems, a practice must carefully review each system's features before choosing one.

An automated claims system must be able to handle the referral process by flagging any referral requirements in advance of services rendered and match the referrals with the appropriate claims to ensure proper reimbursement. A state-of-the-art claims system must also be able to handle claims no matter what the format or media because claims can originate from a wide variety of sources.

If budgetary constraints will not allow for an in-house claims system, then outsourcing to a centralized claims clearinghouse may become a viable option.

Internet-based claims processing systems: Internet-based claims processing is rapidly emerging as a viable and inexpensive method of electronically processing claims across all payers, although early "per click" electronic claims fees of $0.30 to $0.50 per transaction have been too expensive for many groups. A recent trend is to charge a flat fee per month regardless of the number of claims transmitted and processed via the Internet. Thanks to encryption, data sent via the Internet can be as safe as data submitted in more traditional ways.

HIPAA standard electronic transactions have advanced the use of Internet-based claims processing. HIPAA 5010 standards were implemented in January 2012, adding more power to the functionality of electronic claims submission, claims status inquiries, electronic remittance advice, and eligibility checks. Some payers are testing real-time claim adjudication.

Electronic remittance processing: Remittance processing can be extremely labor intensive when done manually. It is now possible to automate this data-entry nightmare. A fully integrated electronic remittance system must be able to automatically post payments, edit the remittance to verify that it balances, store and retrieve the rules for posting remittances from each payer, and report on the transactions for that period (including what was posted and what was rejected).

Cash reconciliation is an important function between the FIS and practice management system. The software should provide electronic cash tracking and reconciling for multiple facilities, allow for various levels of user security, offer interfaces for electronic fund transfers from banks, and produce highly detailed reports.

CONTRACT MANAGEMENT

A contract management system can either be an adjunct module to patient accounting and finance or a separate software product obtained from a third-party payer that interfaces with the current financial system. Electronic tracking of each payer's fee schedule and contractual requirements is much more efficient than manual processing. It provides a centralized database across all payers that should automatically reconcile line-item charges with their contractual adjustments. It should also track the start and termination dates of any contract to ensure that coverage is available when the need arises. This module is available to users throughout the practice and provides simultaneous updates that maintain database integrity. Some practice management systems store contracted fee schedules, making it possible to run an "underpayment report" for payments posted. Comparing actual payments against the contracted allowable amounts ensures that your payer contracts are being fulfilled.

Additional features of this module include automatic, on-screen flags when authorizations and referrals are required, when certain services are not covered under the plan, or when mandatory procedure modifiers are missing. These flags can appear when the appointment is scheduled, during the actual encounter, or during the billing process. Some of this information is also captured in the patient accounting system. Group practice administrators should carefully evaluate contract management software to avoid investing in unnecessary software or features.

Contract management software must be user friendly, adaptable, and flexible enough to allow customized definitions of each insurance carrier's plan. This module needs to include the list of approved providers by specialty, covered services under the plan, and approved facilities. Debra C. Weissman[3] suggests looking for several capabilities in a contract management module:

- User-defined limits by dollar amount or number of visits
- Storage of projected values for dollars per visit, per limits, per 1,000-member month, and per referral (these projected values can be used to compare the practice's actual performance and the plan's expected utilization)
- A separate schedule of approved amounts to be used for plan referrals or specialist referrals or for primary care physician payments to the specialists

If an organization has any third-party payer contracts, regardless of FFS or full-risk capitation, contract management software needs to be able to determine the profitability of such contracts. Reports that indicate the ratio of charges to collections by payer, the denial rates and write-offs by payer, and the ratio of actual payments to the payer fee schedule are all basic and fundamental to contract management. In an FFS market, practice administrators need to be able to compare the costs for providing services to the reimbursement offered for those services by each payer. The software should also be able to report and analyze both direct costs and total costs for patient care within the practice. When considering a capitated contract, the practice is well advised to determine if the revenue per RVU will cover the practice-specific cost per RVU. Signing a contract without this basic knowledge is extremely risky.

PRACTICE MANAGEMENT

Practice management systems include the functions of appointment scheduling, medical transcriptions, purchasing and supplies, meeting the demands of managed care, and providing clinical support. Because the patient record contains information that can potentially be linked to many other clinical and financial records, it is mentioned first in the following introduction of the selected practice management functions. While the descriptions are only intended to offer a brief overview, they will illustrate that some of these functions overlap with other IS components. These paragraphs emphasize the need to critically examine the functions of each potential FIS purchase and to determine how to completely integrate its components.

Claims Management

Claims management software, or "scrubbing" systems, check outbound claims for errors that may cause rejections or delays during the adjudication process. Built-in workflow rules and interfaces with coding software recognize possible errors, such as coding relationships, Medicare and commercial edits, CCI edits, modifiers, CPT to ICD-9 crosswalk, gender, units, and other potential causes of claims denials. Real-time use alerts give the physician or billing staff the opportunity to correct errors instantly instead of waiting for the claims to reject during the revenue cycle. Use of claims management software increases the percentage of claims paid on the first submission.

Practice Management Dashboards

Practice management systems with dashboard reporting features enable the practice administrator to view their practice data daily and monitor activity to make swift business decisions. Key indicators such as monthly charges, payments, RVUs, and visits can indicate a lag in charge capture or coding. Revenue cycle key indicators, such as days in A/R, gross collection rate, net collection rate, and percentage of A/R greater than 90 days, can be monitored. Appointment information, such as the number of new patients, missed appointments, and available appointment slots, can also be viewed on the dashboard.

Dashboards can be customized to the user. The role of the operator will determine what information is displayed on his/her dashboard. Physicians would see clinical and appointment data, billing staff would see billing workflow and tasks, and the front desk would see data related to their duties.

EHR

Meaningful use and practice relationships with hospitals and ACOs are driving the increase in EHRs at an accelerated rate. The utilization benefits are quickly realized through better patient care when staff can quickly access the EHR and provide faster and more accurate answers. To maximize efficiency, practice administrators must push for a commitment to eliminate all paper medical records. Otherwise, dual systems will be maintained indefinitely, and the full potential of the EHR may never be realized. A complete shift toward a paper-free EHR may also include an investment in network fax software (to allow faxes to be sent directly from the software program) and EKG imaging software.

The following is a brief description of some of the various EHR components. Not all are required initially, but financial managers should be aware of how they interface with each other and the features available with each module.

Master patient index: This master patient index interfaces with the appointment scheduling and profiling modules. The critical function of this index is to eliminate duplicate patient records by using a single unique patient identifier. It also facilitates patient tracking throughout the system at different points of entry and at various sites, which plays an especially important role for medical group practices within large, integrated systems. The master patient index is a centralized registration system that contains basic patient demographics (name, age, sex, phone number, zip code), insurance plan coverage, and employer information. It should cross-reference the membership identification number used for each patient by each payer to the unique patient identifier used in a system. Use of a centralized registration system permits simultaneous and system-wide updates on basic patient information, ensuring database integrity, an accurate history, and an audit trail.

Central data repository: As the foundation of the EHR filing system, the central data repository stores critical information compiled from various system sources for immediate access. This core component is akin to the hub of a wheel in that it is connected to all the other patient record components, and it acts as a general, all-purpose patient record database. Especially effective for meeting the needs of small medical groups, the central data repository module may be part of an off-the-shelf relational database. The cloud-based products available today simplify administration; eliminate IT staffing, software, and hardware costs; and provide access to a variety of outside entities such as pharmacies, labs, and hospitals. Cloud-based systems are always up to date, eliminating future investment in new versions of the product.

Clinician order entry: This module is used to log clinical test and examination results and electronically connects the healthcare provider with the pharmacies for prescription requests, with a laboratory for various tests, or with radiology for X-rays. Integrated systems can receive lab results, track unfulfilled tests by noncompliant patients, flag abnormal results for follow-up, and create charts to track lab result trends in the patient record. Electronic prescribing software can check for drug-to-drug interactions, duplicate therapy (by checking other drugs ordered by other prescribers through a hub), and provide prescription history, giving the physician valuable information for quality care. A library of patient education materials can be printed through the electronic prescribing system, ensuring patient understanding and raising patient compliance.

CLINICAL DASHBOARD

Meaningful use of dashboards can be invaluable in attaining certification for the stages of the Meaningful Use Incentive Program. Each core measure is tracked against the requirements to guide the user toward achieving certification.

Notes Module

A patient-visit documentation module provides clinicians with a standard, electronic method of documenting patient encounters for the computerized patient record. This module should also be capable of handling a physician's dictation and transcription. It is well worth the investment to also ensure that the module is adaptable and flexible enough to integrate customized templates for physician use. Templates may include communicating patient diagnosis, treatment plan, and progress between the specialist and the referring physician. A well-designed and implemented patient documentation module eliminates paperwork, saves time and money, and improves the quality of care by providing faster, more accurate communication.

A popular feature of EHRs is the ability to create specific templates for visit types. For example, a "well woman exam" template can be created to document a preventive visit for a female. The elements of the history; review of systems; and past, family, and social history can be formatted into a standard template for completion.

Exam templates can be created to assist in the documentation of problem visits. The assessment and plan portion can be template guided, as well. Beware of the "cloned notes" that can be inadvertently created by introducing the use of too many templates, or a "cut and paste" feature. Copying notes from one patient to another, or carrying forward the exact note for a patient from one date of service to another, is not allowed. Each note should be authentic to the patient visit and date of service. The use of "auto-negative" for review of systems and physical examination elements can lead to over documentation and may raise a red flag for up-coding.

Initially, only hand-held computers and desktop modules were commercially available. Internet-based software has expanded the choice of hardware to include laptops, tablets, and smart phones. Because of the increased portability of these devices, it is imperative to provide patient confidentiality and privacy by limiting access to the electronic files through security measures such as passwords and physical safeguards. The important features for this module are that the user interface be extremely intuitive and that the system be credible to ensure accuracy and integrity of the record. Portable and wireless point-of-care (POC) computing technology captures clinical data for physicians. At the start of each day, the physician downloads the current clinical patient information from the main computer terminal for all the patients that he or she will see that day. During the day, providers document their activities and upload the information back into the main computer terminal every few hours. POC is fast, efficient, and effective because it is easy to use and drastically decreases the manual labor involved with charting patient care. Consequently, healthcare providers can spend more time with patients and less time documenting the visits. In addition, the POCs are carried by each provider, so fewer computers are required, and physicians can dial in from their homes or offices, log in using their passwords, and immediately access patient data, such as test results, in real time.

Practice management systems can interface with POC technology, capturing the CPT and ICD-9 codes along with the provider identity, date of service, and place of service. This feature enables charges to be automatically created, eliminating lost charges for services provided outside the physician's office.

Appointment Scheduling

Used by small and large groups alike, this key component allows onscreen scheduling and appointment viewing across all departments within the practice(s). It is critical to integrate the appointment scheduler with the master patient index to provide immediate and complete information on the patient.

This component does far more for most practices than simply electronic scheduling. It also tracks and monitors network referrals and patient appointment history (including no-shows and recurring visits), generates automatic appointment reminders, and monitors resource utilization for not only the physicians and staff, but also for the examination rooms and various equipment. A useful appointment-scheduling module also allows for customized daily and weekly schedules to meet individual practice needs.

Using an automated appointment schedule can reduce patient no-shows with the integration of automated appointment-reminder technology. Several vendors offer phone calls for patient appointment reminders and confirmations, calls to remind patients due for recalls, and general office communications, such as new service offerings.

Integrating the appointment schedule with the billing system enables the practice to check eligibility with payers for patients with upcoming appointments. The increase in high-dollar deductibles makes it necessary to check the status of a patient's deductible, particularly early in the year to make decisions about time of service collections and payment arrangements.

PATIENT MANAGEMENT

Patient management includes quality assurance through productivity measurement and analyses, monitoring the number of encounters, tracking diagnosis code frequency and other utilization rates, tracking the treatment plan patterns by physician, monitoring referrals and management of referrals, and tracking outcomes. With the advent of PQRI and now the PQRS, there is increased focus on the quality of care versus the quantity of care. Physicians have been able to receive bonuses from Medicare for tracking quality measures on their patients. Many insurance companies have offered quality programs for their network providers, as well.

Physicians must be both effective and efficient while maintaining patient satisfaction. Insurance companies closely monitor the prescription patterns of physicians, the admission rates, and the average length of stay per patient as part of the overall patient management provided by a practice. Proving a practice's track record in efficiency and effectiveness requires quantitative documentation over a period of time. Quality data will become increasingly important as ACOs are formed and payment is driven by quality measures and outcome data, rather than FFS.

Productivity Tracking

Running a practice requires critical decision making. Software, such as Web-based business intelligence solutions, provides important data for medical practices. It allows you to quickly and easily analyze your internal data as well as compare your practice to others. This enhanced understanding helps you improve the quality and efficiency of your business processes and physician performance. A medical group practice needs to know how its provider productivity compares to its peers. Physician compensation is often based on work RVUs (wRVUs). MGMA-ACMPE offers a wide variety of surveys that can be used by a medical group practice for benchmarking. The two most popular are the Cost Survey and the Physician Compensation and Production Survey, which are briefly described in chapter 2. If a practice's physicians and/or mid-level providers need to change their practice styles to become more efficient, then the practice may consider determining goals and incentives to induce change. Some of the more popular indicators used to track productivity include the following:

- Encounters/FTE
- Unique patients/FTE

- Procedures/FTE
- Procedures/Unique patient
- Procedures/Encounter
- RVUs/Procedure
- RVUs/FTE
- RVUs/Encounter
- RVUs/Unique patient

The difference between encounter and unique patient is that an encounter is a documented, face-to-face contact between a patient and a provider who exercises independent judgment in the provision of services to an individual, whereas a unique patient is a single person who receives medical services within a specified amount of time (usually one year). Thus, the unique patient count aggregates the number of persons seen in a practice, not the number of visits. Although certainly not an exhaustive list, the combination of these key indicators offers a starting point to understanding each physician's case mix, level of procedure complexity, and case complexity, as well as productivity measures. A practice could also track procedure frequency, which would indicate a practice's volume and physicians' practice style. It is helpful, however, to monitor each provider's coding habits to detect improper coding of services. Tracking diagnosis code frequency (such as ICD-9 codes) also indicates the types of illnesses within a given patient population. A high frequency of certain diagnoses, such as diabetes, could result in the development of specialized programs geared toward case management. Performance indicators are also discussed in chapter 5.

Referral Tracking

Referrals can be a cause of claims delays if they are not tracked efficiently. Primary care practices often are required to obtain referrals before referring the patient to a specialist or for diagnostic testing services. Specialists may be required to obtain a referral before seeing a patient of certain insurance plans. Tracking the referral process can be time consuming and, therefore, costly. Practice management systems that have a referral module can track both outgoing and incoming referrals. Referral information such as date range, number of visits, or dollar amount of the authorization can be linked to the claims with which they are associated.

Insurance companies closely track the referrals physicians make. They know the frequency of referrals, the types of services provided during the referrals, and to whom patients are being referred. Since referrals are most often made to specialists, and since services offered by specialists are often more expensive than those offered by primary care physicians, insurance companies are very interested in the management of referrals. If a medical group practice generates a considerable amount of revenue from capitated contracts, a practice might decide to take a closer look at the referral patterns of individual physicians to curb potential financial losses.

Patient Satisfaction Surveys

Patient satisfaction surveys, some of which may require identifying patients by insurance or diagnosis, are likely to become more important. This will affect IS requirements and require reports to identify patient populations. With an increasing portion of total revenues coming from managed care contracts, it is advisable that medical group practices of any size at least examine the nonautomated versions of the patient satisfaction surveys. After all, if patients are not satisfied with the level of care that they are receiving within a medical practice, they are less likely to remain patients of their current healthcare provider. The increase in financial responsibility due to high deductibles makes the patient a more active consumer. Patient satisfaction, like the "shopping experience," is an important aspect in the marketing of a practice.

Simply tracking the number of forms distributed versus the number collected is not sufficient because of the bias created by patient self-selection. This means that those patients who had a bad experience or those who routinely fill out all types of surveys are likely to respond. Clinics should aim for response rates of at least 30 percent of all patients that were surveyed to ensure that their analyses are based on a representative cross-section of both patients and providers.[4] Practices will also want to track the satisfaction scores by insurance carrier. This type of tracking may not require sophisticated technology and can be handled through a spreadsheet program if the needed information is relatively simplistic in nature. When using more sophisticated patient satisfaction systems, clinics often include patient satisfaction scores in physician compensation calculations. Aided by these analyses, practices glean quantitative information on how to reward their physicians whose patient care has had high patient satisfaction. Because patient satisfaction surveys usually include questions on the patient's self-reported health or functional status, it is also often used as a health outcomes measure for quality of care and for physician profiling purposes.

Use of a patient portal through the practice's Web site can provide easy access for patient satisfaction surveys, completed electronically, and the results can be easily retrieved and sorted by unlimited criteria for analysis. Portals also allow patients the convenience of checking their account balance, reviewing their statement, making online payments, requesting or rescheduling appointments, updating demographic information, and seeing clinical information, such as test results.

Patient Flow

Tracking the amount of time it takes patients to complete their office visit can help to improve efficiency. The analysis of such statistics will especially help larger practices with a high volume of managed care plans to optimize their operations. Reports on patient flow reflect the percentage of appointments kept, the length of appointment wait times (from phone call to actual visit date), and the amount of time spent in the waiting room before the patient sees the healthcare provider. Waiting time has been shown to influence patient satisfaction; thus, patient flow and patient satisfaction reports may be linked together to increase the potential for report analysis. Practice management systems with appointment schedules often have the capability to "click" on the patient name as they check in, are taken back, and check out. These "clicks" are time stamped and create reports on wait time and patient-visit duration. Practices using the Lean Six Sigma methods to increase efficiency depend on patient flow data to reduce waste and cost. A lean organization focuses its key processes to continuously increase patient value. The ultimate goal is to use evidence-based process discovery for improvement.

DATA/DECISION SUPPORT SYSTEMS

The data/decision support system (DDSS) is a central depository database, which ensures that critical financial, clinical, and operational data are readily accessible when needed. For those entities with risk-sharing arrangements, it accurately reports the extent of services provided as well as the profit and loss associated with each of the services.

The DDSS has traditionally been installed in large integrated delivery systems. Massive amounts of data are stored in what are commonly referred to as data warehouses. While storage has not been a problem, accessing the needed data for a particular purpose has been. Even though large systems have a long history with DDSS, communications technology becomes increasingly important for healthcare organizations of all sizes. Even smaller groups need to invest in at least the off-the-shelf relational databases to contain the clinical and financial information to provide a common thread between contractually linked risk-sharing organizations. A relational database is a database in the form of tables that can be cross-referenced and linked together to create the desired data/report layout. Changes in one table result in the appropriate and simultaneous updates in the other "related" tables.

Vendors are partnering with physicians, hospitals, and other healthcare providers to work together to improve patient care by hosting a registry that encompasses large amounts of patient data for decision making. Evidence-based chronic and preventive care protocols identify and notify patients due for care while tracking compliance and measuring quality and financial results. These solutions focus on population health improvement by enhancing patient engagement from reactive to proactive. The result is a focus on maintaining good health for all patients, not just the acutely ill population.

As a rules-based system, the DDSS allows management to predetermine the actions to be taken on any option by embedding their business rules into the decision-support software. In other words, this software functions as the data analysis tool for decisions within the practice and includes all its clinical and financial data. Use of DDSS will prepare practices for new healthcare initiatives, such as meaningful use, patient-centered medical home, and accountable care.

Registries: Sandy Graham wrote an article on patient care systems in the March 2012 issue of *MGMA Connexion*, "Know Your Data. Know Your Patient."[5] Registries help practices provide effective, efficient care. The article explained what registries can do by providing key tools for improving and reporting performance across many practices. Patient health data will play an increasingly important role as payers reward practices for patient outcomes. A registry can improve care both for populations of patients and individuals, said Deb Maltby, health informatics consultant for HealthTeamWorks, formerly the Colorado Clinical Guidelines Collaborative. A good registry does four things:

1. Helps with outreach
2. Provides clinical support
3. Tracks quality
4. Helps practices educate patients[6]

SIX KEY FACTORS IN SELECTING IS COMPONENTS

FIS purchasers should remember that they are choosing an information system, not a stand-alone or off-the-shelf program. They will need to think in terms of the components that will integrate and comprise the entire system for a practice. The selection process should include careful consideration of these six factors:[7] functionality, scalability, support availability, flexibility, cost, and integration capability.

Functionality: What are the FIS needs? Answers evolve around the functionality of the components. The functionality should include an intuitive user interface that allows clinicians and other users to learn the new system quickly. If it is too complicated to learn, the system will not be used to its fullest potential. The purchaser should remember that the group does not need to automate everything at once. Instead, it is advised to separate the needs from the wants and to then prioritize the needs. Most groups begin with the patient billing and A/R systems and build their system from there. Considering SaaS and purchasing modules incrementally will keep costs down by avoiding multiple capital investments. This model often has built-in upgrades, so future purchases of new releases is eliminated.

Scalability: When building a system from individual components, medical group practices should make sure that the system is upgradable for future requirements. The technical, open-system architecture should allow for customization, expansion, and easy maintenance and should be upgradable when new technology merits further resource investment.

Support availability: Purchased or leased equipment must include sufficient and available support. Reliability is a key attribute for any system; however, even the most expensive equipment breaks down eventually. Administrators should check the track record of the vendor and the equipment before signing the contract. Due to the long-term nature of the relationship with a vendor, the availability of training and vendor system support is important. Good vendor support means everything from ensuring that the initial installation is fully tested and operational and providing toll-free telephone support for basic questions to emergency, onsite service when critical systems fail. Checking references and customer satisfaction is very important. Ask the vendor for references, and schedule site visits to spend time in practices using the system.

Flexibility: Flexibility refers to being able to customize the reports and to change minor settings to adapt the system to particular practice needs. System users should be able to create templates or screens to run ad hoc reports without having to go back to the vendor and pay additional fees.

Cost: Is the selected system affordable? How much time and money are available for investment in automation processes? A medical group practice must have the capital to cover the initial cost of the components and the expense of ongoing maintenance and upgrades. Also, groups need to provide the staff with a significant amount of time to learn a new system and convert files to another system.

Integration capability: How will the FIS function within the current practice environment? Purchasers do not want to be stuck with components that cannot be integrated into either the current or future system components. To get the most value out of the system, every component needs to be able to integrate with the others to avoid double data entry. Practices should learn about current IT initiatives at the hospitals at which they practice, and with what other stakeholders they will need to exchange data in the future, such as ACOs.

SECURITY ISSUES

Administrators are justifiably concerned about external hackers gaining access to confidential patient medical records. However, most of the security violators are usually within the organization. It is unlikely that implemented standards will ever stop the truly professional hackers intent on entering an organization's system, but there are security measures that are quite effective against internal hackers.

In March 2011, HIMSS and MGMA-ACMPE collaborated to protect patient health information by creating a Privacy & Security Toolkit for Small Provider Organizations. Practices of all sizes are responsible for ensuring that the privacy and security of their patients' health information are maintained. Not all physician groups have the internal resources to put the required safeguards in place. The toolkit includes these seven sections:

1. Introduction
2. CMS Meaningful Use — Stage 1 Privacy and Security
3. ARRA/HITECH — New Privacy and Security Requirements
4. HIPAA
5. Guidance and Resources
6. Research/Data
7. Information for the Executives/Key Decision Makers

"This toolkit will prove invaluable for medical groups seeking assistance in traversing the demanding landscape of HIPAA privacy and security," stated Robert M. Tennant, senior policy advisor for MGMA-ACMPE. As these groups increasingly transition to electronic health records, they are finding that the challenge of complying with the privacy and security regulations has escalated significantly. The HIMSS-MGMA Toolkit, with its focus on the new privacy requirements mandated under HITECH and the security component of meaningful use, will be an important resource for those groups implementing new or revised policies, procedures, and technical solutions.[8]

Introducing the concept of password-protected files offers additional security. The philosophy on how to assign passwords should mirror a practice's corporate culture. That is, a practice may choose to focus on security to fend off outside hackers but opt for global access once the user enters the network. On the other side of the continuum is the option of a detailed password system that gives specific rights to individual users. Known as "roles based" authorization, giving specific rights to individual users based on their "need to know" meets the "minimum necessary" requirement under HIPAA. Each time an operator views, enters, corrects, or deletes data, a record is made of the transaction in the system. Operator reports should be run and reviewed by the administration or security officer on a regular basis. Unauthorized or unnecessary access to patients' records should be addressed. Policies and procedures on disciplinary measures for security breaches should be documented and broadcast throughout the practice.

Another viable option is to assign or hire a health information security officer. Although a relatively new concept, the demand for this position will soon expand as technology reaches further into unexplored and unfamiliar territories like the Internet. HIPAA forces healthcare providers to find new ways to protect the confidential data being transmitted electronically. These security officers are charged with "developing and implementing strategies for protecting the security, privacy, and confidentiality of individual patient information in a rapidly changing market and technological environment."[9]

OUTSOURCING OPTIONS

Outsourcing the noncore functions can be very cost effective for many groups and can free up internal resources for greater efficiency in other areas. Another reason for outsourcing would be to gain specialized expertise because of the lack of qualified individuals in the labor force to fill those difficult and demanding jobs. However, experts usually caution against outsourcing any mission-critical function. Even outsourcing the noncore functions, such as member enrollment and eligibility, shifts significant responsibility to the vendor; thus, medical group practices should ensure that the vendor is indeed capable of handling it.

Smaller groups that cannot afford an automated claims system can outsource this function to a medical billing company, thus eliminating the huge investment in technology and training required for implementation of a complete claims processing system. The trade-off is that the medical group loses some of the control over the claims process but gains the medical billing company's existing experience and can save start-up costs.

When investing in a new software product, managers must assess whether the program addresses all mission critical tasks of the practice. Some customization is often necessary to make a product meet a specific practice's needs, but managers should carefully consider the types and degree of customization necessary. Extensive customization can lead to higher maintenance expenses and an increased need for quality control. Changes in one software function can impact data flow in another, and if the software is modified beyond its intended application, the vendor's standard customer service may become insufficient because the vendor no longer understands the system. Thus, higher-level costlier support becomes necessary.

KEY STEPS IN SELECTING IS COMPONENTS AND VENDORS

Although each organization has unique requirements, several standard processes and questions apply no matter what type of computer system is needed. Results of a 1998 survey conducted by *Modern Healthcare* has shown that the biggest hurdle in purchasing an IS today is to obtain value and tangible benefits for the investment.[10] Of course, these values and benefits will differ for each medical group, so it is necessary to assess what is important within one's particular organization. While the most beneficial sequence of the following list may differ from group to group, it is important to carefully complete all suggested steps. This may take several years from the beginning of the process through the completion of installation and training.

Developing a vision: The long-term vision should be based on the organization's business strategy of its technology needs five years into the future. The workflow linkages between business and clinical processes should be considered when developing this vision. If the practice leadership has not updated or revisited its long-term business strategy, it should be done before making a huge investment in computer technology.

Gaining management's buy-in: Executive management ownership of this project is critical to the successful selection and implementation of a new or largely upgraded FIS. In addition, administrators should seek the full support of all physician leaders prior to investing resources in this lengthy process. Without such fundamental support, administrators will face a challenging situation.

Nominating a selection committee: A multidisciplinary selection committee of all major computer users within an organization will ensure adequate input from each of the major groups. Its participants will support what they help create, so the key players of this committee must be sure to allow a forum for everyone's needs and concerns to be heard and considered.

Completing a market analysis: The organization not only needs to know where its business is now, but it should also carefully plan where it is going based on market trends. How will the organization be affected by managed-care penetration? Are patient sources expanding or declining? Where will patients come from in the future? Are patient populations shifting in age or in site of service? What trends do the experts forecast? What is the competition doing and planning? Will the organization be merging or acquiring another group? Will the merger or acquisition be horizontal or vertical? How does the strategic business plan address the changes? This analysis is critical for proper technology planning.

Undertaking an internal needs assessment: An internal needs assessment can determine the current and near-future needs for information technology to achieve the practice's strategic goals. The selection committee should ensure that all departments have sufficient input in this phase to address their current and anticipated future needs and concerns. An assessment of the current computer system helps to determine which additional resources are needed and to ensure that future systems can be fully integrated. If the current system is antiquated or will soon be antiquated, it may be time to replace it rather than sinking resources into integrating it with the new systems. The needs assessment will be used as a "measuring stick" against potential new system solutions.

Researching available technology: Administrators must research the latest technology that can help address issues as they relate to the functions and needs on the internal assessment checklist. A formal assessment and comparison of each system component's capabilities should follow this. Features and functions are top considerations, but administrators must also understand how well the product can interface with the existing system. This is especially important if one of the potential scenarios is to integrate a new IS component into an already existing system or if a significant amount of current and historic electronic data must be transferred to a new software product.

Developing a budget: A reasonable budget for the various components of the new IS is an integral facet of the planning process. Most importantly, planners should keep in mind that they are buying for the future as well as for the present. The IS budget should reflect anticipated major growth or organizational changes. Planners will also need to budget for system maintenance, upgrades, and potential capital cost in the coming years. If possible, the selection team should consider budgeting for a full-time IS professional staff person. Having someone on staff who knows the system well and can handle the minor IS issues (short of system failure) is a wise investment.

Creating a shopping list: The shopping list includes a list of core components based on business needs, functionality, and the long-term vision. This checklist will initially contain both mission-critical needs for each department as well as a wish list. Separating the needs from the wants and prioritizing the list to ensure that the critical functions are identified and properly budgeted will streamline the next step for selecting an IS.

Performing due diligence: Due diligence should be performed on each system component using the shopping list as a guide before selecting a vendor. However, very few vendors have successful products that work well across the entire spectrum of healthcare practices. Typically, vendors will focus on long-term care, ambulatory care, or acute care settings rather than trying to satisfy all markets. Selecting a system solely on price is unlikely to serve a practice well in the long run, so the selection committee should spend as much money as it takes to get a system that will improve the current situation and will allow for future growth. The September 1997 issue of the *Federal Register* lists useful questions that FIS purchasers should ask vendors when considering their computer systems.[11] Exhibit 4.2 incorporates some of these considerations, but medical groups, amidst a selection process, would be well advised to read the complete article.

Developing technology requirements: The next step is to develop detailed technology requirements for the request for information (RFI) or the request for proposal (RFP). The biggest challenge will be to precisely and concisely communicate the organization's needs on paper. Enlisting the assistance of an unbiased, trusted technical expert will go a long way in preventing the frustration that often occurs when trying to communicate in technical jargon. In addition, this expert will be invaluable in augmenting the list of questions that should be asked of each vendor and in providing the organization with the feedback needed to assess the vendor's answers.

Identifying selection process and methods: The selection committee should determine the process and methods for choosing the new system and its vendor. Advance agreement on what will constitute the determining factors and criteria in the final selection will help avoid bickering within the committee when it comes time to pare down the list of possible options.

Developing an RFI or an RFP: The RFI or RFP must detail the organization's needs and should include technical requirements as well as a comprehensive list of questions that all potential partners must answer in writing. Once the entire RFI or RFP is completed, it should be distributed to numerous qualified vendors for bid.

Selecting a vendor: To safeguard against unpleasant surprises, medical groups are well advised to deal only with reputable professionals who have been in business at least five years and who have a substantial installation base of customers. New or small vendors may not be able to stay in business due to the highly competitive nature of systems technology. Technology is rapidly changing, but financial, technical staff, and management stability within the organization are the keys. The selection committee must carefully check out the marketplace reputation of all bidders. This includes some background checking on the bidders' integrity and problem resolution. How much experience do their technicians have with various components of the system under consideration? What is the history of the product's development? (e.g., Was it the result of a merger, or did the vendor create it through research and development over time? Where is the product in relation to its life cycle?) How many of the vendor's customers are currently using these system components? In general, medical group practices should only invest in extensive field-tested hardware and software.

(Text continues on page 117)

EXHIBIT 4.2 ■ Selecting a Billing Service Questionnaire

Are you considering a transition from an in-house billing department to a billing service, or thinking of replacing your current billing service? This checklist will help you get started in evaluating vendors. Christina Moschella, consultant, Medical Division, Edelstein & Company, LLP, Boston, and Nominee in the American College of Medical Practice Executives assisted in creating this tool.

Review your current billing service contract

- Pay special attention to:
  - Inadequate notice and potential penalties
  - Ownership of data and data formats
  - Automatic contract extensions
  - Written notice requirements
  - Termination options
  - Continuation beyond termination date

Evaluate companies

- Ask for recommendations from other practice managers
- Decide on using an in-state or out-of-state company
- Find at least three companies to interview
- Use the questionnaire for each company interviewed

On-site visit

- Narrow your search to two companies
- Visit each one and:
  - Ask to meet some of the staff who will work on your account and talk about what they do and how
  - Ask the staff and management similar questions and compare answers
  - Get a feel for the company and workflow. Do you feel comfortable with the people and procedures?
  - Check references
  - Make decision

Finalizing the commitment

- Review the contract carefully before signing it
- If you are replacing a billing service, compare your old contract with the new one. Does it have all the provisions you want?
- Have your practice's lawyer review the contract before signing it

(Exhibit 4.2 continues on the next page)

EXHIBIT 4.2 ■ **Selecting a Billing Service Questionnaire** *(continued)*

General Questions

Company Name _____

Date _____

How many years have you been in business?

    Years _____

Have you been in business under any other name?

    ☐ Yes   ☐ No

If yes, what name?

    Business name _____

Do you have a compliance plan in place?

    ☐ Yes   ☐ No

Do you have the necessary Health Insurance Portability and Accountability Act regulations in place?

    ☐ Yes   ☐ No

Has your company ever been investigated in a fraud or abuse case?

    ☐ Yes   ☐ No

If yes, what was the outcome?

_____

_____

_____

What is your in-house audit system?

_____

_____

_____

General Questions

Do you have periodic audits done by an outside firm?

☐ Yes ☐ No

Is there a current auditor's report or summary available?

☐ Yes ☐ No

How many certified coders are on your staff?

Certified coders _____

What type of training do you provide your staff?

_____

_____

_____

How often is training done?

_____

_____

_____

What is your hiring and background-check policy?

_____

_____

_____

Do you carry errors & omissions insurance?

☐ Yes ☐ No

Do you offer bookkeeping services?

☐ Yes ☐ No

How many clients do you have with my specialty?

Clients _____

(Exhibit 4.2 continues on the next page)

EXHIBIT 4.2 ■ **Selecting a Billing Service Questionnaire** *(continued)*

Billing Questions

Company Name   _____

Date   _____

What insurance companies do you bill electronically?

    Companies   _____

Are insurance payments posted electronically?

    ☐ Yes   ☐ No

If yes, from what companies?

    Companies   _____

How is the information transmitted back and forth between the practice and billing service? Is the information sent on paper, disk, or electronically?

_____

_____

_____

How is the work load distributed? Is one person responsible for an account or do several people work on it?

_____

_____

_____

Are there any billing processes that your company does not supply?

    ☐ Yes   ☐ No

If yes, what are they?

_____

_____

_____

Do you handle all billing-related and ancillary documentation to insurance companies and private-pay patients?

    ☐ Yes   ☐ No

Billing Questions

If no, what is not handled?

_____

_____

What is your procedure for deposits — lockboxes or other?

_____

_____

How often do you submit claims to insurance companies?

Timeframe for submission   _____

How often do you send statements to patients?

Timeframe for submission   _____

Who is responsible for:

CPT coding   _____

HCPCS coding   _____

ICD-9 coding   _____

What is the process/policy for handling problems, such as incomplete billing information?

_____

_____

How are electronic rejections handled?

_____

_____

How are charges batched?

_____

_____

Are charges confirmed against a service log?

☐ Yes   ☐ No

(Exhibit 4.2 continues on the next page)

EXHIBIT 4.2 ▪ **Selecting a Billing Service Questionnaire** *(continued)*

Payment Posting/Follow-up Questions

Company Name _____

Date _____

How are returned claims and statements handled, and who is responsible for them?

_____

_____

Are payments posted line by line or by the total amount of the claim?

Type of posting _____

How are zero payments (deductibles) posted?

_____

_____

How are denied claims posted and tracked?

_____

_____

_____

How often are reports run for credit balances?

Timeframe _____

Do you prepare a report for abandoned property?

☐ Yes   ☐ No

Who reviews the reports and makes the decisions regarding bad debt, write offs, etc.?
What standards do you follow?

_____

_____

Is there a threshold below which a balance is not billed?

☐ Yes   ☐ No

Are small balances kept on the books or are they written off?

Small balances _____

Data Entry Questions

Company Name   _____

Date   _____

What is your data entry process?

_____

_____

_____

_____

Is there a required format for encounter forms?

☐ Yes   ☐ No

What types of forms and data are the practice required to submit to you?

_____

_____

_____

_____

Can you provide a sample of the types of forms the practice needs to complete?

☐ Yes   ☐ No

How do you verify and audit data entries?

_____

_____

_____

From the time you receive the data, what timeframe do you need to process the claim?

_____

_____

_____

Who has ownership of the data if the contract is terminated?

Ownership   _____

(Exhibit 4.2 continues on the next page)

EXHIBIT 4.2   ■   Selecting a Billing Service Questionnaire *(continued)*

Reports Questions

Company Name   _____

Date   _____

What types of standard reports do you provide?

_____

_____

_____

_____

_____

Can you provide customized reports?

☐ Yes   ☐ No

Can an aged report be completed by "billing date" and "date of service"?

☐ Yes   ☐ No

Can the practice access the computer terminal to perform queries, update records, schedule appointments, generate demand reports, demand statements and superbills?

☐ Yes   ☐ No

Can one report (same page, tabular style) be generated showing a patient's name, insurance provider, charge, payment, adjustment, and balance?

☐ Yes   ☐ No

Can you provide a report showing the names, amounts, and reasons for bad debt, write-offs, and full adjustments?

☐ Yes   ☐ No

Costs Questions

Company Name   _____

Date   _____

How do you determine your fees?

_____

_____

If payment is by percentage, is it determined by the amount billed or by the amount collected?

Payment   _____

Is there an additional charge for paper claims?

☐ Yes   ☐ No

Is there an extra cost for adding a new physician to the system?

☐ Yes   ☐ No

Do you handle physician credentialing?

☐ Yes   ☐ No

What is the conversion process and the costs involved?

_____

_____

Approximately how long will the conversion process take?

_____

_____

Do you provide a conversion schedule?

☐ Yes   ☐ No

Do you handle any old A/R from the previous billing company?

☐ Yes   ☐ No

Does the practice generally require additional staff to handle the conversion?

☐ Yes   ☐ No

(Exhibit 4.2 continues on the next page)

EXHIBIT 4.2 ■ **Selecting a Billing Service Questionnaire** *(continued)*

Computer/Software Questions
Company Name   _____
Date   _____

What is the security system and who has access?

_____
_____

Do you have regularly scheduled virus checks?
☐ Yes   ☐ No

When is the system backed up and where are the back-ups stored (on-site or off-site)?

_____
_____

How are yearly computer system updates handled for:
   CPT codes   _____
   HCPCS codes   _____
   ICD-9 codes   _____

How would the system handle the following situation? A patient changes insurance companies and there are outstanding balances on Plan A and new charges on Plan B.

_____
_____

Can the system handle two primary insurances and differentiate which needs to be billed by date of service?
☐ Yes   ☐ No

Is the practice required to pay for a software license?
☐ Yes   ☐ No

Does the practice have to pay for any software or hardware updates or maintenance?
☐ Yes   ☐ No

Is the practice required to pay for any hardware?
☐ Yes   ☐ No

If so, does the practice retain the license and hardware if the agreement ends?
☐ Yes   ☐ No

Do you use the latest version of the billing software?
☐ Yes   ☐ No

Collections Questions

Company Name   _____

Date   _____

Do you have a seperate department that handles collections?
☐ Yes   ☐ No

Can you generate reports showing the patient's name, the service provider, insurance company, charges, and reason for insurance rejection?
☐ Yes   ☐ No

Describe the collection procedure for private-pay patients.

_____

_____

Do you call patients with past-due balances?
☐ Yes   ☐ No

If the practice does not provide the service with information in a timely manner, is the account written off as a bad debt or as an insurance adjustment?

_____

_____

How do you document services provided but not billable due to timeliness?

_____

_____

Is there a charge to document services not billable to the insurance company or patient?
☐ Yes   ☐ No

Can you provide a sample of collection letters used?
☐ Yes   ☐ No

What process do you follow to turn an account over to collections?

_____

_____

If you turn an account over to a collection agency, are the "regular rate" fees subtracted from the amount due to you when payment is collected?

_____

_____

(Exhibit 4.2 continues on the next page)

EXHIBIT 4.2 ■ Selecting a Billing Service Questionnaire *(continued)*

References Questions
Company Name _____

Date _____

Has the billing service carried out its commitment?
☐ Yes   ☐ No

Was the conversion process handled smoothly?
☐ Yes   ☐ No

Have you encountered any hidden costs or surprises?
☐ Yes   ☐ No

Does the customer service department meet your needs most of the time?
☐ Yes   ☐ No

How helpful is the company to your individual needs?

_____
_____
_____
_____

What, if any, problems have you experienced?

_____
_____
_____
_____

Does the company stay up-to-date on industry changes?
☐ Yes   ☐ No

Would you recommend the service?
☐ Yes   ☐ No

Checking vendor references: The selection committee is advised to check references and to test-drive the new system prior to signing the contract. In addition, the committee should request the entire user group list from the vendor instead of accepting only a preselected list of references from any vendor. The purchaser will have a better chance of hearing unsolicited testimonies from randomly called clients. Reference checks should include testimony from several organizations similar to one's own in size and needs. If the vendor cannot supply such a list, it may be a red flag that this vendor is not very experienced with similar groups. If feasible, the selection team should visit a few of these current vendor customers who have been using the system to see the components at work in real time. The selection team may also request a live demonstration in the medical group's offices using the medical group's own data.

Negotiating a contract: Medical group practices should never accept a standard contract from a vendor. This is a big investment, and it should be treated that way. The cost estimate as determined by the vendor should address all the organization's RFP requirements without extraneous bells and whistles. Depending on the scope of the pending contract, highly experienced legal counsel specializing in acquiring healthcare information technology can be valuable throughout the contract process. A technical expert can also be valuable at this stage. The negotiation process will indicate the vendor's style as future issues arise. Computer system vendors are in a highly competitive market; therefore, they should be willing to negotiate the best possible deal to meet a medical group's needs.

Identifying implementation guidelines: The selection team must develop a realistic timeline for system conversion and implementation. It often takes twice as long as originally thought to work out the kinks that come with every new installation.

FUTURE TRENDS IN HEALTHCARE TECHNOLOGY

Most patient-related documentation (e.g., EMR, X-rays, prescriptions, insurance information, appointment reminders, etc.) is transmitted via the Internet. One of the reasons for the Internet push is that it only takes a Web browser and does not require complicated, expensive technology to link one medical group with another facility. In addition, as more healthcare professionals require access to financial and clinical information, further expansion into Internet-based communication may occur.

Another service now widely available is a Web-based system that allows patients to view their medical records online. One of the major issues is how to present the data in such a manner that a reader cannot misinterpret it. An unresolved question in this new area is deciding what part of the medical records should be available online. It opens a Pandora's box of ethical and legal issues, so it may be three to five years before this option is widely available.

The current trend to integrate the various information system modules is likely to continue. Integration will not only refer to linking financial management modules to one another, but will also move toward the integration of clinical data with the financial management systems. This will include further development of population-based disease management systems, profiling, and EHR systems. FIS might change its focus from the historical review of financial transactions to management reporting to predicting future financial status based on current financial and clinical data. This development will be motivated by both technology advances and the realities of the managed-care health delivery environment. With healthcare providers having to take on more risk, the demands on IS will increasingly take some of the uncertainty out of a medical practice's future.

Progress in hardware and software technology, decreasing hardware costs, and consolidation among healthcare software providers are likely to continue. Matched with the significant changes within the healthcare industry, practice managers will face more challenges in planning for their groups' information needs. Mergers and the development of more integrated systems will also pose difficulties in FIS planning.

In summary, financial managers will experience further expansions in their expected areas of expertise. As their profession evolves further, they will have to follow the industry's trends for increased sophistication in automating their practice's data flow to mirror the clinical, financial, and industry integration and consolidation processes.

To the Point

■ A financial information system (FIS) is any formal process that provides managers with the financial information to interpret their organization's activities as well as to support their decision-making processes.

■ Information systems (IS) need to be aligned with the overall strategies of a medical group practice.

■ Medical group practices need not invest in complete systems all at once but can incrementally invest in their information systems to enhance and protect their mission-critical functions.

■ Medical group practice managers will continue to be faced with the challenging task of integrating financial data with clinical data.

■ Financial management systems include general and cost accounting, patient accounting, and contract management. A tailored chart of accounts (COA) organizes all financial and tax report information within a financial management system.

■ Practice management systems include subsystems such as EHR, patient financial management, appointment scheduling, medical transcriptions, purchasing and supplies, and inventory control functions.

■ EHR systems include patient history, medication history, and an interface to e-prescribing technology, including test orders; lab, X-ray, and EKG results; visit notes; operative notes; and all documentation to support services rendered and billed.

■ Patient management systems include quality and productivity tracking, as well as referrals, clinical outcomes, patient satisfaction modules, and patient flow analysis.

■ The IS characteristics as described through functionality, scalability, support availability, flexibility, cost, and integration capability should be closely examined when making IS investment decisions.

■ Selecting IS components and vendors is a multistep process. Some of the most important steps are gaining management's buy-in, completing a market analysis, undertaking an internal needs assessment, developing a budget, developing technology requirements, identifying selection process and methods, checking vendor references, and negotiating a contract.

■ Outsourcing of FIS functions is often very cost effective and can significantly augment the practice's capabilities. However, once outsourced, internal staff must still closely monitor these functions.

REFERENCES

1. Medical Group Management Association. 2011. *Chart of Accounts, 5th Edition*. Englewood, CO: MGMA.

2. Finkler, S.A. and Ward, D.M. 1994. *Essentials of Cost Accounting for Health Care Organizations*. Gaithersburg, MD: Aspen Publishers.

3. Weissman, D.C. 1997. "Tips on Selecting a Computer System to Manage Managed Care." *Journal of Medical Practice Management,* 131(1): 45–47.

4. Malloy, D. and Cyr, P. 1998. "Patient Satisfaction and Physician Profiling." In *Physician Profiling: A Source Book for Health Care Administrators*, edited by N.F. Piland and K.B. Lynam. San Francisco, CA: Jossey Bass.

5. Graham, S. 2012. "Know Your Data. Know Your Patient." *MGMA Connexion*, March.

6. Ibid.

7. "Picking the Right Managed Care Software." 1998. *Executive Solutions for Healthcare Management*. Gaithersburg, MD: Aspen Publishers. March: 20–21.

8. Medical Group Management Association. 2011. "HIMSS and MGMA Collaborate to Protect Patient Health Information." Press Release, March 29. Retrieved from www.mgma.com/press/default.aspx?id=1248398.

9. "Do You Need a Health Information Security Officer?" 1998. *Strategies for Healthcare Excellence for Healthcare Resources*, September 11(9): 5–8.

10. Morrissey, J. 1998. "Data Systems' Tangible Benefits Still a Hard Sell." *Modern Healthcare*, February 23.

11. Medicare Program: Meeting of the Practicing Physicians Advisory Council. 1997, September 22. *Federal Register 62* (168): 45823–45823.

CHAPTER 5

Reporting Financial Results

Edited by Lee Ann Webster, MA, CPA, FACMPE

After completing this chapter, you will be able to:

- Explain the contents and arrangements of the income statement and the revenue and expense measurement principles followed in preparing this statement.

- Describe the components of the balance sheet and the various classifications appearing on this statement.

- Identify the elements of a model set of financial statements, and illustrate the interrelationship of the income statement and the balance sheet.

- Explain and demonstrate how the major types of operating reports used in medical group accounting present the results of operations and the financial status of the group.

- Summarize and describe the key indicators of performance, which are critical success factors to be monitored and used for appraising the financial and nonfinancial activities of group operations.

Determining the financial accomplishments of a medical group's operations during a designated time period is important to the success and continuance of the group practice's mission and goals. The objective of the next four chapters is to present the basic financial reports that convey a composite picture of the financial results of practice operations and the underlying concepts and systems that support the development of these reports. Chapter 5 covers the income statement and the balance sheet and presents a framework for reporting relevant financial data to the governing body. Chapter 6 examines in detail the major expense categories incurred by medical groups and introduces basic concepts and terminology about the nature of costs and the methods used to accumulate and allocate costs for various internal uses. Chapter 7 shows how costs are accumulated to determine the full cost of medical services and highlights the fundamentals of cost accounting systems. Chapter 8 focuses on the cash flow statement and the interpretation of its contents along with some practical techniques to manage the lifeblood asset of a group, which of course is cash.

THE INCOME STATEMENT

The income statement reports earnings or revenues and expenses; each refers to the same measurement of operating activities. In chapter 3, the differences between the cash, modified cash, and accrual bases of accounting were explained. As stated, since the accrual basis of accounting provides more complete and meaningful information, it will serve as the accounting basis for the majority of the examples in the next chapters.

The income statement provides information to answer the key question, "What are the results of operations for a given period of time?" This statement conveys information about the accomplishments of the practice, measured in dollars. It matches revenue to the costs incurred in generating revenue. By preparing and comparing income statements for several consecutive periods, significant trends in the components of the statement can be identified, and projections can be made of the practice's future earning power.

The discussion of elements appearing on the income statement follows the breakdown shown on the Income Statement of the East Slope Family Practice, P.C., in Exhibit 5.1. (East Slope Family Practice, P.C., is a fictitious practice.

EXHIBIT 5.1 ■ Income Statement — Accrual Basis

East Slope Family Practice, P.C., Income Statement	20X1	20X0
Revenues:		
Patient service revenue (net of contractual allowances and discounts)	$7,100,000	$6,590,000
Provision for bad debts	(100,000)	(90,000)
Net fee-for-service revenue	7,000,000	6,500,000
Capitation revenue, net	200,000	220,000
Other	110,000	90,000
Total medical revenue	7,310,000	6,810,000
Operating Cost:		
Support Staff Costs:		
Staff salaries	1,680,000	1,600,000
Payroll taxes	160,000	153,000
Employee benefits	260,000	230,000
Total support staff cost	2,100,000	1,983,000
General Operating Cost:		
Information technology	190,000	200,000
Drug supply	250,000	252,000
Medical and surgical supply	170,000	175,000
Depreciation	120,000	70,000
Professional liability insurance	90,000	85,000
Other insurance premiums	11,000	10,500
Building and occupancy	620,000	610,000
Administrative supplies and services	103,000	105,000
Professional and consulting fees	70,000	75,000
Clinical laboratory	260,000	240,000
Radiology and imaging	90,000	80,000
Promotion and marketing	32,000	30,000
Total general operating cost	2,006,000	1,932,500
Total operating cost	4,106,000	3,915,500
Total Medical Revenue after Operating Cost	3,204,000	2,894,500
Less: NPP cost	690,000	600,000
Total Medical Revenue after Operating and NPP Cost	2,514,000	2,294,500
Less: Physician cost	2,350,000	2,200,000
Net Income (Loss) after Provider-Related Expenses	164,000	94,500
Other Income (Expense):		
Interest expense (net)	(150,000)	(90,000)
Unrealized gain on marketable securities	15,000	—
Gain on disposal of equipment	20,000	—
Interest expense (net)	(115,000)	(90,000)
Income before Provision for Income Taxes	49,000	4,500
Provision for (reduction of) Income Taxes	12,000	1,500
Net Income (Loss)	37,000	3,000
Retained Earnings, Beginning of Year	400,000	397,000
Retained Earnings, End of Year	$437,000	$400,000

Any similarities to any existing practice are purely coincidental.) The discussion will also refer to the 2011 edition of the MGMA-ACMPE *Chart of Accounts*. This chart is designed to be flexible enough to allow it to be used by a wide variety of medical groups, including large and small groups, various ownership models, and specialties. Another advantage of using this chart is that its organization facilitates completion of the MGMA-ACMPE Cost Survey and benchmarking against the related indicators.

Revenue Measurement and Disclosure

Revenue is the inflow of assets, usually cash or receivables, during a period from performing a service (i.e., treating a patient) or delivering a product or other activities that constitute the ongoing operations of a business entity. As seen in the analysis of transactions in Appendices 1–12 on pages 574–585, revenues increase net assets and owners' equity on the balance sheet. Revenue realization rules establish when this increased value (related to the output of services) should be recognized (entered into the accounts as revenue). Two logical alternatives for a medical group are to realize this increase in value when cash is collected (cash basis of accounting) or when services are rendered (accrual basis of accounting).

Accrual basis income statements consider the revenue created when the service is performed if two conditions are met:

1. The earning process is substantially completed by providing the professional service.
2. Objective evidence exists to show that the asset (receivable) will be collected.

Total medical revenue (this line item may also be called "net revenue") is the final revenue amount and, on the accrual basis, represents earned revenue for the operating period. The "total medical revenue" or "net revenue" amount represents the amount of revenue an accrual practice expects to collect from its medical operations conducted during the accounting period. (For cash basis practices, this is the amount the practice actually did collect during the accounting period.) This amount is after subtracting all write-offs and adjustments for contractual write-offs, charity care, bad debts, and other amounts that the practice will not collect from total gross charges.

Patient service revenue: Generally accepted accounting principles (GAAP) require all healthcare entities to present the patient service revenue net of contractual discounts and any charity care. A 2011 GAAP update requires healthcare entities that *do not* assess the patient's ability to pay when they recognize patient service revenue to present the provision for bad debts as a reduction in the patient service revenue on the income statement, as is shown in Exhibit 5.1. Those healthcare entities that *do* assess ability to pay when recording patient service revenue should include the provision for bad debts in operating expenses.

Capitation revenue: GAAP requires that revenues earned from providing services to prepaid patients on a capitation basis be shown separately if material. These revenues, referred to as either "capitation revenue" or "premium revenue," should be realized in the time period in which services are made available to plan participants. Professional services contracted for outside the group should be accrued as expenses and recognized in the same period in which the related patients are served.

On the income statement shown in Exhibit 5.1, capitation revenue is presented net of subcapitation payments. It is also acceptable to present the gross capitation revenue in the revenue section of the income statement, with the related subcapitation costs being included in operating expenses. Management needs to consider which presentation best fits the organization. The reason that East Slope Family Practice uses the "net" presentation of capitation revenue is that the MGMA-ACMPE Cost Survey uses this method in computing its capitation revenue benchmark ("net capitation revenue"), which is also included in the total medical revenue benchmark. Thus, using this presentation better facilitates comparison with the MGMA-ACMPE Cost Survey data for net capitation revenue, total medical revenue, and the many MGMA-ACMPE Cost Survey benchmarks that are based on a percentage of total medical revenue.

Other revenue: Charges to patients for the sale of medical equipment and optical goods should be segregated from gross charges for professional services. Nonoperating revenues, such as interest revenue, rental income, or gain on the sale of used equipment, do not appear with the operating revenues but rather toward the end of the income statement under the category "Other Income (Expense)."

Revenue cycle disclosures: The notes to the financial statements should disclose the practice's methods and policies for revenue recognition of patient service revenue, capitation revenue, and any significant other revenue. Although not required, the practice may also wish to disclose its gross charge volume related to its net revenue, but it may not refer to gross charges as "revenue," nor should it include these items in a column that adds up to net income or loss.

In 2011, the FASB added a requirement that healthcare entities that recognize significant amounts of patient service revenue at the time of service without assessing the patient's ability to pay include disclosures regarding their policy for assessing the timing and amount of uncollectible patient service revenue. These disclosures should identify major sources of revenue and how the practice assesses credit risk and accounts for these in its accounting system.

GAAP also requires that the notes to financial statements disclose management's policy for providing charity care and the level of charity care provided. This disclosure should include the direct and indirect costs of providing charity care, the methods used to estimate cost, and any funds offsetting charity care.

MGMA-ACMPE Chart of Accounts: The MGMA-ACMPE *Chart of Accounts* includes revenues and adjustment accounts in the 4000 to 4600 series. The accounts for purchased services for capitation patients and subcapitation payments are in the 7810 to 7839 series.

Expense Measurement and Disclosure

Expenses are resources (assets) consumed or used in the process of generating revenue. Operating expenses are defined as expenses incurred in the process of providing healthcare services to patients. These expenses are used to determine net operating income. Groups following the accrual basis of accounting should match expenses to revenues to derive net operating income, regardless of when collections or payments occur.

The major categories of operating expenses provided in the MGMA-ACMPE *Chart of Accounts* are:

5000	Support staff costs
6000	General and administrative expenses
7000	Clinical and ancillary services
8000	Physician and nonphysician provider costs

Each category contains numerous detailed accounts for specific types of expenses. East Slope Family Practice presents operating expense categories for 20X1 as follows:

	Total Amount
Support staff costs	$2,100,000
General operating cost (which includes all general and administrative expenses and the clinical and ancillary expense)	$2,006,000
Nonphysician provider cost	$690,000
Physician cost	$2,350,000

In an incorporated medical group that is a C corporation, all salaries, including those of physicians, are considered operating expenses. In a partnership or limited liability entity (such as an LLC), partners'/owners' (physician) salaries are generally treated as a distribution of net income, while similar payments to nonowner (employee) physicians are considered operating expenses. S corporations typically follow a hybrid approach in which all physicians receive salaries classified as operating expenses, with the owner physicians also receiving amounts accounted for as distributions of profit. East Slope Family Practice includes physician salaries and other physician-related expenses, such as payroll taxes, health insurance, retirement contributions, continuing medical education, and related travel, as a separate item below operating expenses ($2,350,000 in 20X1), although it is organized as a corporation (see its balance sheet in the next section of this chapter, on page 130). The reader should take special note that physician salaries may be presented in a variety of ways in medical groups' income statements. For comparisons between groups (including those with different legal structures) and between years in the same group, separate disclosure of physician cost helps management and outside advisors assess the progress and potential of the group.

Support staff costs include all costs associated with nonprovider staff. These include but are not limited to salaries, related payroll taxes, retirement plan contributions, health and disability premiums, education, travel, and so on. Nonphysician provider costs include similar costs related to the nonphysician providers.

Because metrics involving costs for physicians, nonphysician providers, and support staff are some of the key indicators in evaluating practice financial and operating performance, these costs need to be tracked. Thus, it is important that the practice separate these costs in its accounting records. The best way to do this is to set up separate general ledger accounts for physician, nonphysician provider, and support staff amounts for salaries, payroll taxes, retirement plan contributions, health insurance costs, and so on. The MGMA-ACMPE *Chart of Accounts* does this, and even allows for a more complex structure, for example, further dividing these costs between administrative and clinical support staff.

General and administrative expenses include amounts for depreciation and amortization. Depreciation is the systematic assignment of a portion of the cost of a building or piece of equipment as an expense to the accounting periods that benefit from the use of these assets. Amortization is similar to depreciation; however, it pertains to allocating the cost of leasehold improvements or intangible assets, such as copyrights, or an expense to accounting periods that benefit from the acquisition of that asset. Even though they do not reduce cash or working capital, these items are expenses and reduce the book value of noncurrent assets, such as buildings, equipment, and amortizable intangible assets. GAAP requires a general description in the financial statements as to the method of depreciation by major classes of assets, the balances of these major classes, and the accumulated depreciation taken to date by class and in total.

General and administrative expenses also include items such as rent, supplies (clinical and administrative), utilities, insurance, property taxes, maintenance, repairs, and cost of goods sold to patients. Creditors may be interested in details about cost of goods sold, maintenance, and repairs. If the medical group sells durable medical equipment or other items, it is useful to know both the revenue from and the cost of these items to determine their contribution to net income. To a certain extent, maintenance and repairs can be deferred or accelerated under either the accrual or cash basis because there is some discretion on the part of management with regard to their timing. Thus, it is important to compare one period's expenditures for maintenance and repairs to that of others. Another item included in service and general expense is professional liability insurance, which is a highly sensitive and often significant amount. Other expenses in this category pertain to office supplies, legal expenses, accounting expenses, and various administrative expenditures.

Nonoperating Income and Expense

Nonoperating expenses arise from activities not associated with the rendering of services to patients. Examples of these expenses are research expenses and those related to the management of long-term expenses or to the management of long-term investments and endowments. In the income statement, these expenses, together with nonoperating revenues, are presented after "Net Income (Loss) after Provider-Related Expenses" in a section titled "Other Income (Expense)." It is also common for the "Other Income (Expense)" section to appear after a subtotal called "Net Income from Operations."

In the MGMA-ACMPE *Chart of Accounts*, these items appear in the 9000 section of accounts:

9000   Nonmedical revenue and expenses; Income taxes and related

Note that East Slope Family Practice shows nonoperating revenue (gain on sale of equipment of $20,000 and unrealized gain on marketable securities of $15,000) and nonoperating expense (interest expense of $15,000) separately from the total operating expenses. By disclosing interest expense separately, a group using large amounts of debt financing can compare financial performance with a group financed by owner's equity. Interest expense is deductible in arriving at both accounting net income and taxable income.

In preparing the income statement, whether it is on a monthly, quarterly, or annual basis, presenting prior years' results assists in comparing the current period with the previous year. If the statement shows the monthly or quarterly results, it should include additional columns showing the year-to-date totals as well as similar totals for the prior year. Large groups having several locations might prepare a separate income statement for each location and a combined statement for the entire practice. Small medical practices may prefer to develop fairly simple financial statements that might also contain various operating statistics in a one-sheet format. A more in-depth discussion about expenses will be provided in chapter 6.

Subtotals on the Income Statement

GAAP allows for a certain amount of flexibility regarding the arrangement of the expense accounts and various subtotals on the income statement. The income statement in this chapter includes a couple of subtotals that are consistent with MGMA-ACMPE Cost Survey profitability indicators. "Total Medical Revenue after Operating Cost" shows the amount of net operating income before paying both physician and nonphysician providers. "Total Medical Revenue after Operating and NPP Cost" shows the net operating income after all operating costs except for the physician costs.

Net Income

The "bottom line" or final item on the income statement is called net income. It represents the residual amount after all expenses — operating and nonoperating —

have been deducted from net operating revenue and nonoperating revenue. For the corporate form of a medical group, physician compensation would be classified as an operating expense; thus, net income would be the remainder after all expenses have been covered. For example, East Slope Family Practice shows a net income of $37,000 in 20X1.

STATEMENT OF CHANGES IN EQUITY

The financial statements must disclose all changes to equity accounts during the period, including retained earnings and other stockholders' equity or capital accounts. This may be accomplished by presenting a separate statement of changes in equity, or it may be done through disclosures. Frequently, the income statement will incorporate a statement of changes in retained earnings to fulfill this requirement. Combining these two statements allows less chance of overlooking these changes and also stresses the relationships between revenues, expenses, net income, and retained earnings. More will be said about retained earnings in the next section.

Due to the issuance of additional stock during 20X1, East Slope Family Practice will need to disclose information regarding the changes in its common stock and contributed capital in excess of par in its notes to financial statements, as it is not presenting a separate statement of changes in equity. Groups with many significant changes to their equity accounts would most likely opt for preparing a separate statement of changes in equity.

THE BALANCE SHEET

The question "What is the financial position of the medical group at the end of the year?" will be answered in the balance sheet. In fact, the balance sheet is also called the statement of financial position or the statement of assets and liabilities. As discussed in an earlier chapter, the balance sheet lists the medical group's assets, which in the traditional arrangement of this statement are balanced by the liability claims of creditors and owners' residual equity.

Similar to the income statement, a comparative balance sheet adds to the informational content of this report. Viewing current and prior-year amounts side by side provides a more useful basis for analysis and insight.

The fact that assets equal the sum of liabilities and owner's equity is shown in the East Slope Family Practice's Statement of Financial Position in Exhibit 5.2 as follows:

$$\text{Total assets} = \text{Liabilities} + \text{Stockholder's equity}$$
$$\$1,509,000 = \$647,000 + \$862,000$$

This example will be used to discuss the elements of the balance sheet.

EXHIBIT 5.2 ■ Balance Sheet — Accrual Basis

East Slope Family Practice's Statement of Financial Position	20X1	20X0
Assets		
Current Assets:		
Cash	$200,000	$240,000
Marketable securities	115,000	—
Patient accounts receivable, net of allowance for doubtful accounts of $50,000 in 20X1 and $47,000 in 20X0	640,000	590,000
Accounts receivable — other	2,000	3,000
Deferred tax debits — current	—	—
Prepaid expenses	12,000	10,000
Total current assets	969,000	843,000
Investment:		
Land held for future clinic site	150,000	150,000
Property and equipment, at cost:		
Leasehold improvements	75,000	65,000
Equipment	625,000	575,000
	700,000	640,000
Less: Accumulated Depreciation and Amortization	325,000	500,000
Property and equipment, net	375,000	140,000
Other Assets:		
Goodwill	15,000	15,000
Total Assets	$1,509,000	$1,148,000
Liabilities and Stockholders' Equity		
Current Liabilities:		
Notes payable	$—	$95,000
Current maturities of long-term debt	66,000	—
Accounts payable	60,000	56,000
Accrued payroll, benefits, and taxes	210,000	201,000
Claims payable	16,000	13,000
Claims payable — incurred but not received	3,000	2,000
Income taxes payable	2,000	1,000
Deferred taxes	15,000	5,000
Total current liabilities	372,000	373,000
Long-term Liabilities:		
Long-term debt, less current maturities	260,000	—
Deferred taxes	15,000	10,000
Total long-term liabilities	275,000	10,000
Total Liabilities	647,000	383,000
Stockholders' Equity:		
Common stock, $1 par, authorized 200,000 shares: issued and outstanding 100,000 shares	100,000	90,000
Contributed capital in excess of par	325,000	275,000
Retained earnings	437,000	400,000
Total stockholders' equity	862,000	765,000
Total Liabilities and Stockholders' Equity	$1,509,000	$1,148,000

Assets

In order for the balance sheet to be useful to owners, creditors, and other concerned parties, assets and liabilities must be classified by type; disclosures in notes to the statements must describe these elements more fully. The most common type of classification is to set out the current (short-term) portions of assets and liabilities from the noncurrent (long-term) accounts of each of these.

The specific breakdown of assets in the MGMA-ACMPE *Chart of Accounts* is arranged into four categories as follows:

1. Current assets
2. Investments and long-term receivables
3. Property, furniture, fixtures, and equipment
4. Intangibles and other assets

The statement of financial position of East Slope Family Practice contains these categories:

	Total Amount
Current assets	$969,000
Investments	$150,000
Noncurrent tangible assets (furniture, fixtures, and equipment)	$375,000
Other Assets	$15,000

Current assets: Current assets include cash and other assets that will be converted into cash within one year through the normal operations of the medical group. This definition excludes restricted cash and investments, which, although highly marketable, are not available to finance operations. Classifications of current assets and current liabilities are intended to show the group's liquidity at the date of the financial statement. Current liabilities are subtracted from current assets to measure working capital. Changes in working capital give some indication of ability to pay debts and finance new opportunities.

The East Slope Family Practice example illustrates the typical types of current assets that medical groups reflect in their balance sheets. They are:

	Amounts
Cash	$200,000
Marketable securities	$115,000
Accounts receivable less allowance	$640,000
Accounts receivable, other	$2,000
Prepaid expenses	$12,000

Complete descriptions of these items are shown in the *MGMA Chart of Accounts*.

Marketable securities: Marketable securities include investments in debt or equity securities that have readily determined fair market values and can be sold easily; although, if management positively intends to hold such debt securities to maturity, it may elect to include them in long-term investments and account for them as discussed under "investments and long-term receivables" below. Medical practices on the accrual basis should record these marketable securities at fair market value and recognize any unrealized gains or losses in income. Groups that report their financial statements using the cash basis used for income tax reporting will report these items at cost and not recognize income or loss until they dispose of the securities. East Slope Family Practice's financial statements include marketable securities with a $115,000 value, including a $15,000 unrealized gain.

Accounts receivable: Note that the practice's A/R is presented net of the allowances for contractual adjustments, bad debts, and charity care. The A/R are usually recorded in the general ledger using the gross charge amount, while the allowances for the anticipated write-offs are recorded in contra-accounts, which offset the gross accounts receivable to reduce it to the net anticipated amount to be collected, which is the $640,000 amount shown in the balance sheet. For example, East Slope Family Practice had the following balances in the A/R section of its general ledger:

AC#	Account Title	Amount
1310	Accounts Receivable — Fee-for-service (FFS) (recorded at gross charge amount)	$1,000,000
1331	Allowance for Bad Debts — Patients	(40,000)
1332	Allowance for Contractual Adjustments	(285,000)
1333	Allowance for Bad Debts — Third-party payers	(10,000)
1334	Allowance for Charity Care	(25,000)
Net	Net Accounts Receivable (as shown on balance sheet)	$640,000

By the offset of these allowances ($360,000) against total A/R, the A/R will be carried on the balance sheet at an amount that the group expects to collect from its patients and third-party payers ($640,000). The balance of the allowance for bad debts, also referred to as the allowance for doubtful accounts, must be disclosed on the financial statements in the manner shown for 20X1 on the balance sheet in Exhibit 5.2. Note that this amount ($50,000) is the combined total of the allowance for bad debts from patients ($40,000) and the allowance for bad debts from third-party payers ($10,000).

The notes to financial statements should include information regarding material changes in the allowance for doubtful accounts, including major changes in estimated amounts, self-pay write-offs, third-party payer write-offs, underlying assumptions, or any other unusual items.

Accounts receivable, other: This category includes receivables that do not arise from the practice's normal business operations. These amounts on East Slope Family Practice's balance sheet represent amounts due from employees.

Prepaid expenses: In accordance with the matching principle, groups must match expenses with the related revenue generated. Just as the group must recognize a liability for expenses that it has incurred but not paid, it must also record an asset for expenses that have been paid but not incurred. The prepaid expense on East Slope Family Practice's balance sheet represents professional liability premiums paid in advance of the related coverage period. Because they recognize expenses when paid rather than when incurred, cash basis practices would not have prepaid expenses on their balance sheets.

Investments and long-term receivables: These investments are segregated from current assets because they are held for purposes other than conversion into cash to finance current operations; thus, they are not available for use in current group operations. Their acquisition may use cash that would otherwise be available as a current asset. Items comprising this category of assets are:

- Long-term receivables
- Long-term debt securities, which the practice intends to hold to maturity
- Equity securities with no readily determinable value
- Investments in affiliates
- Property held for future use

A for-profit practice would report these amounts at cost. For debt securities purchased at a discount or premium, an accrual basis practice would use amortized cost. Not-for-profit practices report all debt and equity securities with a readily determinable market value at fair market value.

Investments in an affiliate represent an investment that is held to exercise control of or to significantly influence a closely related entity. A third type of investment involves holding property that is not used currently but may be used in the future. East Slope Family Practice's balance sheets include land acquired for a future clinic site as an investment at its cost of $150,000.

Property, furniture, fixtures, and equipment: This classification includes tangible, long-lived assets used in group operations. Examples of these assets are:

- Land
- Land improvements
- Buildings
- Furniture, fixtures, and equipment
- Capital leases

For all asset groups in the above list except land, the process of depreciation or amortization applies. For the latter, amortization is a process like depreciation in that the capitalized cost of a lease or leasehold improvement is written off or amortized over the life of the lease. As mentioned earlier, depreciation expense is recognized each year as an allocation of the item's original cost. Each year's depreciation amount is accumulated in a separate account that appears as an offset or contra to the related asset account. For example, the cost of a building would be carried in the buildings account and the accumulated depreciation taken to date on the building would be carried in the contra account, accumulated depreciation — buildings. Thus, there would be an accumulated depreciation account related to each of the three depreciable assets accounts above:

1. Land improvements
2. Buildings
3. Furniture, fixtures, and equipment

East Slope Family Practice does not have a building, but it does have the other types of assets listed above: leasehold improvements ($75,000) and furniture and equipment ($625,000). The combined cost of these assets is $700,000, and this cost is reduced by the accumulated depreciation and amortization ($325,000). The difference between these two amounts of $375,000 is called the net book value of property and equipment.

Intangibles and other assets: This fourth category of assets, intangibles and other assets, are few in number in medical group balance sheets. Items that might appear in this category include:

- Organization costs
- Goodwill
- Trademarks
- Trade names
- Deposits

Organization costs include legal and accounting costs to incorporate. Because the Internal Revenue Code requires that such be written off over a 60-month period following the organization date, many cash and tax basis practices include these amounts on their balance sheet and amortize them over a five-year period. Because GAAP requires that these amounts be expensed when paid, an accrual basis practice will not have these amounts on its balance sheet.

Goodwill is an intangible asset that is recognized only when another medical practice is purchased for a purchase price that is greater than the value of the tangible assets acquired. The excess amount is called goodwill. GAAP previously required that goodwill and certain other intangible assets with no definite life, such as trademarks, be written off in no more than 40 years. Changes to GAAP in 2001 require that rather than being amortized, goodwill is to be evaluated annually for impairment and written off if necessary. Intangible assets with a finite life, such as copyrights, are to be amortized on the straight-line method over their useful lives.

Intangible assets cannot generally be sold separately from the entire medical group or major segments of it; therefore, they have no cash value. This fact explains why credit grantors traditionally put little weight on intangibles when they are considering assets as security for a loan.

Liabilities

The *MGMA Chart of Accounts* designates two major types of liabilities: current liabilities and long-term liabilities.

Current liabilities: Current liabilities are obligations arising from past transactions that must be paid within one year from the balance sheet date by using current assets or by creating other current liabilities. The accounts that comprise this category on medical practice balance sheets include:

- Accounts payable
- Claims payable
- Notes and loans payable
- Long-term debt — current portion
- Payroll withholdings
- Accrued payroll liabilities
- Accrued vacation, holiday, and sick pay
- Accrued liabilities — nonpayroll
- Patient deposits
- Claims payable incurred but not reported
- Deferred revenue — capitation or prepaid plan
- Deferred income taxes — current portion

Most of these accounts are self-explanatory, except for the four described below.

Accrued liabilities — nonpayroll represents amounts due for services that have been received and used by the group in operations prior to the supplier's billing date, which fall in the next accounting period. Thus, it is necessary to adjust for this item by recognizing the amount of services received as an expense in the income statement and showing an unpaid liability (accrued liabilities — nonpayroll) on the balance sheet.

The account **claims payable incurred but not reported** represents claims for outside referrals and hospitalization of prepaid patients not yet invoiced to the group. These must be estimated and recorded as an expense during the period and as a liability at the end of the period. Later, when the invoice is received, the claim should be transferred to contract claims payable.

Deferred revenue — capitation or prepaid plans represents payments received by the group in advance of the period in which the group is to provide services. Just as an accrual basis practice must book the asset "accounts receivable" to recognize income that it has earned but not received, it must also book a liability to properly record revenues received but not yet earned.

Long-term debt — current portion is classified as a current liability if current assets are to be used to satisfy the debt. The current portion of long-term debt should include only the principal amount that will be repaid during the next year plus the interest expense that has accrued as of the balance sheet date.

East Slope Family Practice's balance sheet shows eight current liabilities totaling $372,000: current maturities of long-term debt, accounts payable, accrued payroll, benefits and taxes, claims payable, claims payable — incurred but not received, income taxes payable, and deferred taxes. Note that the payroll- and benefit-related liabilities have been combined into one line item to simplify the number of line items on this balance sheet.

Long-term liabilities: This second type of liability is an obligation that will not mature and will not require the use of current assets until after one year from the balance sheet date. The current portion of this debt was mentioned above under "current liabilities." In the notes to the financial statements, disclosure should be made of the interest rate, repayment schedule, security covenants, and other material information. The types of long-term liabilities usually found in groups' balance sheets are:

- Long-term notes payable
- Mortgage payable
- Construction loans payable
- Capital lease obligation — long-term portion
- Deferred income taxes — long-term portion

The first three items above seem to be self-explanatory. Capital lease obligations and deferred income taxes require further comments.

Leases are agreements between two parties for the rental of a facility or property. One party, the lessor, owns the property, and the second party, the lessee, pays rent for the use of the property or facility. Under GAAP, certain noncancellable leases that meet one or more specified criterion must be recorded as a capital lease obligation by the lessee. That is, the amount of the future payments must be recorded as a long-term asset and a long-term liability on the balance sheet of the lessee. The criteria are:

- Lease transfers ownership to the lessee during or at the close of the lease term
- Lease contains a bargain purchase option
- Lease term (including any bargain renewal options) is 75 percent or more of the estimated economic life of the property
- Present value of the minimum lease payments (excluding executor costs, for example, maintenance, taxes, and insurance) equals or exceeds 90 percent of the fair value of the leased property

Once capitalized, the asset and lease liability are accounted for separately. The asset is depreciated, using an acceptable depreciation method over its useful economic life, and the lease liability is treated like any other installment liability.

Leases that are noncancellable, but do not meet any of the four criteria cited above, are called operating leases. In this case, the lease payments are expensed as rent as the payments are made, and the lessee's balance sheet shows no capital assets or liabilities. For all noncancellable leases, capital or operating, a general description of the noncancellable leasing arrangements should be included in the notes to the financial statements.

Deferred income taxes represent the amount of future income taxes due that result from differences between taxable income and income before income tax reported on the income statement. Certain items are required to be treated in a specified way for income tax purposes that are at variance with how they are treated under GAAP. Thus, the amount of income tax payments due currently is based on the corporate income tax return and may differ from the amount of tax expense reported in the income statement. These differences, called temporary differences, may need to be allocated between accounting periods depending upon the nature of the items creating the difference. Temporary differences require that the amount of the tax liability be computed at the end of each year and that the proper amount of the current and postponed (deferred) liability be recognized. At the end of any year, an entity could have a deferred income tax liability or a deferred income tax asset, depending on the direction of the aggregate temporary differences.

A purchase of an X-ray machine, for example, would involve the use of straight-line depreciation on the books and the use of accelerated depreciation on the tax return. This situation results in a timing difference in depreciation expense, causing income tax expense in the income statement to be different (more) from the actual income tax payable on the tax return during the early years of an asset's life. The deferred income tax resulting in this case would be a liability. On balance sheets, most of the deferred income tax liability is shown as long term, while the current portion to be applied during the next period would be reflected in the current liability section.

The Equity Section of the Balance Sheet

The equity section of the balance sheet will vary somewhat, depending on the type of entity. Corporate entities, limited liability entities, and partnerships all have slightly different accounts in the owners' equity section.

Partners' Equity

If the medical practice is organized as a partnership, the owners' equity will be called partners' equity. Partners' equity or partners' capital represents the ownership interest of the partners in the group. It consists of two elements:

■ Contributed capital
■ Undistributed earnings

Frequently, these two elements might be lumped together, because the partnership agreement, rather than a state incorporation statute, governs any distributions to owners. General partners have unlimited liability with respect to debts of the partnership, so the record of contributed capital is not as important to creditors as it would be in a corporation.

Members' Equity

Although a limited liability entity has limited liability characteristics like a corporation, it is treated like a partnership for tax purposes. The owners of a limited liability entity are referred to as "members." The equity section for a limited liability entity is similar to that of a partnership, except that it is called "members' equity," rather than "partners' equity."

Stockholders' Equity

Stockholders' equity represents the ownership interest of the stockholder owners of a medical group that is established as a corporation. The terms comprising stockholders' equity may be somewhat confusing because they contain a mix of legal and accounting terminology that has not been fully standardized. Some examples are *par value*, *stated value*, *capital contributed in excess of par*, and *restricted or appropriated retained earnings*. A stockholders' equity includes the following accounts:

- Contributed capital
  - Preferred stock
  - Common stock
  - Capital contributed in excess of par
- Retained earnings
  - Unappropriated
  - Appropriated
  - Treasury stock
- Donated capital

Contributed capital: When a stockholder (physician) invests money in a corporation, both assets and owners' equity increase. If the amount invested exceeds the par value (or stated value) indicated on the shares issued, the excess is recorded in a separate account, called capital contributed in excess of par. The par or stated value of the stock is recorded in the capital stock account (common or preferred) and represents the legal or stated capital that provides creditors a financial cushion. Unless state incorporation laws provide otherwise, the stockholders' equity in total may not be reduced below this legal or stated capital amount by declaring dividends or re-acquiring owners' shares. Par value, then, is nothing more than the legal capital per share and serves as the minimum consideration that the corporation must receive to issue the shares as fully paid. Once so issued, any holder's liability is limited to the amount invested.

Preferred stock has certain preferences and limitations written into the contract between the corporation and the preferred stock shareholders. Typical preferences include dividends up to some specified percentage, if declared, and accumulation of dividends in arrears for years in which these were not distributed. If the latter characteristic exists, the stock is called cumulative preferred. Dividends must be declared by the board of directors before they are considered to be a liability, and preferred dividends must be paid before any dividend can be declared on common stock. Another preference for the preferred shareholders is a prior claim on assets over common stock if the corporation is liquidated. Limitations of preferred stock contracts commonly include foregoing the right to vote for directors and to participate in dividends beyond a given percentage or a set dollar amount per share.

With both common and preferred stock, the number of shares authorized, issued, and outstanding must be disclosed in the financial statement, along with the number of shares re-acquired but not canceled. The re-acquired shares are called treasury stock, and they are usually subtracted from total stockholders' equity when displayed on the balance sheet. If treasury shares are reissued above their acquisition cost, the excess is added to an appropriate contributed capital account, such as "capital contributed from treasury stock transactions." This gain (or any other dealing in the corporation's own stock) must never be included in retained earnings. If the treasury shares are issued at less than cost, this difference may first be applied to reduce capital contributed in excess of par. If the difference is larger than this latter account, retained earnings will be reduced for the remainder in a manner similar to a dividend transaction.

Retained earnings: Retained earnings are the component of stockholders' equity that accumulates the net income or loss of the entity net of dividends paid. When an entity reports net income for a period, that amount appears as an increase to its retained earnings (a net loss would be a decrease in retained earnings); and, when the entity declares a dividend or distribution of earnings, that dividend amount reduces retained earnings. Thus, at any point in time, the balance of retained earnings on the balance sheet will be the accumulation of lifetime net incomes offset by net losses and also reduced by the amount of dividends declared and distributed to stockholders to date.

When a cash dividend is declared, retained earnings are decreased and a current liability, dividends payable, is recognized. A stock dividend payable in the medical group's own stock, however, does not result in the recognition of a liability, but is recorded as a decrease in retained earnings and an increase in the contributed capital caused by the issuance of more shares.

Retained earnings may be restricted by statute, creditor's contract, or action of the board of directors. State law may require the restriction of retained earnings equal to the cost of any treasury stock. Thus, once the cost of treasury stock acquired is equal to the total retained earnings, no more treasury stock may be acquired or dividends declared, because to do so would reduce total stockholders' equity and net assets below the legal capital. The board of directors may also "appropriate" retained earnings by shifting them to one or several restricted retained-earnings accounts, such as "retained earnings — appropriated for expansion." This restriction does not affect net assets, nor does it earmark any asset for a special project. It merely indicates that the amount appropriated is not available for dividend distribution. If a special fund is to be established, then specific assets will be set aside, and this fund will be labeled as a "fund for expansion" without affecting any portion of retained earnings.

Donated capital: Donated capital is a legitimate description to use when assets have been contributed to the medical group as a gift, such as a piece of equipment or a plot of land on which to erect a medical clinic. This account is part of contributed capital because a gift of assets does not give rise to earnings retained as a result of successful operations. It is disclosed separately, because no stock is issued in exchange for the assets received.

Note that East Slope Family Practice shows three accounts in the stockholders' equity section of its balance sheet that total $597,000.

INTERRELATIONSHIP BETWEEN THE INCOME STATEMENT AND THE BALANCE SHEET

In the early development of accounting, individual transactions were not recorded. At the end of a period of time (not necessarily every month), assets and liabilities were listed, and income for the period was determined by the change in net assets (assets minus liabilities), adjusted for withdrawals or contributions by the owners. This change in net assets was net income and was balanced by increasing owners' equity. Today, each transaction is recorded as illustrated in chapter 3 and in Appendices 1–12 on pages 574–585. Transactions related to operations that increase net assets are generally recorded in a revenue account(s), although occasionally as a decrease or credit in an expense account. Likewise, transactions that decrease net assets due to operations are generally recorded in an expense account(s), although occasionally these may be a decrease (or debit) to a revenue account. The difference between revenues and expenses is the net income shown on the income statement, and this amount also increases the owners' equity on the balance sheet.

Thus, the current period net income must be added to retained earnings (or a capital account for noncorporate entities) in order for the balance sheet to balance. This is the secret to balancing the balance sheet. This account relationship of net income (loss) between the income statement and the balance sheet is called the articulation of the two financial statements.

SUMMARY

Thus far, this chapter has developed the construction and contents of two important financial statements that present the status of the group's operations: the income statement and the balance sheet. The income statement serves as a progress report on how well or poorly operations have been conducted from a financial point of view for a specific period of time. The balance sheet shows the financial picture of the practice at the end of a specific time period. The items on these statements, as well as other detailed financial data that underlie the aggregate numbers, will serve as the basis for analysis and comparison when we begin to use the data to identify strengths and shortcomings in the financial operations of the practice in later chapters. Next, we will examine some major financial measures that tell the story of how well a medical practice is doing.

KEY FINANCIAL OPERATING REPORTS AND INDICATORS

Success and survival in today's ever-changing healthcare environment depend largely on the attention of financial managers to the results and trends in operating statistics of the group's practice. Being informed and monitoring operations require constant vigilance and an understanding of the data that is collected and summarized in the accounting and financial management system. Large medical groups will generally have greater sophistication in their financial management information system. Also, they usually will have more staff to prepare various types of operating reports and to carry out the detailed analysis necessary to glean important insights from the financial data. Small medical groups might have only one individual — the administrator or a business manager — who must be a manager for the total operations of the practice, covering both financial and nonfinancial matters. Regardless of the group size, familiarity with and the ability to use various operating reports is a prime requirement for the effective fulfillment of the financial management role.

The following two lists of operating reports present the types of financial and nonfinancial data that should be produced by the practice's information systems. The reports must be used in the management of the practice, be it an FFS or a combined FFS and prepaid environment. These are most likely not complete lists of reports since the function of any information system is to provide the kinds of reports that fit the specific needs of the group. Also, smaller practices and those without capitation may not need to prepare all reports on the lists because of the mix of their patient loads between FFS and prepaid.

Financial Operating Reports

- Income statement
- Balance sheet
- Cash flow statement
- Cash report
- Operating budget (actual versus budget)
- Accounts receivable analysis (by type)
- Accounts receivable analysis (by age)
- HMO — cost per-member per-month (for practices with capitation arrangements)
- Incurred but not reported claims (IBNR)/lag report (for practices with subcapitation arrangements)

Both the income statement and the balance sheet were covered in the first part of this chapter.

Cash flow statement: This financial statement provides a picture of the cash flows within the medical group for a specific time period, as mentioned in chapter 3. The statement presents the various kinds of cash inflows and outflows, classified by operations, investing, and financing. Its informational content is historical in nature; that is, it shows the cash flows for the last indicated time period, such as the last month, quarter, or year. But the historical cash flows can be used as the basis for predicting future cash flows, which is a vital tool in cash management. More will be said about this statement and cash management in chapter 8.

Cash report: The cash report is very important to the financial manager since it is issued daily (usually) and serves as a sensitive indicator to monitor the adequacy of the amount of cash available for satisfying forthcoming obligations. It shows the sources of cash receipts and the types of cash payments that were made each day. The beginning and ending balance of cash are also shown together with the balances of the checking account(s). Comparisons of this daily cash report can be made with the forward-looking cash plan, and deviations from the planned cash flows can be identified. An indicated cash shortage will require actions such as shifting cash from one bank to another, selling or purchasing short-term investments, or borrowing or repaying short-term debt from the group's line of credit source(s). An example of the cash report and further coverage of cash management is included in chapter 8.

Operating budget: An operating budget is a quantified financial expression of the practice's operating plan for the next year. It serves as a basis for determining the practice's ability to attain predetermined tools, and it provides a tool for monitoring progress and evaluating operating performance. The operating budget, if developed on a comprehensive basis, will consist of a series of informal projections and a number of formal statements. The components may include a profit plan with detailed breakdowns of revenue and expenses, a cash budget, a capital expenditures budget, and a projected balance sheet.

When the operating budget has been developed, approved, and disseminated within the medical group, it becomes the blueprint for action and is followed by group members in planning and carrying out their activities. Periodically, each month or quarter, a report of actual results is prepared that compares the actual amounts with budgeted amounts to determine whether operations are on target with the plan. Such a comparison enables management to alter the activities of the group or adjust its plans to achieve the desired outcomes. The entire area of budgeting will be covered in chapter 11, and examples of this report will be illustrated.

Accounts receivable analysis: Two types of reports are helpful in analyzing and keeping track of accounts receivable balances. One type is a listing of all accounts and their balances arranged by type of payer, such as private pay, insurance companies, Medicare, Medicaid, and contractors. A second kind of report is the same account balances arranged by an aging of each balance, such as 0–30 days, 31–60 days, 61–90 days, and so on. These reports are typically prepared at the end of each month. Chapter 9 provides more information regarding these reports and receivables management.

HMO — cost per-member per-month: This report tracks the actual cost per-member per-month (PMPM) of visits for enrolled members. The calculation of the PMPM cost may be determined by multiplying the number of enrolled patient visits by the unit cost per visit and dividing the product by the number of enrolled members. The PMPM cost may be compared to the monthly capitation amount for services within the group to determine if revenue (capitation) is greater or less than the cost of care. In addition, both of these amounts can be compared with the planned costs of the PMPM cost. The frequency of this report can vary — either monthly or quarterly — and should be available prior to the negotiations of a continuing or new prepaid contract. Chapter 7 provides an example of calculating the PMPM cost for a practice.

Incurred but not reported (IBNR) claims/lag report: The IBNR claims/lag report portrays a list, by source, of the charges from referral healthcare providers (nongroup physicians, hospitals, and laboratories) that have not yet been reported by these providers to the medical group who referred these patients or to the prepaying organizations to which patients belong. This report should contain estimates of these claims, which are used to accrue expenses and liabilities by the medical group and the prepaying organization (HMO). Reports pertaining to these claims are included in chapter 9.

Nonfinancial Operating Reports

- Utilization: medical report
- Utilization: lab report
- Utilization: X-ray report
- In-house referrals report
- Outside referrals report
- Hospitalization report
- Physician profiles
- Patient satisfaction summaries
- Compliance status report

Utilization reports: These reports present a summary of the various services provided by the group to its patients for a period of time. Three major areas covered by utilization reports pertain to medical services, laboratory testing, and X-ray results. Details of each of these services should be shown, such as patient, type of medical procedures and treatments rendered, responsible physician, type of test, and if appropriate, applicable costs. The reports may also present year-to-date cumulative totals for each service area and may also be arranged to include previous totals for comparative analysis.

Referral reports: Patients who are referred to other physicians within the group should be listed on an in-house referral report. Patients who are referred to outside healthcare providers should be included on an outside referral report. Both of these reports should include the patient identification information, the name of the referring physician, the type of treatment or procedures ordered by the group, and the services received from the referred party, as well as any applicable charges for the provided services.

Hospitalization report: This report contains a summary of the hospital services provided to the group's patients for specific periods of time. Information on this report should include patient identification data, referring physician, surgical services performed, hospitalization duration, and the delineation of all types of charges by source.

Physician profiles: Internal and external pressures are motivating medical practices to develop clinical work profiles for physicians and practice specialties so that they can use these profiles as a management tool to meet requirements for improved accountability. The pressures driving medical practices include:

- Healthcare plans striving to control costs while maintaining quality of care
- Consumers who desire better access and broader choices
- Employers and purchasers seeking quality information to augment their purchasing decision-making process

Physician profiling is an analytical tool that uses epidemiological methods to compare practice patterns of providers on dimensions of cost, service, use, and/ or quality (process and outcomes) of care. Profiles can be at the level of the individual practitioner, the group practice, or the healthcare organization as a whole. The profiles will use practice administrative and clinical data, as well as practice and provider demographic data. An important facet of profiling is to provide good benchmarking data on physician practices.

Patient satisfaction summaries: The trend to build successful patient–physician relationships has evolved toward gathering information directly from patients about their perceptions of the quality of service they received from their provider and clinical entity. This focus on patient-centered care shows respect for patients' values, preferences, and expressed needs.

The usual data collected relate to bottom-line perceptions, such as access to care, quality of care, rating of the visit, value of the overall medical care, and likelihood to recommend the group to others. Individual items surveyed pertain to the wait time in getting an appointment, convenience of office location, telephone decorum, in-office wait time, time with the physician, and the physician's explanation of care and his or her personal manner. In addition, patient satisfaction surveys often include demographic data.

Many practices conduct continuous patient surveys and use this feedback to monitor changes in weaknesses perceived by patients. These data may take the form of complaints/compliments, which are tracked and monitored closely by practice providers and administrators.

Compliance status reports: Many healthcare providers have implemented compliance programs in response to heightened security and expectations of compliance and as part of settlements following healthcare fraud investigations. This initiative, officially called a corporate compliance program, evolved from the

U.S. Sentencing Commission Guidelines that were adopted under the Sentencing Reform Act of 1984. The act attempts to standardize and increase the predictability of federal court sentences. The guidelines articulate standards and practices that all federal court judges must follow when sentencing individuals and organizations and encourage the implementation of internal mechanisms to prevent, detect, and report criminal conduct.

It is recommended that medical practices design a corporate compliance program that meets the U.S. Sentencing Commission's Guidelines. These steps, together with an expanded discussion of this program, will be covered in detail in chapter 16. Management of medical practices must prescribe a report to be provided by implementers of the program for their entity. This report should describe the status of efforts to establish the program in compliance with the mandated guidelines. Also, once established, there should be a series of ongoing reports showing that enforcement and discipline procedures are operative to ensure consistent enforcement of the compliance standards.

CHARACTERISTICS OF EFFECTIVE OPERATING REPORTS

Information included in all types of operating reports must possess certain characteristics in order to convey the intended message and to serve as the catalyst for action. The qualities that usually promote this response can be summarized as follows:

■ Accuracy
■ Brevity
■ Clarity
■ Timeliness

Accuracy

Data contained in reports should be accurate. Inaccuracies in amounts, calculations, or narrative statements will destroy the credibility of the preparer and the presentation itself. Furthermore, the information presented must be defensible to others in the medical group. Awareness as to how the data were developed and a check of the "sensibility" of the data are steps that the preparer and presenter must complete. Finally, an objective review of the basis and supporting evidence of any conclusions in the report should be made.

Brevity

No report presentation is effective if it takes more time for users to comprehend than they are willing to invest. It is the preparer's responsibility to be brief and concise. Extraneous material that does not convey the essence of the report should be omitted. Caution should be taken not to cover too many key points in a single report. The attention span of the reader should be estimated, and the scope and length of the report should be developed accordingly. However, factual support should not be sacrificed for the sake of brevity. It is better to gain a solid understanding of half of the message than to have an incomplete understanding because of information overload.

Clarity

To achieve clarity, the preparer must know the user's background and level of understanding on financial matters. With this knowledge, reports can be tailored with the appropriate language and presentation style to ensure that content is understood. If additional explanations and a review of key concepts are essential to gain understanding, these elements should become part of the report. Avoiding the use of acronyms and technical accounting and financial jargon is an absolute necessity for most nonfinancial audiences. The use of specific examples and graphic presentations are received extremely well by most individuals.

Timeliness

No report is worth the effort to prepare if issued in an untimely fashion. Old or dated information is of little value to managers who need relevant and current data to gain an understanding of their operations. If compiling and assembling information for certain reports takes a great deal of time, a system of flash reports showing key items or critical indicators should be devised so that timeliness of disseminating these important data elements is achieved. In the next section, key indicators of operating performance for medical groups of all sizes will be covered.

MAJOR INDICATORS OF PERFORMANCE

The operating reports described in an earlier section represent the important periodic reports that provide the clearest picture of the group's operating status for the time periods they cover. Beyond these reports, a series of key indicators can denote highlights of performance. Some of these indicators are financial in nature, and others are nonfinancial. Their importance lies in the fact that they consist of a condensed aggregate number that can be used in several ways:

- ▓ To be tracked over a time period to ascertain a trend and any changes in a defined trend line
- ▓ To be compared with local, regional, and national statistics, such as those published in the MGMA Cost Survey and Physician Compensation Survey, to indicate how a specific medical group compares with medical groups of similar size or make-up

While there are a great many such indicators, this section of the text will describe only a limited number considered to be the most critical measures of the practice's operations, financial status, and clinical composition. Other performance indicators will be included in chapter 12.

In certain indicators, the term "FTE physician" is used. FTE refers to "full-time equivalent" and is employed in order to form a common base for calculating certain monetary and nonmonetary aggregates per physician across all groups. The number of FTE physicians in a medical group is a combination of full-time and part-time physicians. A physician cannot be counted as more than 1.0 FTE regardless of the number of hours worked. The minimum number of weekly work hours for a 1.0 full-time equivalent is the number of hours that the medical group considers to be a normal work week, which may range from 35 to 40 hours. The FTE of a part-time physician can be computed by comparing the time a physician spends working in the practice or in a hospital on behalf of the group to that of a full-time physician; for example, a physician who works 20 hours compared to a normal work week of 40 hours would be classified as a 0.5 FTE.

Most of these indicators are only useful if compared with other practices' indicators or with a practice's own historical results. Without this comparison, indicators will only offer current status information, and an objective evaluation of a practice's performance becomes difficult. The key indicators are arranged by the following categories:

- Financial
  - Practice performance
  - Operating costs
  - Accounts receivable
- Nonfinancial
  - Patient data
  - Group medical staff and administrative support
- Prepaid services

Financial

Practice performance

(1) Total Gross Charges per FTE Physician

$$\frac{\text{Gross FFS Charges} \; + \; \text{FFS Equivalent Charges (for Capitation Plan Patients)}}{\text{Total FTE Physicians}}$$

This indicator identifies the average amount of gross charges generated per group physician. It provides an overall picture of the financial productivity of the group. Gross charges include FFS charges and the FFS equivalent charges for services provided to patients who are covered under capitation contracts between the practice and HMO.

(2) Total Medical Revenue per FTE Physician

$$\frac{\text{Total Medical Revenue}}{\text{Total FTE Physicians}}$$

This indicator identifies the average amount of actual medical revenue per group FTE physician. Total medical revenue includes revenues from all medical sources. This indicator is an important measure of the financial stability of the group and a means of comparing relative productivity and profitability between practices.

(3) Total Operating Cost per FTE Physician

$$\frac{\text{Total Operating Cost}}{\text{Total FTE Physicians}}$$

This indicator identifies the allocation amount of operating cost incurred to provide patient care per FTE physician. For the purposes of this metric, operating costs include the salaries and benefits paid to the practices' support staff and the general operating costs but do not include salaries and benefits paid to physicians and nonphysician providers (NPPs). It can be used to monitor efficiency and cost effectiveness of operations. When used with other indicators, it can identify the potential financial resources available for provider income and/or group profits.

(4) Total Operating Cost and NPP Cost per FTE Physician

This is similar to the immediately preceding metric, "Total Operating Cost per FTE Physician," except that this indicator adds the NPP cost to the numerator. Thus, the numerator not only includes all the costs in the operating costs in indicator 3, but also includes the salaries and benefits for NPPs. Having two separate cost indicators, one that includes NPP cost and one that excludes NPP cost, provides an opportunity for more insight into the group's costs and profit potential.

(5) Total Medical Revenue after Operating Cost per FTE Physician

$$\frac{(\text{Total Medical Revenue}) - (\text{Total Operating Cost})}{\text{Total FTE Physicians}}$$

This profitability indicator identifies the amount of net income available for provider compensation and/or future reinvestment in the practice after deducting operating cost (as defined above). It provides information that groups can use to plan and budget. This indicator also identifies a group's cash flow (particularly for cash basis groups), which can be used to measure the group's liquidity.

(6) Total Medical Revenue after Operating Cost and NPP Cost per FTE Physician

$$\frac{(\text{Total Medical Revenue}) - (\text{Total Operating Cost} + \text{NPP Cost})}{\text{Total FTE Physicians}}$$

This profitability indicator is similar to indicator 5, except that it focuses on profit after subtracting both operating cost *and NPP cost* from total medical revenue. It identifies the amount of net income available for physician compensation and/or future reinvestment in the practice after deducting operating cost and NPP cost.

(7) Gross Collection Ratio

$$\frac{\text{Net FFS Revenue or Collections}}{\text{Gross FFS Charges}}$$

This ratio indicates the FFS collection margin for the group. Collection margin is the amount of actual revenue collected as a percentage of the practice's gross charges. This ratio is used to estimate the amount of services that must be provided to patients to achieve a particular level of revenue for the group. It is also useful for projecting future cash flows based upon recent charges. Because this indicator is dependent upon the practice's fee schedule (and these vary considerably among various groups and specialties), this indicator is not useful for assessing billing office efficiency.

Operating costs

(8) Total Operating Cost as a Percentage of Total Medical Revenue

$$\frac{\text{Total Operating Cost}}{\text{Total Medical Revenue}} \times 100\%$$

This indicator identifies the group's overhead ratio, meaning the percentage of total medical revenue that is being spent to cover operating costs. When subtracted from 100 percent, it identifies the proportion of total medical revenue that will be available for physician compensation and/or future reinvestment in the practice.

(9) Total Support Staff Cost per FTE Physician

$$\frac{\text{Total Support Staff Cost}}{\text{Total FTE Physicians}}$$

This indicator identifies the average support staff cost per FTE physician. As discussed previously in connection with other indicators, this cost includes not only salaries paid to support staff, but also the related payroll taxes and benefits. Salaries, payroll taxes, and benefits for physicians and nonphysician providers are not included in this cost. This metric indicates how cost efficient the group is in establishing employee compensation. When used with other indicators, the ratio can identify what proportion of operating cost is attributed to support staff cost and whether these expenses are being recouped by the group.

(10) Total Medical and Surgical Supply Cost per FTE Physician

$$\frac{\text{Medical and Surgical Supply Cost}}{\text{Total FTE Physicians}}$$

This indicator identifies the average medical and surgical supply expense allocated to each physician. It indicates whether supply costs are reasonable and if the group is using supplies efficiently. Similar metrics can be computed for other line-item costs, such as drug costs, building and occupancy costs, and information technology costs.

(11) Total General Operating Cost per FTE Physician

$$\frac{\text{Total General Operating Cost}}{\text{Total FTE Physicians}}$$

This indicator identifies the average general operating cost (or nonpeople cost) per physician. It can be used to assess whether these costs are reasonable. When used with other indicators, it can help identify what proportion of operating cost is attributable to general operating cost and whether these expenses are being recouped by the group.

(12) Total NPP Cost per FTE Physician

This indicator tracks the cost of the nonphysician providers per FTE physician. As previously discussed, the NPP cost includes not only the salaries paid to the nonphysician providers, but also the related payroll taxes and benefits. This metric can be used to assess whether NPP costs are reasonable. In connection with a review of best practice data, it can provide guidance as to the optimum levels of NPP staffing for practice efficiency and profitability.

Accounts receivables

(13) Accounts Receivable per FTE Physician

$$\frac{\text{Accounts Receivable}}{\text{Total FTE Physicians}}$$

This indicator provides an average measure of the group's charges that are outstanding per FTE physician. When used with other financial indicators, this information can assist in determining potential problem areas in the group's billing and collection procedures. This metric can measure the A/R at its gross value as expressed in gross charges or at its net expected collectible value as reflected on an accrual basis balance sheet. Whichever method the practice uses for valuing its A/R, it should use it consistently when making internal comparisons. When comparing against external data, the practice should ensure that it is valuing its A/R consistent with the method used for valuing the external benchmarks.

(14) Adjustments as a Percentage of Gross FFS Charges

$$\frac{\text{Contractual Adjustments} + \text{Charity Care}}{\text{Gross FFS Charges}} \times 100\%$$

This indicator identifies the percentage of gross FFS charges that will not be collected for rendered services due to contractual adjustments and charity care. This percentage figure is the result of contractual or regulatory adjustments made by HMOs, PPOs, governmental agencies, and other payers, as well as charity care. This indicator assists the group in estimating its future collections and in monitoring and controlling the extent of services for which it will not be reimbursed.

(15) Bad Debts Due to FFS Activity as a Percentage of Gross FFS Charges

$$\frac{\text{Bad Debts Due to FFS Activity}}{\text{Gross FFS Charges}} \times 100\%$$

This indicator provides information identifying the percentage of total gross charges that will not be collected for rendered services as a result of bad debts arising from FFS activity. These are the amounts that are theoretically collectible but that the practice failed to collect. Do *not* include contractual adjustments or charity care in the numerator of this indicator. This metric assists the group in monitoring and controlling its ability to collect payment for services rendered.

(16) Adjusted Collection Ratio

$$\frac{\text{Net FFS Revenue or Collections}}{\text{Adjusted FFS Charges*}}$$

*(Adjusted FFS Charges = Gross Charges – (Contractual Write-offs + Charity Care Write-offs)

This ratio indicates how effective and efficient the group is in collecting its adjusted FFS charges. This ratio measures effectiveness and efficiency by comparing the amount of revenue the practice actually collects with the amount that it theoretically should collect. High ratio values indicate high effectiveness and high efficiency; low values indicate low effectiveness and low efficiency.

(17) Months Revenue in Accounts Receivable

$$\frac{\text{Net Accounts Receivable}}{\text{Annual Adjusted FFS Charges}} \times 1/12$$

This indicator identifies a relative measure of the average number of months that a group's charges are outstanding, pending collection by the group. It also assists the group in monitoring and controlling its collections for outstanding receivables.

(18) Days Revenue in Accounts Receivable (also known as "Days in A/R")

$$\frac{\text{Net Accounts Receivable}}{\text{Annual Adjusted FFS Charges}} \times 1/365$$

This indicator is similar to the previous indicator, except that it measures the average number of days that a group's charges are outstanding, pending collection by the group.

"Adjusted" versus "Gross" Charges to Compute Days or Months in A/R: The above examples show these indicators computed based on the *annual adjusted charges* and the current A/R balance, also computed at its net adjusted charge basis. That is, the balance of the charges and the A/R are presented net of the anticipated contractual adjustments, charity care adjustments, allowance for doubtful accounts, and other adjustments. The advantage of this presentation is that it gives a better indication of what the accounts receivable is actually worth to the practice.

Just as the "Accounts Receivable per FTE Physician" in indicator 13 can also be presented using gross charges, the "Days or Months in A/R" metrics can be (and frequently are) computed using gross charges and the "gross" value of A/R before any adjustments or write-offs. This is often easier to compute for many practices, particularly those on the cash basis that record these adjustments when the account is collected or deemed uncollectible and do not generally compute contractual adjustments and other write-offs or adjustments relating the current balance of A/R. For example, to compute "Days in A/R" based on annual gross charges, use:

$$\frac{\text{Gross Accounts Receivable}}{\text{Annual Gross FFS Charges}} \times 1/365$$

To compute "Months Revenue in A/R" based on annual gross charges, use:

$$\frac{\text{Gross Accounts Receivable}}{\text{Annual Gross FFS Charges}} \times 1/12$$

Using shorter periods of time to compute the "Months or Days in A/R" metric: Because much of the outside survey data for these metrics are computed based on annual data, a practice should use annual data when benchmarking against such data. For internal purposes, however, the practice may wish to use shorter periods of time. This is because seasonal fluctuations in volume affect the balance of A/R. During periods of high volume, practices will have higher charges and a higher balance of A/R reflecting those charges. Some practices have lower activity during December due to the holiday season slowdown and have a correspondingly lower balance in A/R at that time. To take that lower A/R balance that reflects primarily December charges and compare it against an average daily or monthly charge amount that averages in activity from higher volume periods leads to a days or months in A/R indicator that is deceivingly low. Many practices compute the days or months in A/R metric internally using a two- or three-month period. For example, assuming a two-month period, gross days in A/R would be computed as follows:

$$\frac{\text{Gross Accounts Receivable}}{\text{Gross FFS Charges for the Most Recent Two Months}} \times 1/60$$

To compute the metric for months revenue in A/R, change the "1/60" (indicating 60 days) to "1/2" (indicating two months). To compute these metrics on a "net" basis, use net A/R and net FFS charges, rather than gross A/R and gross FFS charges.

Nonfinancial

Patient data

(19) Ambulatory Patient Encounters per FTE Physician

$$\frac{\text{Physician Ambulatory Patient Encounters}}{\text{Total FTE Physicians}}$$

This indicator measures overall group physician productivity by identifying the average number of outpatient encounters per FTE physician.

(20) Hospital Admissions per FTE Physician

$$\frac{\text{Hospital Inpatient Admissions}}{\text{Total FTE Physicians}}$$

This indicator identifies the average number of inpatients admitted by each physician. When used in conjunction with the indicator "Hospital Inpatient Professional Service Gross Charges as a Percentage of Total Gross Charges," it also provides a general indication of the extent to which clinical practice occurs in the hospital.

(21) New Patient Registrations per FTE Physician

$$\frac{\text{New Patient Registration}}{\text{Total FTE Physicians}}$$

The survival of a group practice usually depends on attracting and retaining new patients. This indicator allows a group practice to monitor the amount of services attributable to new patients. It also provides some basis for examining productivity data since new patients tend to require more provider time than returning patients.

Group medical staff and administrative support

(22) Total FTE Medical Support Staff per FTE Physician

$$\frac{\text{Total FTE Medical Support Staff}}{\text{Total FTE Physicians}}$$

This indicator identifies the utilization of the group's medical support staff. The medical support staff consists of registered nurses, licensed practical nurses, medical assistants, medical receptionists, medical secretaries/transcribers, and medical records personnel. Comparing this metric with external data is useful in helping practices achieve the right level of staffing.

(23) Total FTE Administrative Staff per FTE Physician

$$\frac{\text{Total FTE Administrative Staff}}{\text{Total FTE Physicians}}$$

This indicator identifies the utilization of the group's administrative staff to perform general administrative, business office, and managed-care administration and maintenance activities. Comparing this metric with external data is useful in helping practices achieve the right level of staffing.

(24) Total FTE Laboratory Staff per FTE Physician

$$\frac{\text{Total FTE Laboratory Staff}}{\text{Total FTE Physicians}}$$

This indicator identifies the productivity and utilization of laboratory employees. Comparing this metric with external data is useful in helping practices achieve the right level of staffing.

(25) Total FTE Radiology/Imaging Staff per FTE Physician

$$\frac{\text{Total FTE Radiology/Imaging Staff}}{\text{Total FTE Physicians}} \times 100\%$$

This indicator identifies the productivity and utilization of radiology/imaging staff. Comparing this metric with external data is useful in helping practices achieve the right level of staffing.

Prepaid Services (Commercial, Medicare, and Medicaid Contracts)

(26) Average Number of Prepaid Plan Members

This indicator identifies the average number of prepaid plan members for the reporting period. This information allows a group to monitor the growth or decline of membership in the prepaid plan.

(27) Net Capitation Revenue as a Percentage of Total Medical Revenue

$$\frac{\text{Net Capitation Revenue}}{\text{Total Medical Revenue}}$$

This indicator identifies the percentage of total net revenue attributable to capitation contracts. This information can help the group in identifying how much of its operational cash flow is dependent on capitation contracts for each reporting period and can be used for budgeting and planning activities.

(28) Net Capitation Revenue per-Member per-Month (PMPM)

$$\frac{\text{Net Capitation Revenue}}{\text{Average Number of Prepaid Plan Members}}$$

This indicator identifies the average revenue per-prepaid member per-month to determine whether capitation payments are appropriate. It also can be used for budgeting and planning activities.

(29) FFS Equivalent Charges (for Capitation Plan Patients) PMPM

$$\frac{\text{Annual FFS Equivalent Charges (for Capitation Plan Patients)}}{\text{Average Number of Prepaid Plan Members}} \times \; 1/12$$

This indicator identifies the average monthly FFS equivalent gross charges generated per prepaid member. This information, when used with revenue/ membership-related indicators, can help determine if capitation payments are appropriate. It also can be used for negotiation of capitation rates between the group and the HMO.

(30) Net Capitation Revenue as a Percentage of FFS Equivalent Charges

$$\frac{\text{Net Capitation Revenue}}{\text{FFS Equivalent Charges}}$$

This indicator identifies the relationship between prepaid income and the work performed, measured as FFS equivalent gross charges, on behalf of prepaid plan members. If this percentage is greater than 100 percent, there is greater prepaid income than FFS equivalent charges. This indicates, for the time period, that capitation payments, copayments, and risk-sharing revenues exceed the charges for care provided to prepaid plan members. If this percentage is less than 100 percent, FFS equivalent charges are greater than prepaid income. When used in conjunction with indicators 27 and 28, this indicator can help determine if capitation payments, copayments, and risk-sharing contracts are appropriate for care provided to prepaid plan members.

To the Point

- ▪ The income statement conveys information about the accomplishments of the practice, measured in revenue dollars, matched with related efforts, measured by goods and services consumed, called expenses. By comparing income statements for several consecutive periods, significant trends in statement components can be identified and projections about the practice's future earning power can be made.

- ▪ Revenue is the inflow of assets, usually cash or receivables, from performing medical services or other activities that constitute the major ongoing operations of the business entity.

- Expenses are resources consumed or used in the process of generating revenue. Operating expenses are those resources consumed in the process of providing healthcare services to patients. These expenses are matched with net revenue to determine net operating income. Nonoperating expenses are those expenses arising from activities not associated with rendering patient services.

- Net income is the residual amount after all expenses — operating and nonoperating — that have been deducted from net revenue and nonoperating revenue.

- The balance sheet lists the medical group's assets balanced by the liability claims of creditors and the residual owners' equity.

- Current assets include cash and other monetary assets that can be converted into cash within one year through normal operations of the medical group. This group includes unrestricted cash, marketable securities, A/R less allowances, supplies, and prepaid expenses.

- Investments are comprised of restricted cash, long-term receivables, investments in securities, investments in affiliates, and property held for future use.

- Intangibles and other assets may include organization costs, goodwill, deposits, and other long-term assets not included in other categories.

- Current liabilities are obligations arising from past transactions that must be paid by using current assets or by creating other current liabilities. The major kinds are accounts payable, claims payable, notes and loans payable, long-term debt — current portion, payroll withholdings, accrued payroll liabilities, accrued vacation, holiday and sick pay, and accrued liabilities — nonpayroll, patient deposits, contract payable incurred but not reported, deferred revenue — capitation or prepaid plan, deferred income taxes — and current portion.

- Long-term liabilities are obligations that will not mature and will not require the use of current assets within one year of the balance sheet date. The major types are long-term notes payable, mortgage payable, construction loans payable, capital lease obligations — long-term portion, and deferred income taxes — and long-term portion.

■ If a medical group is organized as a partnership, the owners' equity is called partners' equity and is comprised of two elements: contributed capital and undistributed earnings. If a medical group is organized as a limited liability entity, the owners' equity is called members' equity and consists of those same two elements. If a medical group is established as a corporation, ownership is referred to as stockholders' equity and includes accounts for preferred stock, common stock, capital contributed in excess of par, donated capital, retained earnings — unappropriated, retained earnings — appropriated, and treasury stock.

■ A list of typical operating reports for management information in the financial area includes: income statement, balance sheet, cash report, cash flow statement, operating budget (actual versus budget), and A/R report. Practices with capitation income would also be interested in the incurred but not reported (IBNR) claims/ lag analysis (by type and age) and various capitation analyses. In the nonfinancial area, some documents are utilization, referral, and hospitalization reports; physician profile and patient satisfaction summaries; and compliance status reports.

■ Information contained in operating reports must be accurate, brief, clear, and timely to be effective.

■ Key indicators denote performance highlights of significant aspects of the practice. Some of these are financial in nature, others are nonfinancial.

CHAPTER 6

Understanding Operating Expenses and Cost Accounting

Edited by Lee Ann Webster, MA, CPA, FACMPE

After completing this chapter, you will be able to:

- Recognize the distinction between costs and expenses and explain the basic rules of measuring and reporting costs and expenses in operating reports.

- Relate the nature and purposes of responsibility accounting, the types of responsibility centers used, and how the chart of accounts can be used to establish responsibility accounting within medical groups.

- Describe the types of expenses used in accounting for medical groups' activities and the logic of classifications in the chart of accounts.

- Define the basic cost terms, concepts, and applications used in the management accounting context.

- Distinguish between the various types of patterns in costs when activity levels change and how these cost classifications can be estimated for medical groups.

While chapter 5 presented the major categories of operating expenses as outlined in the *MGMA Chart of Accounts*, chapter 6 elaborates on these breakdowns and discusses the composition of these expenses more fully. It also explores the underlying basis for the cost and expense principles and measuring rules followed in accounting. A system for incorporating costs and expenses in reports for internal decision making — responsibility accounting — is explained. The use of various types of organizational arrangements for collecting and reporting relevant accounting information is illustrated for segments of a medical practice.

This chapter introduces cost accounting, a major area of management accounting, by covering the basic terms and concepts of this important discipline and the major uses of cost information. It discusses the many ways that costs are classified, described, and illustrated. Finally, this chapter describes the behavior of costs when the level of activity changes and illustrates this concept with examples.

THE NATURE OF COSTS AND EXPENSES

Earlier chapters described the historical cost principle as one of the cardinal tenets of accounting. We defined expenses as resources used up in the generation of revenue and cost as the amount of resources consumed to acquire an asset. For example, in the purchase of a new piece of equipment for $10,000, the asset cash ($10,000) is exchanged for another asset (equipment), and the $10,000 becomes the carrying value of the equipment in the accounting records. Cost is used as the valid measure of value for two reasons: It is the result of an exchange between buyer and seller, and it is an objective amount subject to independent verification. Thus, we attribute this cost principle as the basis of measurement for all assets acquired in an exchange transaction, and, for that matter, liabilities incurred, as well.

What happens to costs after they become assets that are consumed or used up in the process of producing benefits for the business? Historical costs of assets become expired costs when they are used to generate revenue, and we can refer to them as expenses. To understand the nature of expenses, it is useful to distinguish the several ways that costs become expenses. They are:

▪   When expenses are closely related to the production of revenue, such as wages paid to the medical staff for providing patient services or when a product is sold to a patient, the costs are recognized as an expense in the same period when revenue is reflected. This represents the matching principle cited earlier. In this case, expense recognition is tied to revenue recognition.

■ When it is difficult to associate a cost with generating revenue, a "rational and systematic" allocation policy may be developed to approximate the matching principle. This type of expense recognition pattern involves assumptions about the benefits as well as the costs associated with those benefits. One example could be an accounting policy that dictates allocating the cost of a long-lived asset (such as equipment) over all of the accounting periods during which that asset is used because the asset generates revenue through its useful life. This process, as mentioned previously, is called depreciation.

■ When no apparent connection exists between a particular cost and revenue or a future benefit, costs are charged as expenses — or losses — to the current period. Examples include marketing and promotion costs to promote the medical practice or assigning occupancy costs to the current period.

In summary, costs are analyzed to determine whether a relationship exists with revenue. Where this association applies, the costs are expensed and matched with revenue in the period when the revenue is recognized. If no connection appears between costs and revenue, an allocation of cost on some systematic and rational basis might be appropriate. Where, however, this method does not seem desirable, the cost may be expensed immediately.

As indicated in the previous chapter, operating expenses are defined as expired costs incurred in the process of providing services to patients. These expenses are used to determine net operating income. Nonoperating expenses are those expired costs generated by activities not associated with rendering services to patients. Further, operating expenses can be classified and summarized into various totals to provide different dimensions of operational activity within the medical group. The typical classification of expenses most frequently followed is the natural classification.

When costs are used for internal management decision making, the accounting system needs to contain a flexible arrangement of accounts such that costs can be traced to various segments of operations. This system is called responsibility accounting, and it is presented next.

RESPONSIBILITY ACCOUNTING

The Nature of Responsibility Accounting

The previous sections on the makeup of the financial statements present the prime reports that satisfy the information needs of both internal users (group management and physician owners) and external users (creditors and others). Often these reports are not detailed or in-depth enough to be useful in the daily operations of a medical practice. Besides their highly condensed and aggregate nature, the manner in which the information is formulated and presented may not be in the most useful and relevant format. For example, the income statement shows the results for a past period of time, and the balance sheet depicts the financial position for a date in the recent past. Financial managers and decision makers would like to have more details about various revenues and expenses, which would help them plan future operations. Furthermore, breakdowns and different aggregations of financial data are needed to provide insights into what has occurred in the practice so that action can be taken to alter certain procedures and establish different policies to control future activities. Thus, we need a specific framework for accounting data accumulation, classification, and reporting; this is the role of responsibility accounting.

Responsibility accounting is the establishment of a system of accounts aligned with the organizational structure of the medical group so that information can be collected and reported to managers responsible for the practice's operations. This concept is most useful for large-sized groups that have individuals with responsibility for specific areas of the practice. Structuring the accounting data in this way is also helpful to smaller groups, even though only one or a few individuals are responsible for all phases of operations. Having information in detail enables management to know what is occurring in the practice and how to best respond to the changing environment.

Responsibility accounting does not require different accounts from those provided in the *MGMA Chart of Accounts*. This chart contains many useful categories and arrangements that recognize the concept of responsibility accounting and is expandable to accommodate group practices of all sizes.

Responsibility accounting is founded on the premise that the accounting system should support the planning and control efforts of the organization. As a system, it attempts to provide managers with information to help them perform their tasks and attain established goals. Thus, responsibility accounting is at the heart of the management control process. Management control is defined as a process or system by which managers ensure that resources are obtained and employed efficiently and effectively in achieving the organizational goals and objectives.

For medical groups, greater awareness and specific application of management control processes in the operation of their practices are greatly needed in today's uncertain healthcare environment. The delivery of medical care must be accomplished in the most efficient and effective modes that the industry can develop and follow. Let's spend a few moments on the terms *efficiency* and *effectiveness*.

Efficiency refers to the relationships of inputs (costs) and outputs (revenues and quality care). If output in terms of revenue dollars is satisfactory or reasonable, and the quality of care is the best it can be and is delivered incurring the least possible cost, then we know that the group has been efficient in the discharge of its medical responsibilities. *Effectiveness* is a concept relating to the relationship of an organization's results with its goals and objectives. A medical practice is considered effective if it is able to achieve all its stated goals and objectives. If it fails to reach these ends, then the practice would be deemed ineffective. A practice may be effective but also be inefficient if it achieves its ends but does so at a financial loss to its owners. Medical groups need to adopt a management control approach and establish policies and practices to plan and control their overall operations and to satisfy the desired efficiency and effectiveness outcomes.

Responsibility Centers

A key concept and tool of responsibility accounting is the designation and use of responsibility centers. Responsibility centers are identifiable organizational units headed by a designated individual through which the activities of a medical group are performed. Usually, the manager of a responsibility center has decision-making authority and exercises some measure of control over a segment of a group's practice. Each responsibility center consumes some resources of the medical group and provides some benefit, directly or indirectly, to patients. In organizations, responsibility centers may be an activity, a department, a function, or a specific geographic location. They may consist of the activities of a single employee or of an entire department.

The basic operations of a responsibility center are reflected in Exhibit 6.1. Using inputs or costs of resources, the responsibility center transforms inputs into outputs or revenues from patients and paying agencies. Responsibility accounting provides information about these inputs (costs) and outputs (revenues). The two purposes for accumulating and reporting financial information on this basis are (1) to provide information to control revenues and costs and (2) to provide information for decision making.

Responsibility centers consume inputs or costs and produce outputs or revenues. However, the measure of outputs is not revenue for all centers. In medical groups, revenue can only be used to measure outputs of departments or functions that deliver medical services directly to patients. For responsibility centers that do not treat patients directly, such as the accounting department or the human resource department, the output cannot be stated by patient revenue dollars. Nevertheless, services to others in the medical group are the output of these indirect centers, but they are not valued or considered as services rendered directly to patients. Furthermore, these intragroup services cannot be measured in objective financial terms because of the absence of market-based transactions. These distinctions will be apparent when we describe the types of responsibility centers that can be set up when expense allocation procedures are discussed in the next chapter.

EXHIBIT 6.1 ■ Resource Flows — Responsibility Center

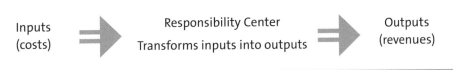

Inputs (costs) → Responsibility Center — Transforms inputs into outputs → Outputs (revenues)

EXHIBIT 6.2   ■   Types of Responsibility Centers

Type of responsibility center	Traceability of financial data	Nonfinancial measures of performance	Financial measures of performance	Evaluation criterion
Expense or cost center	Expenses: total expenses; expenses per unit of output	Time spent and quantity of resources consumed per unit of output	Amount of expenses: actual vs. previous period, actual vs. planned, actual vs. other comparable groups	Minimize expenses: minimize dollars of expense per unit of activity
Profit or contribution center	Revenues and expenses: total revenue, total expenses, profit or contribution	Number of patients served, time spent, and quantity of resources consumed per unit of output	Amount contributed by responsibility center to cover common costs and generate income for physician	Maximize profit or contribution
Investment center	Revenues, expenses, assets employed	Number of patients served, time spent, and quantity of resources consumed per unit of output	Return on assets employed (also measures cited above)	Maximize return on assets

For purposes of financial management, three types of responsibility centers can be identified: (1) expense or cost centers, (2) profit or contribution centers, and (3) investment centers. Each type is summarized in Exhibit 6.2. These centers differ in the types of financial information that may be generated by each and the degree of emphasis on the element of the resource flows that is implied by the type designation. Basically, they differ in the criteria by which their performance can be evaluated.

Expense or Cost Centers

Expense or cost centers measure and report expenses or costs incurred as their primary operating statistics. These centers do not serve patients directly, but costs are traced to them and reported in total for each cost center. Cost centers are evaluated on their ability to minimize costs either in total dollars or in cost per unit of service. Some examples of cost centers in medical groups are medical records, reception and appointments, and occupancy.

Profit or Contribution Centers

Profit or contribution centers perform a service to patients. Revenues and direct costs related to each patient's care are traced to them, and a measure of profit or contribution is determined and reported for each profit center. The profit or contribution centers are evaluated on their ability to control costs in relation to the revenue generated, produce a satisfactory contribution to cover common costs, and provide the physicians with their desired income levels. The term *contribution* is defined as revenue less direct costs traceable to the contribution center. Examples of profit or contribution centers are the medical group's clinical and ancillary departments, such as family practice, pediatrics, laboratory, radiology, and so on.

Investment Centers

Investment centers are responsibility centers for which the amount of assets employed can be determined, as well as the revenues and costs generated by that center. Profits or contributions produced by these centers can then be related to the amount of assets used to compute a rate of return on investment. This type of center is used for large organizations with diversified operations and multiple products and services. For example, large groups that have independent, self-supporting clinics scattered throughout several markets may use investment-center accounting to determine the rate of return from each of those clinics. Another area in which return on assets is useful is in the evaluation of an ancillary department that has a large investment in equipment. In this case, the ancillary department could establish fees to generate a desired rate of return on assets employed.

Most organizations will have other responsibility centers to which financial data cannot be traced. Although revenues and costs cannot be related to these responsibility centers, some types of nonfinancial data are available for all responsibility centers. This nonfinancial data may include time spent, hours of operations, quantity of resources consumed, or some physical measure of output.

ACCOUNTING FOR RESPONSIBILITY CENTERS

As indicated in chapter 4, the fifth edition of the *MGMA Chart of Accounts* provides for immense flexibility in capturing financial data. The chart shown in Exhibit 6.3 provides for four fields. Thus, the segments would appear in the following order:

Entity Field	Basic Field	Responsibility Center Field	Provider Field
XX	XXXX	XX	XXX

EXHIBIT 6.3   ■   *MGMA Chart of Accounts* Fields

Field	# Digits	Purpose
Entity Field	2	Allows a practice with multiple legal entities to "roll up" the individual account balances into consolidated financial reports.
Basic Field	4	This is the core financial statement account, designating the various assets, liabilities, equities, revenues, and expenses that make up the general information-gathering function of an accounting system for financial statements and tax returns. It will also facilitate data collection for the MGMA Cost Survey and a limited amount of cost accounting.
Responsibility Center Field	2	Allows for accumulation of data by administrative cost centers, ancillary service centers, clinical departments, or locations. Can also include providers if the provider field is not used.
Provider Field	3	Allows for classification and reporting of revenues and expenses by provider.

So a practice that was part of a complex group of entities might have the following account:

04.8221.11.114, meaning

04: For entity #4

8221: Physician Insurance — Health

11: For Department #11 (e.g., obstetrics and gynecology)

114: For physician #114 (e.g., Dr. Smith)

Practices that are not composed of multiple entities would not need to use the entity field, so their chart of accounts might have three segments. Smaller practices or those desiring simplicity and/or less detail might use just two fields. For example, a group might include physicians as responsibility centers, along with the billing department and the laboratory, and use only the basic field and the responsibility center field. Finally, in its most basic form, a chart need only include the four basic field digits.

An exhaustive list of possible responsibility centers within all medical practices is beyond the scope of this volume. A list of typical responsibility centers used by small- to medium-sized medical practices is provided in Exhibit 6 4.

EXHIBIT 6.4 ■ Examples of Responsibility Centers

Medicine	Radiology	Medical support services
Family practice		Reception and appointments
Pediatrics	**Other physician**	Medical records
Allergy and immunology	Psychiatry	Medical secretaries
Occupational medicine		Record audit
Dermatology	**Ancillary medical services**	
Obstetrics and gynecology	Laboratory	**Occupancy and use**
	Pathology	Building and grounds
	Physical therapy	Maintenance
Surgery	Optical	Housekeeping
General surgery	EKG	Security
Orthopedic surgery	Allergy	
Thoracic surgery	Psychology	**Administrative services**
Vascular surgery	Radiation therapy	Administration
Ophthalmology	Nuclear medicine	Human resources
Otolaryngology		Accounting
Colon and rectal surgery		Management information systems
Anesthesiology	**Health and rehabilitation**	Purchasing
Plastic surgery	Social worker	Credit and collections
Neurological surgery	Patient education	Business office
	Nutrition	Insurance

BASIC CONCEPTS OF COST ACCOUNTING

Cost accounting is an essential component of proactive management reporting. Accurate cost identification at all levels, most notably at the treatment and procedure levels, provides an effectual basis for practice management, flexible budgeting, cost control, and managed care contract analysis.

Cost accounting systems are information systems and databases that provide medical groups with the so-called true cost of services and products. Prior to the era of prepaid contracts, groups often relied on cost information developed from billing data. The specific prices for services charged to patients were often based on optimizing reimbursement rather than detailed cost analysis. Groups that base their costs on the ratio of costs to fees charged may make incorrect calculations. Thus, managers may assume they are losing money on a diagnosis-related group (DRG) when they are actually making money and vice versa, which can lead to inappropriate business decisions. By knowing the true costs of specific cases, groups will be in a stronger position to negotiate competitive healthcare contracts, market their services, and focus their efforts on the review of unprofitable areas. The use of cost data benefits a practice in several areas, particularly in the following five situations:

1. Income measurement
2. Distribution of income to physicians
3. Cost control
4. Overall planning
5. Decision making

Income Measurement

When general-purpose financial statements are prepared using generally accepted accounting principles, expenses must be matched with revenues to measure income. Fortunately, medical groups do not face the income determination problems found in manufacturing or other businesses that have complex inventory cost measurements. The basic issue in measuring expenses is the choice between the cash and the accrual basis of accounting. We have emphasized that the accrual basis provides the best measure of income for groups today, especially for those with a sizable prepaid component.

Distribution of Income to Physicians

The organization of the practice and the income distribution method chosen by the medical group determine the information needs. Many fee-for-service (FFS) groups use production-based income distribution methods. The billing system and the convenient cash-basis income system provide the information needed for income distribution. With the added emphasis of rewarding for production, FFS medical groups also tend to relate direct costs to revenue produced either by the individual physician or, more commonly, by specialty. In addition to the billing system and income statement for the group as a whole, FFS groups have adopted cost accounting systems that relate direct costs to specialties and departments. In addition to relating direct costs, group management also uses certain techniques of allocating indirect costs to physicians, departments, and specialties so that distributable income can be in the proportions desired by management. For example, when individual physicians are considered as profit centers, an allocation formula may assign larger proportions of indirect costs to specialty physicians, rather than allocate indirect practice costs equally to all profit centers. This would allow primary care physicians to receive a larger share of the group's distributable profits.

Production-oriented income distribution systems are not consistent with prepaid medical care. Rather than treat sicker patients or treat them more often, the motivation is to keep patients well. Assuming that the quality of care remains high, financial incentives favor preventive rather than curative care. In prepaid medical groups, income distribution methods have shied away from a production orientation to compensating physicians by salary with incentives that include care utilization and referral control. In this scenario, information needs include PMPM cost and cost per unit of activity. In some cases, when the distributable income is partially based on the prepaid practice segment, the allocation formula for indirect costs may be designed to charge a larger share of indirect costs to physicians who see more patients than others, in an attempt to influence the treatment behavior patterns of these physicians.

In recent years, we have seen a growing emphasis on quality indicators by both government and private payers. Programs such as the PQRS and the ACO establish at least part of the reimbursement for medical services on quality indicators or reporting. Thus, we may see future physician-compensation models employing a multicomponent pay structure that includes a quality component.

Cost Control

The third major purpose of gathering cost data is to control costs. The first step is determining the relationship between cost and activity. In order to control activities — and ultimately costs — both must be traced to the appropriate responsibility centers of the practice.

The ability to control costs depends on how clearly responsibility center activities have been defined. In many businesses, managers of responsibility centers are held accountable for costs incurred by their centers. In most medical practices, however, the manager of the responsibility center — particularly a physician who heads a specialty — is often expected to carry out the medical activities of the center and leave cost control to the administrator or financial manager. As a result, the administrator or financial manager has responsibility for costs incurred by someone else in the organization. This sharing of responsibility for costs leads to a lack of control, where the responsibility center manager does not want to be accountable for cost control, and the administrator/financial manager cannot exercise control.

In a combined FFS/prepaid medical group, no distinction exists between the delivery of care to patients from either category. For example, a particular lab test or immunization is considered to be the same regardless of the patient. To control costs for the prepaid patient, the group must develop a cost control system for the entire practice. Cost-per-procedure data would then be used to develop the cost PMPM for the prepaid practice. Because the cost system is developed for the entire practice, the FFS component should benefit, as well.

The second aspect of cost control is the ability to evaluate the current level of costs in relation to a benchmark. This is accomplished by the development of a budget consisting of costs that reflect expected conditions and resource usage. Chapter 11 covers the development and use of budgets for planning and control purposes.

Overall Planning

Although medical practices have a planning process, some FFS practices do not use a formal budgeting system. In the past, physicians in an FFS practice have been able to meet increases in expenses and generate higher personal income through higher fees and increased productivity. Now or in the near future, however, fee increases will have to be justified by the cost of services provided. Whenever a prepaid component is added to the practice, budgeting soon follows.

Planning and controlling operations require two dimensions of information: first, knowledge of what happens to revenues and costs as activity changes; and second, knowledge of when cash will be collected and when cash must be paid. Meaningful cost projections must be based on the amount of resources consumed for the amount of services performed. For this purpose, accrual measurement of expenses and knowledge of cost behavior patterns are necessary.

Decision Making

Because decisions involve the future and possible changes in the practice, cost data must be tailored to each specific situation. Some decisions, such as setting fees, are routine and are based on data from the financial information system. Other issues, such as whether to perform a laboratory test in-house or use an outside laboratory, do not come often. These decisions, as the following three examples illustrate, may depend on data from outside the practice.

Setting fees and negotiating capitation: Fees are set to recover the cost of rendering the service and to furnish the provider with a certain level of income. The relevant cost is the full cost of providing a particular service. The full cost of a service is the sum of the costs incurred directly to provide the services plus a fair share of such support charges as occupancy and administration. The resulting cost for a particular service is an aid in setting the fee for that service.

Capitation may be based on either the equivalent of FFS charges or the costs of the services to be provided. The FFS equivalent must be adjusted for collection expenses and bad debts, which are not generally an issue for prepaid services. When FFS charges are used, determining the capitation rate is not substantially different from setting the FFS fees. Ultimately, the fees or capitation payments must cover all costs. Development of cost by procedure and then cost PMPM allows the group to determine areas where costs exceed revenues and may suggest further analysis or action.

When to add a physician: A growing prepaid practice may reach the point at which it is less expensive to add a physician and perform a particular service inside the group than to continue to refer outside. Only the costs of adding the physician and the referral costs are relevant to the decision. Allocated administrative and other fixed costs that will not be affected by adding a physician are not relevant to the decision. However, qualitative factors, such as the practice's long-range goals and its relationship with other providers in the community, should be considered.

Laboratory tests performed in-house or outside: This decision, usually termed "make or buy" in the business literature, should be made by comparing the entire cost of purchasing a test from an outside laboratory with the incremental expenses of performing the test in-house. The full cost (that is, direct costs plus allocated indirect costs) of in-house testing should not affect the make-or-buy decision since indirect costs, such as allocated occupancy and administration costs, will not change as a result of performing the test in-house. The incremental costs (which may contain both variable and fixed costs) can be compared with the cost of purchasing the service outside in order to make a decision.

CLASSIFICATION OF COSTS

Costs can be associated with many things including a service or a product or running a department, promoting a practice, providing credit, and purchasing equipment. Furthermore, costs can be further categorized as historical costs, replacement costs, future costs, joint costs, common costs, direct or indirect costs, and controllable or uncontrollable costs. The point to remember is that the term *cost* must be identified with some degree of specificity. Use of the word *cost* by itself is vague and often confusing. This next section will explain some of the cost classifications. Other types of designations will be mentioned later.

Direct and Indirect Costs

A direct cost is a cost that can be traced to or caused by a particular service, product, segment, or activity of the practice (sometimes referred to as a cost object). For example, direct costs include the identifiable costs of performing a particular procedure, making a product, or managing a department or an office. In treating patients, the direct costs are the salaries of the physician and other medical personnel involved in delivering care, the supplies used, and in some cases, the outside referral costs.

In contrast, an indirect cost is a cost that cannot be traced to a particular cost object — a service, product, segment, or activity of the practice. These costs are necessary to support the total practice. However, they are caused by two or more cost objects jointly but are not directly traceable to either one individually. The nature of indirect costs is such that it is not possible, or at least not feasible, to measure directly how much of the cost is attributable to a single cost object. Examples of indirect costs are the salaries of employees in the business office, malpractice insurance premiums, and occupancy costs such as rent, property insurance, and maintenance expenses. In trying to determine the full cost of medical care, indirect costs are usually allocated to the cost of patient care on some equitable basis. These indirect costs are also referred to as *overhead*.

The notion of direct and indirect applies specifically to the cost objects involved. For example, the salaries of the persons in the business office are treated as indirect costs when focusing on the cost of medical treatment. However, these same salaries would be considered direct costs when one is interested in determining the cost of running the business office.

Full Costs and Differential Costs

Full cost refers to all the resources used for a specific cost object, such as treating a patient or running a specialty department. The full cost is determined by associating the total direct costs of that activity plus a fair share of indirect costs. For example, to determine the full cost of operating a specialty department within a medical group, the direct costs of operating that department (physicians and support medical salaries, supplies, etc.) would be added to an allocated proportion of the applicable indirect costs (such as occupancy costs, business office expenses, etc.) that support that activity.

Differential costs, sometimes referred to as incremental costs, are expenses that always relate to a specific situation. For example, a medical group may decide to have an in-house laboratory to conduct its testing, or it could contract with an outside laboratory. In comparing the cost of laboratory testing, one can derive the differential cost between the two by contrasting the cost of having the tests conducted internally, say $20, versus the cost charged by the outside source, say $25. The differential cost, in this instance, would be $5 in favor of having the work done in-house.

The term *differential* can also be used in the context of differential revenue. Differential revenues are those that are different under one set of conditions than they would be under another. For example, assume a medical group could perform a certain treatment by acquiring a piece of equipment to use in-house and receive a fee of $2,000 because of the faster service. Presently, a patient is referred to an outside medical facility to have this treatment done, for which the medical group charges the patient $1,500. Thus, the differential revenue in this case would be $500 to the group.

Controllable Costs and Noncontrollable Costs

Similar to direct and indirect costs, the classification of controllable versus noncontrollable costs depends on the point of reference. All costs are controllable at some level in any business, but not all costs are controllable at the same level of management. Costs are considered controllable at a particular level of management if the manager has the power to authorize or influence the amount of those costs. For example, a manager of a specialty department is responsible for controlling his or her employees' use of supplies. Supplies expenses are thus controllable costs. However, the manager of a specialty department has little influence over the amount of rent, maintenance costs, and utilities charged to the department except, perhaps, for the percentage allocation of the total occupancy costs. Thus, the occupancy costs would be deemed noncontrollable by the specialty manager. But somebody else in the organization, perhaps the administrator or governing body that makes decisions on rented facilities and utility services, would assume control of those occupancy costs.

This discussion of cost control at specific levels of management is useful in assigning responsibility for incurring costs and reporting the cost data to the appropriate managers. It should be noted that a time dimension applies to the classification of costs as controllable and noncontrollable. Some costs cannot be controlled in the short run but can be controlled in the long run. For example, the group's medical director may not be able to control the premiums on malpractice insurance short-term (say one year), but he or she can influence their long-term control by ensuring quality care is practiced by all members of the group.

Discretionary Costs

Discretionary costs are costs not considered to be absolutely essential to the short-term operations of the practice. For example, the costs of continuing education courses for business office staff are classified as discretionary — they could be foregone without great harm in the short term, except for employees' ill feelings and disappointment. Other examples of discretionary costs are promotion and marketing expenses, management consulting fees, sponsorship of an employee social event such as a group picnic, and charitable contributions to local community organizations.

Group management or the administrator reviews these discretionary costs periodically, usually annually, to determine whether the cost should be incurred or not. These costs are usually the first to be reduced or eliminated during periods of difficult economic times, since their discontinuation does not affect short-term operations or profitability. Because these items could affect the practice over time, however, discretionary costs should be examined periodically to determine their long-term impact.

Sunk Costs

A sunk cost is a cost that has already been incurred and, therefore, cannot be changed. For example, a historical cost, such as the book value of a depreciable asset, is a sunk cost. No decision made today can alter what has already happened. Sunk costs should be excluded from accounting analyses that are prepared to assist management in making decisions about the future, since they are irrelevant. For example, a medical group purchased an expensive piece of equipment three years ago for $100,000. Depreciation to date has been $60,000 (with an estimated life of five years), which makes the book value of the asset $40,000. An advanced model is now available that will perform more efficiently and at considerable annual cost savings of $175,000. The $40,000 book value of the old equipment, which is still productive and usable, should not figure in the decision of replacing the equipment with the new model. The cost savings resulting from the use of the more efficient model, plus the added gains from higher performance levels, are the relevant factors to be considered. The sunk cost of $40,000 should be ignored.

Opportunity Costs

Opportunity costs measure the potential benefits that are lost when one course of action requires that an alternative course be passed up. For example, an administrator has projected excess cash of $200,000 in the practice over the next six months. At the end of this period, the monies will be needed in the practice. Two choices are available for the short-term investment of these funds: a money market account that pays 3 percent or the purchase of a U.S. Treasury bill currently yielding 4.5 percent. If the administrator decides to invest in the money market account, the opportunity cost of not investing in the Treasury bill is $1,500 ($200,000 × 1.5 percent × 1/2 year) or:

Interest earned by investing $200,000 in a Treasury bill for six months at 4.5 percent	$4,500
Interest earned by investing $200,000 in a money market account for six months at 3.0 percent	3,000
Opportunity cost — contribution to net income foregone by using the less profitable alternative	$1,500

Hence, the administrator might consider switching investments to maximize the return to the practice and minimize the opportunity cost.

Opportunity costs differ fundamentally from other classifications because they do not represent a transaction involving a cash disbursement. However, they should be considered in all decisions involving the commitment of resources. For example, in deciding whether a practice should expand to another office location, management should consider the opportunity cost of investing the resources in other activities or alternatives before committing the funds to the new location.

BEHAVIOR OF COSTS

Effective planning and controlling of costs requires an understanding of cost behavior — how a cost element will respond to changes in the level of activity. As the level goes up or down, a particular cost may rise or fall in concert with the change in activity, or it may remain constant. If managers understand how costs behave, they will be able to predict how costs will fluctuate under various operating conditions. A lack of understanding of the effect of different activity levels on costs can lead to dire consequences. For example, if the revenues of a medical practice will be drastically reduced due to the retirement or departure of physicians, the financial manager needs to know what costs will be eliminated completely, which ones will be reduced, and which ones will remain the same. An understanding of cost behavior enables managers to better estimate future costs and improve decision making in many situations. The four basic cost behavior patterns are:

1. Variable
2. Fixed
3. Mixed or semivariable
4. Step-fixed

The relative proportions of each type of cost, referred to as the cost mix, deter-mine the cost structure of the organization. Some businesses — such as oil re-fineries and, for that matter, most medical practicing entities — have high fixed costs and relatively few variable and mixed costs. Others, such as management consulting firms, have more variable than fixed costs. Maintaining a constant awareness of the entity's cost structure can enhance the quality of manage-ment's decisions. Each of these cost behavior patterns will be discussed next.

Variable Costs

Variable costs are items of cost that vary, in total, directly and proportionately with volume or the level of activity changes. Thus, if activity increases 10 percent, the total amount of variable cost also increases by 10 percent. For example, assume a medical practice uses an outside laboratory for a certain test and that laboratory charges $20 per test. The cost of using the outside laboratory for different volumes of tests would be:

Number of Tests	Cost per Test	Total Variable Cost of Testing
1	$20	$20
100	$20	$2,000
1,000	$20	$20,000

Note two aspects of the example. First, the activity measure is specified — the number of tests sent to the outside laboratory. When labeling a cost as variable, the variable activity level associated with the cost item must be clear. Second, the total cost is variable because the total amount of cost changes, but the cost per unit of activity remains a constant $20 in this example. To avoid confusion, remember that the term *variable cost* refers to costs whose total varies proportionately with volume or activity.

Examples of variable costs in a nonmedical setting include the commissions of salespersons that vary with sales dollars generated, labor costs of hourly workers that vary with the number of hours worked, and vehicle fuel costs that vary with the number of miles traveled. In the medical setting, supplies are among the few costs that are variable. The cost of medical supplies varies directly with the number of patient visits and the types of procedures performed. For example, each X-ray procedure requires additional film and other supplies.

In a medical practice, the activity base tied to a variable cost is usually the patient. In a hospital, the base may be the patient or occupied beds. A graphic display of the behavior of variable costs in relation to fluctuations in activity or volume changes is shown in Exhibit 6.5.

Fixed Costs

Fixed costs are costs that remain constant in total regardless of changes in the level of activity. Examples include rent for facilities and equipment, property taxes, administrative salaries, and malpractice liability insurance. These costs may increase over time but they do not vary because of changes in the level of activity within a specified period of time. The important characteristic of fixed costs is the fact that although the total amount remains the same at different activity levels, the fixed cost per unit changes with the levels. As activity or usage increases, the average fixed cost per unit will fall since the fixed cost is spread over more units. Conversely, when the activity level decreases, the average fixed cost per unit will rise since the constant fixed costs are spread over fewer units. To illustrate this phenomenon, examine the $10,000 monthly rental cost for medical equipment and how the average cost per patient changes with fluctuations in volume, as shown in this example.

Monthly Rental Cost	Number of Patients Treated	Average Cost per Patient
$10,000	10	$1,000
$10,000	100	$100
$10,000	1,000	$10

Note the sharp changes in the average cost per patient as production levels change. Also, note that this is an average cost; that is, the total fixed cost is averaged over, divided by the number of patients treated.

Although the term *fixed cost* may imply that cost cannot be changed, that is incorrect. The term refers only to items of cost that do not automatically change with changes in activity. Fixed costs can be changed for other reasons, such as through a deliberate management decision. The term *nonvariable* is, therefore, more appropriate than fixed; but the term *fixed cost* is more widely used.

Fixed costs dominate the type of costs incurred by medical entities. Most of the salaries paid — physician and nonphysician — and related benefits are usually considered fixed. Other fixed costs in medical groups are liability insurance, most general and administrative expenses, occupancy, and interest expense.

A useful distinction for planning purposes is to classify fixed costs into two categories: committed and discretionary.

Committed fixed costs (land, buildings, furniture, and equipment): These costs measure the amount of investment in the fixed assets of the practice. Such costs would include depreciation of buildings and equipment, taxes and insurance on real estate, and salaries of top management and key operating personnel. The notion of commitment comes from the fact that these costs are long term. They cannot be eliminated or reduced significantly in the short run without impairing the continuity and long-term objectives of the practice. Thus, if business should decline and operations must be cut back, the practice would find it difficult to sell off its fixed assets and discharge its key people from a short-term point of view. Most practices prefer to keep this structure and investment intact because the costs of replacing these assets and personnel would be far greater than the short-term savings that might be realized.

Discretionary fixed costs: Sometimes called managed costs, these costs stem from annual decisions by management to spend a designated sum in certain fixed expenditure areas. Some examples are promotion and training expenditures. Since the benefits (gain) from these expenditures are long term and difficult to correlate with attendant costs, management generally decides to spend a stipulated amount each budget year on these items. Although they are somewhat "locked in" to this level of commitment for that year, they can eliminate or reduce these amounts the following year if a reduction appears in order. Actually, firms will even reduce their outlays for these fixed costs during a year if business activity declines significantly. Exhibit 6.5 displays the graph relationship between fixed costs and activity levels.

Summary of variable and fixed cost behavior

The behavior of variable and fixed costs at different activity levels is extremely important for grasping the proper perspective about their use in planning and controlling. Exhibit 6.6 summarizes their behavior well. All managers should keep the impact on total and unit costs for activity-level changes clearly in mind when analyzing costs and their behavior over time and over various situations. Note that the *total* variable costs change with volume or activity level fluctuations, but the *unit* variable cost stays the same. The opposite is true for fixed costs — the *total* fixed costs remain the same with volume or activity-level movements, but the *unit* fixed cost changes.

EXHIBIT 6.5 ■ Illustration of Four Cost Behavior Patterns

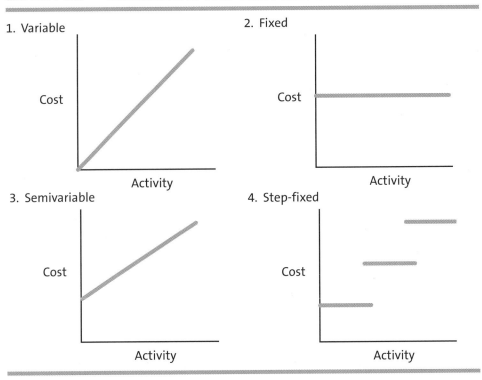

EXHIBIT 6.6 ◼ How Fixed and Variable Costs Change with Changes in Volume

	Total costs	Per-unit cost
Fixed costs	Constant	Changes
Variable costs	Changes	Constant

Mixed or Semivariable Costs

A mixed cost is a cost that includes both variable and fixed-cost elements. Mixed costs seem to have a chameleon-like quality in that at some activity levels, they appear to have characteristics of a fixed cost, while at other levels, they may appear to be a variable cost. The total amount of a mixed-cost item varies in the same direction as, but less than proportionately with, changes in volume. If volume increases by 10 percent, the total amount of mixed cost will increase by less than 10 percent.

An example of a mixed cost is the expense of operating an automobile. As related to the number of miles driven, gasoline, oil, tires, and servicing costs are variable, whereas insurance and registration fees are fixed. A manufacturing example would be electricity costs, which are considered mixed with regard to the volume of goods produced. That is, the cost of powering production equipment is variable while the cost of lighting the premises is fixed. A common example of mixed medical cost is processing patient receivables through a service bureau. The contract with the service bureau may provide for a fixed charge per month plus a charge per entry or per line. Exhibit 6.5 shows the graphic relationship of a mixed cost in the section labeled semivariable.

Step-Fixed Costs

Step-fixed costs are fixed over a range of activity and increase when activity levels go up. They increase again with another higher range of activity in a stair-step fashion. Note this configuration in Exhibit 6.5. In many healthcare situations, personnel tend to be added as levels of certain activity are reached. Thus, as the volume of patient care grows, the group may add another physician, nurse, or receptionist in stair-step fashion as activity levels increase. For example, assume that one physician can support annual gross charges of $900,000. As volume increases beyond this amount, another physician and perhaps another nurse must be added. Actually, as mentioned earlier, medical groups and most healthcare entities have a predominantly fixed-cost structure. Since adjustments must be made in cost when volume increases, we might conclude that the vast majority of medical group costs are of a step-fixed nature.

Relevant Range of Activity

The four cost behavior patterns assume their configurations when both a period of time and a range of activity are considered. As the time period envisioned becomes shorter, more costs become fixed. For example, most costs incurred by a medical practice for an hour or a day do not change regardless of the number of procedures performed. As the time period becomes longer, more and more costs change as activity levels change, so much so that the phrase "all costs vary in the long run" is often used. However, within a specific time period, very few costs are completely variable. In the event of a drastic decrease in volume, management would take action to reduce costs considered fixed, which would not be appropriate if activity continued at a normal level. On the other hand, as capacity within an existing set of facilities is reached, some costs increase disproportionately, such as overtime premiums and the additional insurance that may be required.

Because of these dynamic features of cost behavior, we need to simplify the categorization of variable, fixed, mixed, and step-fixed costs. This is accomplished by examining the cost amounts and activity levels incurred for a time period of one year. Further, although the cost-volume relationships are plotted with straight lines, we are only interested in the range of activity — called the relevant range — that is likely to occur during the given year. For example, a particular cost may be related to the number of patients treated during the year. The range may be from 0 to 10,000 patients for a certain medical group. Realistically, we can omit the lower and upper ends of this range because the probability of patient care being at these levels is very low. Thus, after careful analysis, the relevant range might be set at between 3,000 and 8,000 patients. It would be a mistake to believe that the relevant range extends from zero activity to the full capacity of existing resources. Exhibit 6.7 shows the selection of a relevant range for a step-fixed pattern of fixed costs.

EXHIBIT 6.7 ■ **Fixed Costs and Relavent Range**

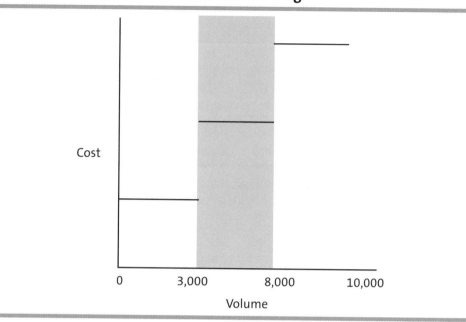

HOW TO DETERMINE COST BEHAVIOR PATTERNS

Two practical means are used to determine the cost behavior patterns: inspection of accounts and the study of past cost behavior patterns. The methods differ in the sources of data used.

Inspection of Accounts

The inspection of accounts method simply involves examining the amount of costs incurred at various levels of activity logged in the group's accounting records. The pattern as to which costs are variable or fixed becomes fairly evident when account totals are examined carefully over time. This method, though, is both intuitive and arbitrary; thus, it is subject to a higher degree of error than other methods. However, in areas where analysis is not very sensitive to a classification error of costs, this method may provide a quick and inexpensive measure of cost behavior.

To illustrate this approach, Exhibit 6.8 presents a list of accounts from the *MGMA Chart of Accounts* with an indication of their probable cost behavior patterns. Caution, however, should be noted since each medical group is different and cost behavior patterns must be determined from staffing patterns, contracts, and style of practice in the group.

EXHIBIT 6.8 ■ Illustration of Inspection of Accounts

MGMA Chart of Accounts # (Basic Field)	Account Title	Cost Behavior
5110	Salaries — Administration	Fixed. These are generally set in advance and are generally dependent on factors other than practice volume.
5150	Salaries — Ancillary Services	Step-fixed. Clinical medical practice personnel are hired in steps, resulting in a stair-step pattern.
6120	Building and Facilities Lease/ Rent	Fixed. Generally set in a long-term lease.
6185	Malpractice Insurance	Fixed. Annual premiums set in advance.
6340	Accounting, Legal, and Actuarial Services	Fixed. Dependent on factors other than volume.
6311	Postage	Mixed. Component related to billing and patient correspondence is variable. Component related to other administrative functions, such as accounting and human resources, is fixed.
7210	Drugs and Medications	Variable. Dependent on volume.
7221	Medical Supplies Expense	Variable. Dependent on volume.
7810	Purchased Services for Capitation Patients	Variable. Dependent on volume.
8112	Physician-Owner Bonuses	Variable. Additional compensation to physicians is generally based on production, although quality factors may play a larger role in the future.
8311	Nonphysician Provider Salaries/Draw	Fixed. Base compensation is generally set in advance and dependent on many factors other than activity level. Any salary based on production should be segregated and classified as variable. For example, the MGMA Chart of Accounts uses AC# 8312 for nonphysician provider bonuses.
8421	Nonphysician Provider Insurance — Health	Fixed. Generally set by contract.
9210	Interest Expense	Fixed. These expenses have no direct relationship to the level of activity.

Study of Past Cost Behavior Patterns

This method is a little more formalized than account inspections. In analyzing past experience, it assumes that data examined are accurate and that future cost behavior will duplicate past cost behavior. When accurate past cost data are available, they provide the empirical evidence to study and develop cost behavior patterns. The issue of accuracy becomes important when accounts are maintained on the cash basis. To avoid a distorted cost behavior pattern, use of resources should be recorded in the period of use rather than in the period of cash payment.

To measure cost behavior patterns from past data, the analyst "fits" a straight line to the data. The assumption is made that these data vary linearly — that is, in a straight line. Mathematically, one may fit a straight line to any set of two or more points. Evaluating the quality of the fit and the reliability of the resulting cost/activity formula requires sound judgment. Exhibit 6.9 illustrates the fit for a mixed cost that contains a certain level of fixed cost plus a variable cost per unit of activity. The three general methods of determining cost behavior patterns from past data are:

■ Scatter graph approach, which relies on a visual fit using a graph;

■ High-low point method, which fits a line to two representative points of data; and

■ Linear regression analysis, which fits a line to several observations using statistical methods.

EXHIBIT 6.9 ■ Illustration of Fitting a Straight Line to Cost and Activity

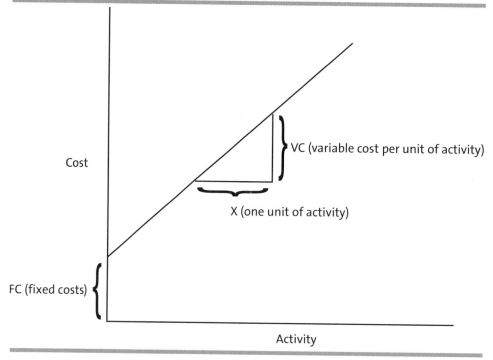

To the Point

■ Cost, the amount of resources given up to acquire an asset, measures value because it arises from an exchange between buyer and seller and functions as an objectively determinable amount subject to independent verification.

■ Expenses are expired costs since they represent historical costs that have been used up in producing revenues.

■ The matching principle is applied in three ways: when costs can be directly associated with the generation of revenues; when no connection can be made between costs and revenues, an allocation of cost to the period's revenues is made; and where neither of these situations prevail, costs are expensed immediately.

■ Cost accounting systems are information systems and databases that provide medical groups with the "true cost" of their services and products. The accumulation of cost data is important for the following types of uses:

  – Income measurement

  – Distribution of income to physicians

  – Cost control

  – Overall planning

  – Decision making in specific situations

■ Because the term cost has many applications, one must describe the object or reference point with which cost is being associated.

■ Direct costs are costs that can be traced to or are caused by a particular service, product, segment, or activity of a practice. Indirect costs are costs that cannot be traced to a particular cost object and are caused by two or more cost objects jointly.

■ Full cost means all the resources used for a specific cost object such as treating a patient or running a specialty department. The full cost is determined by associating the total direct costs of that activity plus a fair share of the indirect costs to reach a combined total.

■ Differential or incremental costs are those that are different under one set of conditions than under another. They always relate to a specific situation.

■ Controllable costs are costs over which a designated manager has some influence to authorize a given level for a particular time period. Noncontrollable costs are those over which a manager has no influence.

■ Discretionary costs are those not considered absolutely essential to the short-term operations of the practice.

■ Sunk costs are those that have already been incurred and cannot be changed by any decision currently being considered.

■ Opportunity costs measure the potential benefits that are lost or sacrificed when the choice of one course of action requires that an alternative course be given up.

■ Cost behavior, a major cost classification method useful for planning and control purposes, pertains to how a cost element will respond to changes in the level of activity. The four basic cost behavior patterns are variable, fixed, mixed, and step-fixed.

■ Variable costs are cost items that vary, in total amount, directly and proportionately with volume or level of activity changes, but unit variable cost stays the same.

■ Fixed costs remain constant in total, regardless of changes in the level of activity, but the unit-fixed cost changes as activity increases or decreases. The two types of fixed costs are committed and discretionary.

■ Mixed costs include both a variable and a fixed element. The total amount of a mixed-cost item varies in the same direction as, but less than proportionately with, changes in volume.

■ Step-fixed costs are fixed over a range of activity and are then increased in a stair-step fashion for a certain period.

■ The relevant range of a cost function involves the activity of costs and volumes likely to occur during a given time period. It also represents the data that should be used in determining the cost behavior of that cost element.

■ To determine cost behavior patterns, two practical means are (1) inspections of accounts and (2) the study of past cost behavior patterns.

CHAPTER 7

Determining the Cost of Patient Care

Edited by Rhonda W. Sides, CPA/ABV/CFF/CGMA, CVA

After completing this chapter, you will be able to:

- Identify the unit of care to be measured (e.g., episode of care, bundle of care, per treatment, per procedure, per diagnosis, and per relative value unit).

- Identify all costs associated with the provision of the unit of care — fixed, variable, direct, indirect, and discretionary.

- Apply these costs to the various revenue sources to understand the true costs of providing services, comparing to payer contract rates, process improvements, budgeting, and other financial management issues.

- Learn the underlying premise of activity-based costing and how to apply this method of costing to a physician practice.

Costs are a moving target, and every resource consumed should be included in a cost analysis. Cost accounting is as important now as it was when cost accounting first became relevant to physicians at the beginning of the managed care era. The benefits of performing a cost analysis are enormous. The obvious benefit is in knowing what it costs to do business — to provide a service, a treatment, or a procedure, or to serve a particular payer mix. But the tangential benefits are just as great: knowing your business, knowing your medical practice, and learning the inner workings of all the tasks and activities that are required to service the end result — the patient.

In this chapter, we will cover how to accumulate various costs, allocate costs to different segments of a practice, and arrive at the cost of a unit of care or the cost of specific medical services. An illustration will show how relative values can be employed to develop a standard costing approach useful to medical group decision makers. Another cost accounting tool, activity-based costing, is described, indicating a way of determining the cost of services with greater accuracy.

For medical practices, the typical costing objectives have historically been revenue-producing responsibility centers and procedures. By developing the full cost of each procedure, services can be summarized into categories that serve as valuable aids in negotiating reimbursement payments, developing budgets, and assisting in other areas of operational decision making. Full costs can also be matched with revenues generated in responsibility centers (profit centers), and the resulting net income can be used to evaluate performance of the physicians/managers responsible for those practice areas.

Revenues and costs are classified, segregated, and traced to specific costing objectives that include time periods, services, and responsibility centers. Direct costs can be traced to a specific activity. Because indirect costs are common to several costing objectives, they cannot easily be assigned to a particular responsibility center without some type of allocation process. This chapter will show how all costs can be accumulated and how indirect costs can be allocated to relate to specific costing objectives.

COST ACCOUNTING SYSTEMS

In the dynamic economic environment of healthcare, medical group management must generate and analyze cost data to determine the operating status of its practice and to implement an effective cost management and profit strategy. In this mature era of managed care and integrated healthcare delivery systems, knowledge of a practice's costs becomes essential if the practice is to compete successfully and be profitable. Cost accounting is essential to these tasks, just as it is in every other business and has been for decades. Physician practices, 20 years after managed care became the dominant reimbursement system, are still lagging in undertaking this exercise and incorporating it as an ongoing management tool.

Cost accounting offers management a system to be used not only in tracking historical information, but also in projecting future performance strategically. The results can be put to a variety of uses, including:

- **Accurate costing:** By utilizing cost accounting data, management can generate "true" costs that are helpful in analyzing business operations, managed care contracting, budgeting, and compensation.

- **Cost control:** A cost accounting system enables management to analyze both variable and fixed costs at different production levels. This establishes optimum output and cost norms that enable actual results to be compared with what costs ought to be.

- **Variance identification:** Once the cost norms are set, management can monitor the relationship between projected costs and actual costs to identify areas where costs may be out of line with desired levels.

- **Asset protection:** An effective reporting system can result in increased efficiency, theft prevention, and decreased waste.

STANDARD COST SYSTEM

A standard cost system uses future or expected costs in conjunction with past costs. While the development of concepts, processes, and applications of standard cost systems have been finely tuned in many other industries, cost accounting remains largely untapped by physician practices. It will continue to adapt to the nuances of medical practices and be an important factor in controlling overall costs, especially with the ever-changing reimbursement patterns and the progression toward a modified or bundled payment system through ACOs. These innovations are also necessary because of the changes in medical and business technology.

What is a standard cost? A standard cost is a measure of how much an item *should* cost rather than a record of how much it actually did cost. Standard cost is used to describe what the cost of one unit of service, such as a treatment or procedure, should be. Standard costs work like a budget. The uses of a standard cost system include the following:

- Determining what medical procedures or treatments should cost, tracking their actual costs to see if the standards have been met, and investigating those situations where there is a difference between standard and actual costs, called a variance.

- Facilitating the preparation of budgets by using the standard costs of various services in responsibility centers.

- Promoting efficiency objectives among the staff by instilling cost and time factors as important variables to consider in delivering services and carrying out activities.

- Assisting in the implementation of responsibility accounting whereby accountability for cost control is assigned to specific managers. The fulfillment of their responsibility is evaluated through performance reports.

Standard costs of individual procedures are the building blocks of what might be considered an "advanced" cost management system for most medical groups. They incorporate a level of detail and accuracy not routinely used in a physician practice. It usually takes a significant effort to develop procedural standards and related costs and then integrate them into a cost system. The effort generally involves careful study and analysis of provider time spent in rendering clinical services and measuring of significant resources consumed in that process. Ample time should be invested in developing these measurements so that standards of resource usage and resource costs can be determined. Physicians and management should carefully evaluate their need for this level of analysis before undertaking the task of establishing standard costs. However, physician practices are encouraged to undertake this step. Here are some general ideas about developing a standard cost system and the issues usually encountered when establishing such a system.

ACTIVITY-BASED COSTING (ABC)

An alternative costing approach, called activity-based costing (ABC), can be applied to physician practices to address the difficulties associated with traditional full-cost allocation systems. ABC is a more sophisticated approach to developing costs, but fully implementing such a system may outweigh the benefits. ABC systems differ from traditional or standard systems by modeling the usage of all organizational resources on the activities performed by these resources and then linking the cost of these activities to outputs, such as procedures, services, or cases.

To apply this method, costs are first assigned to activities as opposed to responsibility centers. Examples of these activities would be scheduling a patient or performing an X-ray. Then the activity costs are assigned to outputs using cost drivers, which "cause" the costs to be at a certain level due to the amount of activity that is performed from start to finish. The identification of cost drivers requires doing an analysis of all activities performed throughout the company to determine the resources used to perform each activity and what "drives" costs to be at a certain level.

To illustrate the ABC approach, let's use the operational task of supply purchasing and management. The following tasks are typically performed in this process:

- ▪ Determining supply requirements
- ▪ Selecting the vendors
- ▪ Ordering the supplies
- ▪ Receiving and inspecting the incoming supplies
- ▪ Stocking the supplies
- ▪ Maintaining the supply inventory records
- ▪ Accounting for the supply invoices
- ▪ Issuing the supplies to the centers

None of the labor used in any of the tasks in this activity is directly related to performing a clinical service for revenue. The cost in a particular activity may be "driven" by the number of supply units handled, by the number of supply orders, or by the weight of the supplies. The financial analyst must decide which cost drivers are the best indicators of the cost relationship and then use those drivers as the bases of assigning the amounts in each cost pool to the output.

ABC systems report more accurate costs than a traditional standard costing system because they clearly identify the costs of the different activities performed in the organization. They assign the costs of these specific activities to outputs using measures that represent the types of demands that individual outputs — for instance, revenue service lines — make on these activities. ABC recognizes that activities cause costs to be at certain levels.

ABC is forward thinking, whereas traditional cost accounting is based on historical data. Traditional cost accounting is a good starting point for those practices just beginning this process, and then the results may be used to transition into more of an ongoing ABC approach to projecting the future and controlling costs.

Furthermore, this type of costing will reveal, in more detail, how resources are consumed throughout the organization. Much of what has been traditionally treated as overhead can now be treated as a direct cost of products or services, and many companies gain a more detailed understanding of why overhead is what it is. Physicians often do not understand why it costs so much to run a practice; this exercise makes it clear. An additional significant benefit comes from discovering which activities add value to the service performed versus known and real added costs. Costs that do not add value are either imperative anyway or candidates for reduction or minimization in the overall process. Some of the specific benefits include performing certain activities more efficiently, substituting more expensive activities with less expensive ones, redesigning processes to eliminate certain activities entirely, and reassigning personnel to alternative duties for better efficiency.

With more accurate production costs, managers can make better decisions about their services and the activities required to perform these services. Such decisions include introducing or discontinuing certain services and setting specific volume levels of services to attain a certain profit level.

The crux of the ABC process is developing a working model of the practice. Practice modeling identifies the resource processes and demands that are unique to the medical practice.

MEASURING FULL COST USING STANDARD COSTING

A series of steps can be used to measure the full cost of a medical service or procedure. Then the total cost of specific types of services can be calculated by taking the full cost of a service — both direct and allocated indirect costs — and dividing it by the units of activities performed by the responsibility center. When procedures differ widely between services, some relative unit of measure may be necessary to define a unit of service. For example, one procedure may involve one unit of service while another involves two or more units of service. In these instances, relative values (covered later in this chapter) are useful.

The steps to measure the full cost of a service or procedure are:

Step 1: Identify responsibility centers. What is it you want or need to measure the cost of (e.g., a unit of care, such as a specific in-office surgical procedure or a revenue, or a cost center, such as radiology)?

Responsibility centers should reflect the group's organizational structure and style of practice adopted by the physicians. Responsibility centers can be based on types of services, physicians' specialties, locations, and other centers that are important measurements for the practice and its owners. The primary consideration in choosing the types of responsibility centers is for the control of revenues and costs. Distribution of income to physicians is important but only secondarily.

Step 2: Trace all revenues and costs to the center responsible for incurring them. This will also be an excellent exercise in determining what costs are not currently tracked accurately or with adequate detail.

Analyze the practice's data for tracing revenue per responsibility center or unit of care by using practice production reports and by using the general ledger to trace practice costs that are used to produce these services.

For each responsibility center, revenue and costs should be identified. Again, the primary consideration in tracing costs should be revenue and cost control.

Step 3: Allocate costs to the responsibility centers — both revenue-producing centers and cost centers that support the practice and the revenue centers. Allocate all costs of servicing the unit of care or responsibility center to determine the full cost of each service line or center. This serves as a baseline only and should be revised for costs that can be or should be modified or challenged.

Several procedural questions are involved in considering the allocation of these costs:

■ Technique of allocation — Should service department costs be allocated directly to revenue-producing responsibility centers, or should they be allocated to other service departments, as well?

- Order of allocation — Which service department's costs are allocated first, second, and so on?
- Basis of allocation — What basis should be used to allocate costs? Some examples are square footage used, number of patient visits, time spent by staff, and volume of revenue.

There is no one right way to answer each of these questions. Allocation of costs is always an arbitrary action, but the process should be fair, equitable, and understandable and be the best choice for each cost allocated relative to practice concerns. However, please note that following a different technique, order, or basis of allocation may produce different results for total allocated costs to a particular responsibility center. (See Exhibit 7.1.)

EXHIBIT 7.1 ■ Example of Allocation Bases for a Laboratory

Cost Description	Cost Behavior	Allocation Base
Laboratory (several revenue centers)	Direct to Revenue	Based on a lab increment measurement that puts all lab tests on the same relative scale with one another and allocated to the three separately identified revenue centers
Building and Occupancy	Indirect to All Centers	Allocated in two steps: First by square footage; second by management for additional usage consumed by information technology energy and infrastructure consumption and lab for additional usage of energy and infrastructure (e.g., cabling and security)
Purchasing	Indirect to All Centers	Estimated based on shipping and supply reports available through accounting records, including supply assignments made to each responsibility center
Information Technology	Indirect to Revenue	Estimated actual usage by IT management — 75 percent of IT costs utilized by lab revenue centers; costs allocated by charge revenue
Information Technology	Indirect to Cost Centers	Estimated actual usage by IT management — 10 percent marketing/sales; 10 percent A/R management; 5 percent other — split by FTEs
Human Resources	Indirect to Revenue	60 percent lab by revenue — arbitrarily estimated by management responsible for hiring to estimate actual usage by each responsibility center

(Exhibit 7.1 continues on the next page)

EXHIBIT 7.1 ▪ **Example of Allocation Bases for a Laboratory** *(continued)*

Cost Description	Cost Behavior	Allocation Base
Human Resources	Indirect to Other Cost Centers	40 percent divided by three, to fin./sales/adm., arbitrarily estimated by management responsible for hiring to estimate actual usage by each responsibility center
Financial Services	Indirect to Revenue	By revenue collected — no accurate allocation — this estimate is based on revenue because those revenue centers with the most revenue typically receive more support from these cost centers
Quality Assurance	Indirect to Revenue	Based on the volume of tests within each revenue center; estimate based on the fact that quality assurance processes support each test relatively the same to one another
Research and Development	Indirect to Revenue	Based on a lab increment measurement that puts all lab tests on the same relative scale with one another
Marketing and Sales	Direct to Revenue	Direct allocation — data available in accounting records, recorded as incurred in segregated chart of accounts
Customer Service and Reporting	Indirect to Revenue	Estimate by FTEs — all tasks performed the same on a per patient/per lab test basis by each FTE in the responsibility center
Medical Billing and A/R Management	Indirect to Revenue	Billing processes per claim are relatively the same regardless of revenue center supported; billing cost center allocated by charge revenue

COST ALLOCATION TECHNIQUES

Several options for allocating costs are commonly used. The two most common are direct allocation and step-down allocation.

Direct allocation: This method is the simplest and requires a minimum of clerical effort. Every medical practice has centers of activity that are revenue-producing. For example, doctors and mid-levels treating patients and charging for their services and nonrevenue-producing (or pure cost) centers whose main function is that of supporting the revenue producers (nurses, front office staff, billing and collections, and accounting). The costs of each service department are allocated directly to revenue-producing responsibility centers.

In a complex organization with many shared services between departments, the direct allocation method is not best. It fails to recognize that services performed by one cost center may benefit another. For example, IT services support a practice's billing department but neither department creates revenue by treating patients. However, that does not mean that the billing department's costs should not include some IT costs before billing costs are allocated out to the revenue centers for which they work.

Step-down allocation: The step-down technique is simple and will lead to a more equitable allocation than the direct allocation in a shared services environment, which is the most likely scenario in a medical practice. A fair result will arise from the order in which service department costs are allocated. The method requires that the costs of each service department be allocated in a predetermined order, each as a separate step. The approach specifies that the costs of the service departments providing the most services to all departments should be allocated first. All remaining service departments' costs are then allocated in descending order, determined by the amount of service they render. Thus, as the costs of a service department are allocated to revenue-producing responsibility centers and remaining service departments, there is a step-down or continuation to the next service department.

Once the costs of a specific cost center or service department are allocated, no subsequent allocations are made to it from other service departments, thus the meaning of "step-down." However, because no subsequent allocations are made to a cost center once it has been allocated, the step-down technique does not produce the absolute full cost of each service department.

This technique is the most widely used method of cost allocation and is reasonably accurate for most purposes, as well as those costs that may not be exact or are support costs — not costs directly attributable to a revenue center. It is also a systematic approach that involves only moderate clerical effort. See Exhibit 7.2, which illustrates an example of step-down allocation for a typical orthopedic practice.

EXHIBIT 7.2 ■ **Example of Step-Down Allocation Method**

Responsibility Centers	Direct Costs	Indirect Costs	Allocate Building/ Occupancy	Allocate IT	Allocate Administration	Allocate Billing/ Scheduling/ Medical Records
Revenue Centers						
Office Visits	$X		$X	$X	$X	$X
Surgeries	$X		$X	$X	$X	$X
Radiology	$X		$X	$X	$X	$X
Cost Centers						
Building/Occupancy		$X	$ZERO			
Information Technology		$X	$X	$ZERO		
Administration		$X	$X	$X	$ZERO	
Billing/Scheduling/ Medical Records		$X	$X	$X	$X	$ZERO

Step 4: Determine the cost per RVU and each procedure code. This is calculated by first dividing the full allocated cost of each revenue center by the number of RVUs performed within the revenue center. The resulting cost per RVU is then used to calculate the cost per procedure.

This step involves determining the unit costs of services or procedures performed by the revenue-producing departments. This amount should be used in establishing billing rates, in seeking reimbursements, and in making financial decisions. To calculate it, the full allocated cost of each revenue-producing department is divided by the measure of service or number of procedures performed. If there is a wide range of services or procedures performed within a revenue center, it will be necessary to use some relative weighting scale, such as Medicare's RVUs, to equate the services or procedures. This is illustrated later in the chapter.

The question arises: What is the best measure of cost? There is no one correct answer since each cost is an arbitrarily determined amount. Care should be taken in identifying responsibility centers, tracing costs to responsibility centers, choosing the order of allocation, and selecting the bases of allocation.

Step 5: Determine the cost per treatment or case by using the cost per procedure or service to determine the cost per episode or unit of care, such as a specific procedure, case, or diagnosis.

Not only is it helpful to know the full allocated cost of providing a particular service or procedure, but it is also increasingly important to know the costs of providing an episode or a bundle of care, especially for a particular type of case, treatment, or diagnosis. And being armed with this information is an increasingly important component of a practice's financial decisions. Physicians need to know their costs of doing business and how that relates to current revenue maximum levels and anticipated payment changes expected from future ACO and other evolving payment arrangements.

ISSUES IN COST ALLOCATION

There are no right or wrong accounting allocation processes. This step in the process is the most important by far and the most challenging. It can be the difference between profit and loss, and many people could be affected by these outcomes. Be aware that there are allocation options that don't work because they do not fairly charge those responsibility centers that consume the resources for what they actually use. There are a number of issues to understand that lead to a fair cost allocation. The needs and characteristics of a particular physician practice should be considered when selecting the allocation technique, the order of allocation, and the basis of allocation. If the cost structure is relatively insensitive to less precise calculations, the financial burden of a precise allocation method would not be justified or reasonably necessary. The sensitivity should be tested, however, for impact on outcomes.

To make the best choice, the following qualitative tests should be applied:

   ■   Is the method fair and equitable?
       –   In terms of how it charges all the cost centers or units of care for the costs that each consumes?

- ▪ Is it understandable?
  - – To all those being charged, is every center that consumes the resource being charged according to the closest reasonable denominator of how the center uses it?
  - – Even if it is fair and equitable, if it is not understood, it will not be trusted.
- ▪ Do the benefits of the allocation methods justify the costs of the allocations to the organization?
  - – If a simpler base will generate a similar result, then the allocation should not require minutia to fairly allocate the costs.

For most decisions relating to the practice's patient volume and mix of services, it is very important for costs to be traced on the basis of how those services actually drive and consume the costs. This is the crux of the analysis. If it isn't properly measured, the results are useless. Arbitrary or average allocations of cost should not be allowed to distort the results. Each responsibility center, whether a revenue-generating center or a cost center, drives and consumes costs necessary to carry out its activities in the practice and should be charged its fair share of the cost burden accordingly.

As mentioned, when establishing an allocation method, responsibility center managers should agree on the technique, order, and basis of allocation before any allocation analysis is performed. These issues should be decided on the basis of fairness, equity, understandability, and cost to implement.

Once these decisions are made, the cost data can be analyzed and the results evaluated. A presentation of alternative methods together with their impact on actual data will often cause managers to shop for the methods that will improve their positions. The final allocation decisions should charge each responsibility center for what it uses regardless of the outcome. Understanding the behavior of how each responsibility center drives certain costs and making allocation decisions based on the expected use will yield the most meaningful result.

ORDER OF ALLOCATION

An order of allocation must be established when the step-down technique of cost allocation is used. Different orders of allocation may produce a significantly different cost for a particular responsibility center. To ensure fairness and equity, begin with the responsibility center that provides the services to other responsibility centers but that also takes the least services from other centers. A good example is building and occupancy costs. Following these guidelines, the general order of cost center allocation for a typical practice would be building and occupancy, administration, information technology, purchasing, reception and scheduling, billing and collections, and medical records.

Keep in mind that the order should progress from the responsibility center that provides the most services to others to the responsibility center that serves the revenue-producing centers only (e.g., billing and medical records).

Factors that should be considered when determining which allocation bases to use include cause and effect, facilities provided, ability to bear the costs, and strategic effects.

Cause and Effect

To reiterate, the most important aspect of cost allocation is that the relationship between the cost to be allocated and the responsibility center receiving the allocation must be clear. Cause and effect is best measured through usage records. For example, the use of an MRI technician or the use of specific chemotherapy drugs may be charged to users directly. The cause-and-effect criterion is a logical framework for ascertaining allocation bases because it normally results in fair and equitable cost allocations that are mutually acceptable to both the provider and user of the service.

For some responsibility centers, such as the administration cost center, there is no sufficient measure of cause and effect. Attempts to measure cause and effect based on the time the administrator devotes to each responsibility center will usually cause more problems than they solve and will still likely not measure the value of the costs to each center based solely on time. There will be some cost centers for which the allocation base will not be accurate but it can be reasonable.

Facilities Provided

The underlying logic is that facility space and related costs are provided for essentially all of the practice's responsibility centers. As a result, each responsibility center should share responsibility in the use of facilities. Occupancy costs are not optional for most responsibility centers. These costs entail not only rent but also utilities, insurance, real estate taxes, janitorial services, maintenance, and so on — costs that are expected to be incurred by the business.

Ability to Bear the Costs

This criterion is arbitrary since costs are allocated on the basis of use and not those centers' ability to cover additional costs. Costs of services are independent of their results. Any allocation scheme that uses revenue, gross charges, contributions, or a similar allocation base without consideration of services provided in roughly the same proportion may be based on the ability to bear, which may be unfair and create a skewed result. This debate sometimes occurs between responsibility center management, but costs should be assigned to users on the basis of consumption regardless of whether the users are profitable.

There may be a good reason for a certain cost, even if it makes a department unprofitable; there may be a reason for a "loss leader," such as a dermatology practice offering free skin screenings or an ophthalmology practice offering free eye exams. This practice is similar to other sales strategies common in everyday commerce, such as when a grocery retailer advertises a low price special on seasonal items like turkeys during the fall holiday season. In that case, the meat department will suffer a decrease in profit during this sale period, but other departments may enjoy increased profits from the holiday selling season, which leads to additional overall sales of extras and impulse buying of items with higher margins.

Strategic Effects

This factor relates to the physicians' desires to reach certain goals and objectives of the group. One example pertains to a goal of obtaining a certain level of distributable profits. In multispecialty practices with physicians in both primary care and various specialties, management may want the responsibility centers of the specialties to bear a larger proportion of the indirect service costs because of their more intense usage of facilities or staff; thus, the group members may agree on a formula to affect this result. In all these instances, allocation bases become a critically important and strategic tool for assisting in achieving organizational goals. Again, the primary goal is that of charging the user for the costs consumed as reasonably and accurately as possible.

ALLOCATION BASES

To select allocation bases for costs, the cost center should be segregated because it requires a basis that would not be the same as those of other centers, otherwise combining cost centers. One allocation basis per cost center provides for acceptable allocation of the costs inherent to that center. Some of the most meaningful and common bases used are:

- Square footage: Derived from the number of square feet occupied by each responsibility center and converted to a percentage of total square feet.

- Utilization: Based on the number of units (hours, dollars, etc.) of usage derived for the individual responsibility centers. Such utilization patterns can be established over a period of months. During that time, records of utilization are kept with the utilization amount estimated for each center, subject to an annual review and revision. Another simpler method is to report actual utilization by each responsibility center on a monthly basis.

- Patient visits: Derived from the number of patient visits to the medical practice or further derived by specialty or service if applicable (e.g., vascular surgery with vein ancillary revenue service, or procedures, such as pain physician and procedure room, etc.).

- Personnel count: Derived from the number of employees in each responsibility center and converted to a percentage of total employees or FTEs. Subdivision can be determined, in which services are provided exclusively for certain physicians based on the cost of services provided only to them.

- Revenue production: Determined by the billing system to indicate the amount of gross charges, adjusted gross charges, number of procedures, CPT code counts, number of cases, or per physician, and so on.

- RVUs: Developed by multiplying the frequency of coded procedures by the relative value scale amounts.

- Direct costs of responsibility centers: Based on detailed general ledger accounting records, costs can be easily allocated directly to responsibility centers as incurred.

- Gross payroll: Determined by job description and payroll records.

- Agreed percentages: Derived by consensus of group members to a stipulated percentage of usage for each responsibility center.

- Specific identification: Established through the use of monthly tally cards, time reports, or number of requisitions.

An important point is that the more costs that can be directly and fairly allocated to the responsibility center at the accounting level, the more accurate the results and the less work required later in allocating costs.

In allocating costs, the main question to answer is whether it makes sense to charge the expense on that basis. The allocation factor for a specific set of costs should be the most relatable and relevant factor for how costs are consumed (i.e., prorated by square footage for rent versus dollars of revenue because rent varies with usage by square foot, not dollars of revenue).

A PRACTICAL APPROACH TO THE INITIAL COST ANALYSIS

Before attempting to develop procedure standard costing, certain decisions should be made so that the entire costing process is easier and significant operational issues will be uncovered early on. These planning decisions include:

1. Responsibility center selection
2. Responsibility center operations documentation
3. Procedure selection
4. Control time period and data selection

Responsibility Center Selection

Standard costs are initially produced for the revenue-producing responsibility centers because these are the centers for which a practice sells services and receives revenue for the provision of those services typically broken down by procedure. It is those areas of the practice that the full cost (direct and indirect) of providing the services should be lower than the revenue received, thus yielding a profit.

In addition to revenue centers, many overhead responsibility centers present opportunities for identifying costs at the procedure level. Examples of these are billing, reception and scheduling, and purchasing. It is easy to focus efforts on the direct costs of revenue-producing centers, but detailed costing of cost (overhead) centers — measuring how they support the revenue centers — is also extremely important.

Responsibility Center Operations Documentation

By documenting the operations carried out by each responsibility center, detailed costing of procedures can be developed. Through this effort, production activities can be examined carefully and inefficient practices uncovered. This may be the first opportunity for management to identify production problems and to adopt cost-saving solutions. The first time is an eye-opening exercise and can help in uncovering inefficiencies and problems that may have gone undetected for some time. Such a focus represents a "value-added" approach to an internal evaluation of a practice's operations.

Operations documentation is best accomplished through the use of interviews, observation, and questionnaires. The content should focus on the following areas:

- Responsibility center's organization
  - Determine the responsibility centers that should be measured separately for both revenue-producing centers and cost centers. Below are some examples of relevant centers for which physicians may wish to measure the cost of providing services and their profitability.
  - Revenue-producing centers
- Office visits
- Surgeries
  - In-office versus performed elsewhere (e.g., surgery center)
- Radiology
  - X-ray versus bone density versus MRI
- Laboratory
- Procedures
  - EKG versus stress test
- Supplies
  - Inventory items billed
  - DME
  - Drugs
  - Cost (overhead) centers
- Building and occupancy
  - Supports revenue and cost centers
- Information technology
  - Supports revenue and cost centers
- Administration and general operating costs
  - Supports revenue and cost centers
- Reception and scheduling
  - Supports revenue-producing centers only
- Billing and collections
  - Supports revenue-producing centers only

For each separate revenue or cost center measurement, the assumption is that all costs within a particular center will be allocated using only one allocation factor. This should be considered when identifying centers to be measured. For example, it makes the most sense to allocate building and occupancy costs on a "per square foot" basis to all other centers because each center would typically consume building/occupancy costs relative to each other on a square-footage basis and, therefore, prorating the costs along this basis would treat each center fairly. It would charge each center for a close approximation of what each actually used or consumed.

An example that would make this assumption incorrect and unfair would be if the practice had an MRI machine, and the MRI machine had additional building and occupancy costs associated with it. These additional costs include the protection that had to be built within the walls and floor of the room that housed the MRI, as well as the extra electricity that the MRI used. On a per-square-foot basis, the MRI consumed more costs than did the other centers. In this case, the MRI's additional building/occupancy costs should be carved out and allocated at a higher cost per square foot.

As discussed earlier, the more costs that can be directly traced to a center through the initial recording of costs in the accounting records, the less allocation decisions and allocation math that must take place later. This not only allows an easier application of the costing system, but it also allows for much more accurate tracking and ongoing monitoring and makes the cost system more valuable as a management tool whose results are available with minimal effort.

- ◼ Estimated current production
- ◼ Estimated minimum staffing requirements: Do any clinical or clerical personnel work for other responsibility centers? If so, for which ones and how much time is usually involved?
  - – Assign each staff member to a revenue or cost center. Some employees may service more than one center. In those cases, the employee's time should be approximated and prorated accordingly among the centers they service.
- ◼ Are any services provided for and/or by other responsibility centers?
- ◼ What are the hours of operation and the hours of highest and lowest activity?
- ◼ What is the typical waiting time a patient experiences?
- ◼ How are supplies recorded in the general ledger? Are they expensed at the time of purchase or inventoried?
- ◼ Is there anything about the operation of the center that negatively affects performance? This might include poor physical layout, lack of sufficient space, or inadequate technology.
- ◼ Also, the questionnaire should address procedures most frequently performed by the responsibility centers. Information should be collected on the procedures with significant volume. Questions should include:

– Do any procedures vary in duration or resource intensity due to the type of patient — pediatric, adult, geriatric, and so on — or acuteness of condition or significant supplies used? If so, are separate CPT procedure code numbers or modifiers used? Can this type of data be mined from the current EHR system or billing system?

– Are any procedures essentially identical except for a major supply item (e.g., contrast used in an MRI test)?

– Are any procedures performed that are charged on a case basis (e.g., obstetrics) regardless of the resources consumed or the actual number of visits?

– Are there any procedures or functions related to patient care that are not billed but that make up a significant amount of the center's activity (e.g., surgery global period for follow-up office visits)?

In addition to providing data for cost determination purposes, operations documentation may also identify certain benefits to the medical practice. These benefits include:

▪ Indication of responsibility center interaction and capacity issues. By revealing how responsibility centers interact, operating documentation can highlight possible coordination problems that may result in inefficient patient services such as scheduling, obtaining proper referral documentation, authorization or precertification data, and patient eligibility.

▪ The documentation of general flow and capacity problems, including physical layout constraints, scheduling/communication problems, and equipment inadequacies, helps to explain why a center operates inefficiently. Once problems are documented, improvements can be more easily identified and costs can be tied to these issues.

This part of the project allows management at all levels to challenge the organizational structure, the operations, and the management information obtained and reported by the transaction systems.

Procedure Selection

In this step, procedures within each responsibility center are identified so that detailed standard costs can be determined. Top procedures can be isolated for costing by using the "80/20 rule" applied to each responsibility center. Standard costs can be determined for those procedures that are significant in volume and expense amount, which usually makes up about 80 percent of a practice's total procedures.

A list of the responsibility center's procedures, including the annual procedure volume, the most recent procedure charge rate, the current reimbursement rate from major payers, and the relative values for each procedure, should be compiled. The group's billing system can easily provide the volume and charge data and, most likely, the contract rate and RVU data. Many billing systems today have this capability. If not, relative values can be obtained from the Medicare Fee Schedule (www.cms.gov), which presents the resource-based relative value scale (RBRVS) of relative values for CPT codes. The fee schedule and the relative value scale are both available for download in a spreadsheet format.

Control Time Period and Data Selection

Data from the control period supplies the majority of the data for the initial system implementation. Whatever period of time is used for measuring revenue production and volume should also be used to measure costs because those would have been the costs that were consumed to produce the revenue during the same period of time.

In selecting the control time period, several factors should be considered. First, the control period should reflect current operations since the most recent data will closely reflect current procedures, staffing, patient types, equipment status, and overhead costs. Second, it is preferable to use data for a full fiscal year. This generally eliminates integrity problems associated with seasonal volume fluctuations, accruals, inventory, and intermittent spending patterns associated with such items as legal fees, vacation time, capital expenditures, and year-end financing and tax strategies.

Once the control period is selected, the following financial and statistical information should be obtained for that period:

- Year-to-date detailed general ledger expenses by responsibility center and account (e.g., medical supplies, drugs and medications, laundry/linen) that show each entry made to each account during the control time period.
  - Reading the general ledger allows for a thorough understanding of routine and typical costs by vendor names, monthly amounts, and so on, and will assist in identifying outliers important in determining the true costs of services, as well as projecting future expected costs.
  - Normalize the costs for any expenses that are believed to be extraordinary or one-time expenses.
- Year-to-date payroll per employee (e.g., productive, vacation, holiday, and benefits)
  - The employee listing should be segregated into the various revenue and cost centers that will be measured. The cost of employees who support more than one center should be prorated to centers on the basis of support provided to each.

A listing of fixed assets by responsibility center should be developed so that depreciation and/or financing costs can be attributed to the centers on the basis of how the assets are used by each. Estimates for common area and administrative assets may be best allocated using the number of employees, patient visit volume, or revenue. Again, the basis of allocation should be the one that most fairly prorates the costs to each center based on how the assets are actually used. Let's take waiting room furniture as an example: Even though the practice may vary widely in the dollar amounts of revenue per procedure that is performed, every patient who visits a practice probably waits in the waiting room for a similar amount of time and uses the same approximate amount of resources (e.g., chairs, TV, magazines, and lighting). Therefore, the fairest way to allocate the cost of waiting room assets may be by distributing the costs to each revenue center based on the number of patient visits. Regardless of which revenue center the patient presents for or which procedure, each revenue center is benefited by the waiting room on no more than a "per patient" basis.

Also at this time, supplemental current period data should be collected that includes:

- Current labor rates by responsibility center, by position
- Current purchase price of supply items used, including description and current unit cost

Once the control period information is collected for both the revenue side and the cost side, the cost accounting analysis can begin and standard costs can be set.

After standard cost data have been developed, medical practices should prepare detailed cost summary sheets to show the summary and composition of the standard cost of an individual or group of procedures. This should include a breakdown of labor, supplies, equipment, and overhead with both a "quantity" and a "rate." By having detailed cost sheets for most procedures in a responsibility center or by revenue center, it is possible to aggregate the sheets for all procedures necessary to treat an illness and arrive at a total standard cost of procedures undertaken. This type of costing will become increasingly important with the solidification of ACOs and new or joint payment methods. Such summary data can be very helpful in contract negotiations with managed care payers, as well as setting fees for joint venture work, planning expansion, and so on.

A cost management system's standard costs should be updated periodically to remain an effective management tool. For existing procedures, this entails updating resource usage and the unit costs of individual procedures. New procedure standard costs should be documented and incorporated into the cost management system database as new services or transaction systems are implemented or as more responsibility centers develop procedure standards.

Generally, it is recommended that standard costs be reviewed and updated annually. In a rapidly changing environment, such as a period of high inflation and certainly changing reimbursement rates and CPT codes, resource unit costs should be updated more frequently. The updating process involves a review of existing procedure standards with the relevant responsibility center manager.

If there is a large difference between average reimbursement and routine costs of a procedure, a set of procedures, or a revenue center as a whole, then a time study to find out why may be cost beneficial and very useful.

A method that uses the concepts of standard costing with less record keeping and application time involves the use of relative values as the basis of standard cost derivation. This is recommended because no matter how long it takes, RVUs are already set, and if there is zero profit, then you can figure out why.

RESOURCE-BASED RELATIVE VALUE SCALES

Over the last decade or so, Medicare RBRVS RVUs have become a standard tool in developing the costs of provider services, in evaluating provider performance within a medical practice, and in comparing with other providers.

RBRVS is a scale of the different values assigned to physician services by CPT code, and the values are designated as RVUs. RBRVS was developed by Medicare to replace the "usual, customary, and reasonable" fees used by physicians.

Furthermore, one CPT code, 99213, was initially used to scale all other CPT codes. For example, the established office visit, level 3 — code 99213, was originally valued at 1.00 with the advent of the RVU scale. This means that the complexity of any other CPT code is valued relative to 99213.

The use of RBRVS as a basis for standard costing allows for the measure of the relative differences in the consumption of resources between various procedures. The three components of RBRVS — work, practice, and malpractice — with their relative weights permit the development of a cost-allocation strategy of an average component cost per unit (procedure).

Let's perform the exercise for how RVUs can be used for developing standard costs for procedures.

The Medicare RBRVS Fee Schedule has three components:

1. A relative value component that adjusts relative payments among services;
2. A geographic component that adjusts payments among different locales across the country using geographic factors that measure differences in the cost of living and in physician practice costs; and
3. A conversion factor that transforms RVUs into dollars.

Although RBRVS are primarily concerned with fees paid by Medicare to physicians for healthcare services, they also provide important data about the resources and work expended in delivering specific services. Thus, the RVUs underlying the fee schedule may be used to determine the cost of services rendered by providers and to measure their financial performance in new ways. For example, the RVUs can be used to evaluate the contributions to profits made by individual physician activities and office staff productivity and to determine estimates of the cost of services provided.

The RBRVS system uses relative values on the basis of the resources used by physicians to perform a particular service. The resources are divided into three parts:

1. Work RVU (physician work) — involving time, technical skill, physical strength, mental effort and judgment, physician stress, and total work

2. Practice expense RVU — such as rent, support staff, and supplies, which vary by the physician's gross revenue, mix of services, and practice location

3. Malpractice expense RVU — varies by code

An example of the RVU breakdown, using 2012 RVUs for a common CPT code, 99213 Established Office Visit code, is shown below.

Work RVU	0.97
Practice RVU	1.07
Malpractice RVU	0.07
Total RVU	2.11

Medicare RBRVS use relative values for most CPT codes. The method then converts these relative values into dollar amounts by applying a conversion factor. Each procedure code establishes a relative weight for physician work and practice expenses, which recognizes the magnitude of resource use for various procedures. Medicare and major insurance carriers typically pay on a per CPT code basis, or as a percentage of RBRVS, which is tied to the RVUs associated with each code.

To carry the above example further, the Medicare reimbursement rate for 99213 would be as follows, which multiples the total RVUs for 99213 by the 2012 Medicare conversion factor (reimbursement rate) of $34.0376. This results in the total Medicare reimbursement payment of $71.82 for providing one office visit for a Medicare patient using CPT code 99213.

Total RVU	2.11
Medicare Conversion Factor	$34.0376
Total Reimbursement	$71.82

Using this approach, a medical group practice can determine the total number of RVUs based on different procedures performed that are generated during a given time period. Since RVUs summarize the relative weights of procedures performed by physicians for all patients, regardless of payer, they form an apples-to-apples basis of work performed and a comprehensive basis of evaluation for the overall financial performance of the practice.

To develop RVUs, the procedure code data from a practice's billing system is correlated with relative value weights for each procedure from the Medicare RBRVS. The RVUs are calculated as shown in Exhibit 7.3 for a typical orthopedic practice.

EXHIBIT 7.3 ▪ **Example of Calculation for Total RVUs Performed**

Code	Procedure	Total CPT Procedures Performed	Total RVUs Performed per CPT Code	Total RVUs Performed
20610	Drain/inject joint	280	1.81	506.65
20663	Application thigh brace	85	10.51	893.59
27244	Repair thigh fracture	40	32.76	1310.27
27253	Repair hip dislocation	80	25.01	2001.04
27310	Exploration knee joint	150	19.44	2915.66
27427	Knee reconstruction	100	19.10	1910.49
27440	Revision of knee joint	75	21.14	1585.66
27487	Knee joint replacement	175	46.88	8203.87
27580	Fusion of knee	35	38.27	1339.41
99202	Office visit, new	500	1.99	995.62
99203	Office visit, new	300	2.87	861.69
99204	Office visit, new	200	4.39	879.00
99212	Office visit, established	150	1.15	172.80
99213	Office visit, established	500	1.94	970.16
99214	Office visit, established	325	2.86	928.62
72170	XR pelvis	300	0.71	212.10
73500	XR hip	200	0.73	146.79
73550	XR thigh	500	0.76	380.44
73560	XR knee	1400	0.84	1178.38
Total annual relative value service units				**27,392.22**

Costing Using RVUs

In lieu of more detailed approaches for developing standard costs, using RVUs provides a way for medical groups of all sizes to establish a practical costing system that will yield information approximating that produced by more sophisticated cost development techniques. The RVU system derived by RBRVS has a rationale that resembles the most accurate method, time, and motion studies because relative values relate directly to the physician work and the overhead resources consumed in performing procedures.

The basic elements required to use the RVU method of standard development for procedures are:

▪   A historical production report of provider activity showing a frequency distribution of all coded CPT codes for a given time period (production time period should be the same as the cost time period);

■ A set of historical financial reports consisting of an income statement, general ledger, or a summary of account balances that identifies total dollar amounts of total costs incurred for the practice for the same time period as the production report;

■ The most current listing of RVUs per CPT code along with the respective geographic practice cost indices (GPCIs);

■ A spreadsheet software package, such as MGMA's DataDive, which allows the user to enter CPT codes, modifiers, the frequency of CPT code procedures, geographic location, place of service, and physicians to calculate total RVUs, total component RVUs, RVUs worked per physicians, total RVUs per CPT, and so on, including graphical presentations of the results. The tool allows exportation of graphs to Excel for management reporting.

Methodology of Calculating RVUs

Step 1: Using spreadsheet software, list each CPT code making up the practice's list of most frequent procedures and assign its relative value for work (w), practice expense (p), and malpractice (m). Adjust each code's separate component relative value by its associated GPCI [(RVw × GPCIw), (RVp × GPCIp), (RVm × GPCIm)].

For example, continuing with the example using CPT code 99213, its 2012 component RVUs for work RVUs, practice RVUs, and malpractice RVUs are .97, 1.03, and .07, respectively. Each component's respective GPCI for the locale of Tennessee for 2012 is .972, .898, and .523. By multiplying the respective RVUs by the corresponding GPCIs, the adjusted relative values for work, practice, and malpractice are .94, .92, and .037, resulting in a total GPCI adjusted RVU of 1.897.

See Exhibit 7.4, which calculates total RVUs by components, including GPCIs, for common codes used in an orthopedic practice. The list of procedures shown here is for example purposes only to illustrate this exercise. A practice's list of most frequent procedures would be more comprehensive.

Step 2: Calculate the total number of RVUs worked for the practice during the selected time period. This involves multiplying the adjusted RVU for each CPT code component by the frequency of the utilization of that code. The total RVUs for each CPT code component are then added to arrive at a total RVU for each CPT code. Finally, the RVUs for all the CPT codes are added to determine the total RVUs produced for the practice during this time period.

Continuing the example, the frequency for code 99213 is 500. Multiplying this frequency by each component's adjusted RVUs and adding up these projects yields the total adjusted RVUs for that code. For code 99213, the total RVUs are 470.00 [(500 × .94) + 480.00 (500 × .96) + 18.50 (500 × .037)]. Total RVUs can also be calculated by multiplying the total adjusted RVU for the code, 1.94, by the frequency, 500, which will also result in 968.50 RVUs.

Step 3: Calculate the cost per RVU per responsibility center. Using an income statement or a list of account balances for the same time period as the frequency

EXHIBIT 7.4 ■ Example of Component RVU Calculation with GPCI Factors

CPT Code	Physician Work RVUs	Work GPCI	Adjusted Work RVUs	Fully Implemented Practice RVUs	Practice GPCI	Adjusted Practice RVUs	Malpractice RVUs	Malpractice GPCI
20610	0.79	0.972	0.77	1.09	0.898	0.98	0.12	0.523
20663	5.74	0.972	5.58	4.83	0.898	4.34	1.14	0.523
27244	18.18	0.972	17.67	14.72	0.898	13.22	3.57	0.523
27253	13.58	0.972	13.20	11.6	0.898	10.42	2.67	0.523
27310	10.00	0.972	9.72	9.68	0.898	8.69	1.96	0.523
27427	9.79	0.972	9.52	9.56	0.898	8.58	1.92	0.523
27440	11.09	0.972	10.78	10.27	0.898	9.22	2.18	0.523
27487	27.11	0.972	26.35	19.75	0.898	17.74	5.34	0.523
27580	21.10	0.972	20.51	17.36	0.898	15.59	4.15	0.523
99202	0.93	0.972	0.90	1.17	0.898	1.05	0.07	0.523
99203	1.42	0.972	1.38	1.58	0.898	1.42	0.14	0.523
99204	2.43	0.972	2.36	2.13	0.898	1.91	0.23	0.523
99212	0.48	0.972	0.47	0.74	0.898	0.66	0.04	0.523
99213	0.97	0.972	0.94	1.07	0.898	0.96	0.07	0.523
99214	1.50	0.972	1.46	1.5	0.898	1.35	0.10	0.523
72170	0.17	0.972	0.17	0.58	0.898	0.52	0.04	0.523
73500	0.17	0.972	0.17	0.61	0.898	0.55	0.04	0.523
73550	0.17	0.972	0.17	0.64	0.898	0.57	0.04	0.523
73560	0.17	0.972	0.17	0.73	0.898	0.66	0.04	0.523

of code utilization, aggregate the total costs for the three RBRVS components — work, practice expense, and malpractice. Additional analysis will likely be required in which the direct costs of each component must be determined. In addition, all indirect costs must be allocated to each component. The direct and allocated indirect costs for each responsibility center are added to reach a total cost per component.

When each responsibility center's total costs have been determined, these amounts are divided by the total number of RVUs performed to produce the cost per RVU per revenue center. For the continuing example of the orthopedic practice, total work, practice, and malpractice RVUs were 13,749, 11,937, and 1,312, respectively, which sums to total RVUs performed. Dividing each revenue center's total allocated cost by its respective RVU total will result in a cost per RVU. Dividing the total practice costs by the total practice RVUs will produce a total overall cost per RVU for the practice and can be immediately

Adjusted Malpractice RVUs	Total Adjusted RVU per CPT Code	Total Procedure Count	Total RVUs Performed	Total Adjusted Work RVUs	Total Adjusted Practice RVUs	Total Adjusted Malpractice RVUs
0.06	1.81	280	506.65	215.01	274.07	17.57
0.60	10.51	85	893.59	474.24	368.67	50.68
1.87	32.76	40	1,310.27	706.84	528.74	74.68
1.40	25.01	80	2,001.04	1,055.98	833.34	111.71
1.03	19.44	150	2,915.66	1,458.00	1,303.90	153.76
1.00	19.10	100	1,910.49	951.59	858.49	100.42
1.14	21.14	75	1,585.66	808.46	691.68	85.51
2.79	46.88	175	8,203.87	4,611.41	3,103.71	488.74
2.17	38.27	35	1,339.41	717.82	545.62	75.97
0.04	1.99	500	995.62	451.98	525.33	18.31
0.07	2.87	300	861.69	414.07	425.65	21.97
0.12	4.39	200	879.00	472.39	382.55	24.06
0.02	1.15	150	172.80	69.98	99.68	3.14
0.04	1.94	500	970.16	471.42	480.43	18.31
0.05	2.86	325	928.62	473.85	437.78	17.00
0.02	0.71	300	212.10	49.57	156.25	6.28
0.02	0.73	200	146.79	33.05	109.56	4.18
0.02	0.76	500	380.44	82.62	261.50	10.46
0.02	0.84	1400	1,178.38	231.34	732.20	29.29
		5,395.00	27,392.22	13,749.62	12,119.16	1,312.02

used to compare to the practice's Medicare reimbursement rates per RVU. See Exhibit 7.5 for a presentation of component RVUs, along with GPCIs applied for the state of Tennessee locale, and the resulting costs per RVU in each revenue center. Below is an illustration of the calculation for converting a practice's fee to a per RVU basis for comparison to payment per RVU.

Converting to RBRVS per RVU:

Practice fee for CPT code 99213	$95
RBRVS RVU	2.11
Fee divided by RVU	$45.02
▪ Compare to Medicare payment/RVU	$34.0376
▪ Compare to payer contract payment:	
• At RBRVS 115% per RVU	
• $34.0376 × 1.15	$39.14

EXHIBIT 7.5 ■ Example of Calculating Cost per RVU

	Office Visits	Surgical Procedures	Radiology	Total
Gross Charge Revenue	$650,000	$1,850,000	$1,000,000	$3,500,000
Net Revenue	$200,000	$990,000	$110,000	$1,300,000
Allocated Direct and Indirect Costs to Revenue Centers	$150,000	$465,000	$85,000	$700,000
Total RVUs	4,807.88	20,666.63	1,917.71	27,392.22
Net Revenue per RVU	$41.60	$47.90	$57.36	$47.46
Cost per RVU	$31.20	$22.50	$44.32	$25.55
Medicare CV per RVU	$34.0376	$34.0376	$34.0376	

EXHIBIT 7.6 ■ Calculation of Cost per CPT Procedure Code

CPT Code	Adjusted Work RVU per CPT Code	Adjusted Practice RVU per CPT Code	Adjusted Malpractice RVU per CPT Code	Total Adjusted RVU per CPT Code	Cost per RVU by Revenue Center
20610	0.77	0.98	0.06	1.81	$22.50
20663	5.58	4.34	0.60	10.51	$22.50
27244	17.67	13.22	1.87	32.76	$22.50
27253	13.20	10.42	1.40	25.01	$22.50
27310	9.72	8.69	1.03	19.44	$22.50
27427	9.52	8.58	1.00	19.10	$22.50
27440	10.78	9.22	1.14	21.14	$22.50
27487	26.35	17.74	2.79	46.88	$22.50
27580	20.51	15.59	2.17	38.27	$22.50
99202	0.90	1.05	0.04	1.99	$31.20
99203	1.38	1.42	0.07	2.87	$31.20
99204	2.36	1.91	0.12	4.39	$31.20
99212	0.47	0.66	0.02	1.15	$31.20
99213	0.94	0.96	0.04	1.94	$31.20
99214	1.46	1.35	0.05	2.86	$31.20
72170	0.17	0.52	0.02	0.71	$44.32
73500	0.17	0.55	0.02	0.73	$44.32
73550	0.17	0.57	0.02	0.76	$44.32
73560	0.17	0.66	0.02	0.84	$44.32

Step 4: Calculate the cost per CPT procedure code. This requires multiplying the adjusted relative value of each CPT code component by the cost per RVU for that component. In the continuing example, the cost of CPT code 99213 is $60.36. Alternatively, the cost per CPT code procedure may be calculated by multiplying the practice total cost per RVU by the practice total adjusted RVUs. An example is shown below and in Exhibit 7.6 of using the cost per RVU results to calculate the full cost, as allocated, of providing each CPT procedure. Keep in mind that Exhibit 7.6 does include GPCIs throughout the calculations.

Converting to RBRVS per CPT:

Cost per CPT code	
$31.20 × 2.11 =	$65.83
Practice fee for CPT code 99213	$95
Multiplied by RBRVS RVU for 99213	2.11
Compare to Medicare RBRVS	
34.0376 × 2.11 =	$71.82
Compare to contract RBRVS 115%	
$34.0376 × 1.15 × 2.11 =	$82.59

Cost per CPT Procedure	Payer A Allowable	Payer B Allowable	Payer C Allowable	MGMA ABC Model Results for Cost per Type of Service
$40.71	$63.87	$75.00	$85.00	$95.53
$236.54	$371.55	$400.00	$350.00	$95.53
$737.03	$1,123.42	$1,100.00	$1,500.00	$514.63
$562.79	$859.13	$900.00	$850.00	$514.63
$437.35	$664.73	$650.00	$700.00	$514.63
$429.86	$654.11	$650.00	$700.00	$514.63
$475.70	$718.58	$750.00	$700.00	$514.63
$1,054.78	$1,613.85	$1,700.00	$1,800.00	$514.63
$861.05	$1,315.36	$1,400.00	$1,200.00	$514.63
$62.12	$67.44	$80.00	$80.00	$40.40
$89.61	$97.59	$100.00	$110.00	$40.40
$137.12	$149.77	$150.00	$135.00	$40.40
$35.94	$39.36	$40.00	$50.00	$40.40
$60.54	$65.75	$75.00	$70.00	$40.40
$89.14	$97.46	$105.00	$95.00	$40.40
$31.34	24.53	$22.00	$20.00	$81.79
$32.53	25.14	$22.00	$20.00	$81.79
$33.73	26.37	$28.00	$30.00	$81.79
$37.31	28.81	$28.00	$30.00	$81.79

There will likely be codes without relative values in a practice's schedule of services. In those instances, the missing RVUs of these codes can be estimated from a group of total RVUs of similar codes.

For costs relevant to each responsibility center, now that total costs have been allocated, various cost denominators can be calculated such as cost per patient, cost per test, cost per physician, cost per location, and so on.

ACTIVITY-BASED COST ANALYSIS

Activity-based costing (ABC) essentially takes a traditional or standard costing system to the next level by breaking down each routine task performed in a medical practice into its own responsibility center.

ABC first requires identifying the primary tasks and activities performed regularly in a medical practice. Examples of these routine activities are (1) purchasing supplies, (2) performing an office visit, (3) providing an injection, or (4) billing a claim. When identifying these activities, tasks that are directly related to performing the activity are assigned to the activity. ABC closely measures what it takes to actually perform a specific activity, from start to finish, whereas traditional costing backs into what the cost actually was and then uses that result as the standard until such time that it changes. The example illustrated in this chapter is really a mix of both traditional/standard costing and ABC.

As emphasized earlier, it is important to know what the practice's costs actually are and, by studying the current operations, determining what costs have been in order to perform the tasks and activities at hand. That information serves a baseline and a starting point. The more cost data that can be directly attributable to a task, an activity, or a cost or revenue center within the accounting records themselves, the more accurate the cost analysis will be. The costs of each activity are determined and then allocated to the activity on the basis of routine and expected consumption.

As was introduced earlier in the chapter, the use of time studies for the practice's primary tasks and activities is an accurate method of measuring and thus allocating costs directly to those activities responsible for creating the need for the costs and consuming them — whether or not it is profitable and efficient. When questioned, providers and staff generally know how long it takes to perform routine tasks, how many supplies are routinely used in carrying out the tasks, and so on. They are a huge asset to gathering information used in allocating costs accurately and should be consulted. It is only through this exercise that management can learn how to improve processes effectively. From that point, management can begin to assess where there may be opportunities for improvement in efficiency and cost savings and opportunities to increase revenue through more effective use of the staff and processes by which the practice carries out its activities.

Exhibit 7.7 illustrates how the ABC model can be used to determine the cost of a routine office visit, including an X-ray, performed at an orthopedic practice.

The example calculates the direct costs of each routine task required in this activity, which includes labor costs and other direct costs associated with providing this service. The activity's estimates of time would be based on time studies, observations, and discussions with staff and providers who regularly perform these services. The result provides a more accurate per-procedure cost that can be used for comparison to reimbursement rates and for operational improvements. However, the ABC analysis only reflects primary direct costs that are consumed in providing the service. It is just as important to allocate the indirect costs as well because the total costs are being paid by the practice and are part of the costs needed to support the overall business. The cost analysis exhibited in this chapter, although traditional and standard in its approach, takes into consideration 100 percent of a practice's costs and emphasizes direct

EXHIBIT 7.7 ■ Example of ABC Costing Activity: Routine Office Visit with X-Ray

Components of the Visit	Direct Costs Consumed	Cost to Provide Service
Patient Check-in		
Includes patient demographic and insurance verification; collecting copays and payments; entering information into billing and/or EHR system		
Salary and benefits cost — labor	$20.00 per hour	
Time used in process	5 minutes	$1.67
Provider Time with Patient		
Consultation with physician		
Salary and benefits cost — labor	$200 per hour	
Time used in process	8 minutes	$26.67
Routine X-ray		
X-ray technician		
Salary and benefits	$30 per hour	
Time used in process	5 minutes	$2.50
Radiology Reading Fees	$15.00 per image	$15.00
Paid to outside radiologist for X-ray		
Patient Follow-up Scheduling		
Patient check-out process of scheduling surgery, further radiology testing, referring physician, etc.		
Salary and benefits cost — labor	$20.00 per hour	
Time used in process	5 minutes	$1.67
* Total Direct Cost of Routine Office Visit with X-ray		**$47.50**

* Does not include two cost factors: (1) indirect overhead and (2) fixed costs incurred between patient visit time and in times of low productivity and high capacity.

allocation and reasonable estimation of how resources are consumed. The physician practice has an advantage over most other businesses when it comes to having a relative benchmark across the industry with which to compare its data: the RVU, as published by Medicare. Because the overall industry standard for work performed under most CPT codes is already established, it serves as a pretty good ABC benchmark already. And whether one agrees with the Medicare-established RVUs as representative of the most accurate amount of work required for a particular service, the RVUs serve as the standard of measurement for reimbursement. Knowing where your practice stands along that benchmark is critical to measuring profitability in the current and future payment systems.

USING THE RESULTS OF A COST ANALYSIS

Once the practice's costs are defined, whether historical as a starting point or estimated using ABC and actual cost data, the results of the analyses can be used for a variety of exercises relating to productivity, profitability, and payer contracting issues. Primary uses include the analysis of profitability of managed care contracts, peer comparison, physician productivity, and various service lines and operational areas.

Managed care contract profitability analysis: Under managed care, physician practices are predominantly receiving payments that are discounted from the practice's fee schedule, based on a fee schedule presented by the payers that may or may not be negotiated. Depending on a practice's location, geographic area, specialty, size, and so on, a practice may not have enough leverage to effectively negotiate and may just be stuck with two options: to participate or not to participate. And not knowing the costs of providing services can be financial suicide in this situation, which is all too common.

Thus, determining the profitability of participation in a practice's plans with significant volume is important. Once a cost per procedure has been developed, the cost per procedure can be multiplied by the frequency of each CPT code performed that has served patients belonging to a particular payer category. In addition to the standard cost per procedure, two other data points are needed. A fallacy of this method is that it assumes patients in all payer categories consume the same resources per CPT code, when certain payer categories may require more work than others, such as Medicare patients of an aged patient base group. But overall, it is an excellent way to see how the practice's total resources are consumed to serve a patient population, whether by payer mix, physician mix, or location mix, provided the practice's data systems can generate reports for CPT frequency within these various mix categories.

The cost analysis's resulting cost per procedure provides a reasonable cost per CPT code. Costs per CPT code can then be grouped with other costs per procedure to develop a total cost per case, per diagnosis, or per treatment such as an obstetrics case, a fracture treatment, or a hypertension diagnosis. To accomplish this, the practice must project the expected utilization by CPT code for the episode of care or treatment. Multiplying the projected utilization for each CPT code by its cost per procedure will provide a total projected practice cost of providing care. This can be used to estimate the cost of providing various services, as well as the costs of serving patients insured under a particular contract.

The charts below illustrate what a practice should do to begin using the results of a cost analysis and to get a handle on how these performance indicators can impact the cost of providing services.

1. Perform a revenue breakdown analysis:
   - Total practice receipts $1,300,000
   - Total receipts from
     - Managed care plans: $1,200,000
   - Percentage derived from
     - Managed care plans: 92%
       - Breakdown by payer:
         - Plan A: 65%
         - Plan B: 25%
         - Plan C: 10%

2. Perform a revenue collection rate analysis:

	Plan A	Plan B	Plan C
Gross Charges	$2,220,000	$895,000	$385,000
Collections	$780,000	$300,000	$120,000
Contractual Adjustments	$1,300,000	$450,000	$260,000
Gross Collection %	35%	34%	31%
Contractual Adjustment %	59%	50%	67%
Net Collection %	94%	84%	98%

3. Perform a managed care fee schedule comparison:

Fee Schedule: Managed Care Planning*				
CPT Code	Practice Fee	Plan A Allowable	Plan B Allowable	Plan C Allowable
1. 99212	$60	$39	$40	$50
2. 99213	$80	$65	$75	$70
3. 99214	$95	$97	$105	$95
4.				
5.				
6.				
7.				
8.				
9.				
10.				

* Include for top 80 percent of CPT Codes

Exhibit 7.6 illustrates how to use the results to compare to payer allowable rates on a per CPT code basis. In this example, notice that the cost of providing office visits is higher than the average Medicare reimbursement rate for the service. The results tell management several things: (1) Profit must come from a blend of more profitable services, (2) studies should be undertaken to find possible efficiencies in the practice's routine processes, and (3) this data can be used to assist in managed care negotiations by allowing management to demonstrate costs with reasonable accuracy when reimbursement rates offered are lower than the industry's median costs. It is important to remember when analyzing costs per CPT to payer reimbursement that the frequency of CPTs should also be considered. The analyst should be careful not to overanalyze a large discrepancy on a CPT that has a low frequency when, in the big picture, the difference on this particular procedure may not be material.

Peer comparison: Physician practices have long used the available MGMA data to compare their key benchmarks to peer practices. MGMA has recently developed an activity-based cost model example that allocates data collected in a multispecialty group to analyze the large group's cost of providing various services. The model calculates the group's total cost per procedure in the following six categories:

1. Medical procedures inside the practice

2. Medical procedures outside the practice

3. Surgery and anesthesia procedures inside the practice

4. Surgery and anesthesia procedures outside the practice

5. Clinical laboratory and pathology procedures

6. Diagnostic radiology and imaging procedures

See Exhibit 7.6 for comparison of MGMA's ABC costs per procedure category as compared to the hypothetical example used for illustration purposes.

Physician productivity: The cost analysis results may be utilized to compare production costs of an individual physician, specialty of physicians, location of physicians, and so on. The data can also be used to break down costs by work RVU as it relates to physician compensation plans that are based in whole or in part on work RVU methods. Comparing the actual cost per procedure of a physician's activity to the expected costs allows monitoring of variances. Investigation of the causes of these variances should be undertaken for possible improvements to the process and to bring actual costs in line with expected costs.

Operations improvements: As mentioned throughout the chapter, a cost analysis, by default, leads to discovery of operational and process information that can be used in a positive way to help the practice not only determine its costs, but also to find cost savings. This is done through observation of activities, interviews with providers and staff, and a thorough review of the accounting records and related documents. This by-product information remains to assist the practice in its overall endeavor to increase profits and remain viable.

With the increasing regulatory and technology challenges of running a physician practice, changes undertaken in a practice can impact costs directly as well as indirectly by affecting routine processes. Practices are currently in the midst of adding EHR systems and increased information technology security and applications, as well as forming joint ventures and adding additional ancillary services and specialties. With the addition of each comes an obvious cost impact (e.g., capital expenses, start-up costs, additional staff and supplies). These costs should be projected and rolled into the projected practice costs of providing services. For large projects, this will assist management in determining the point at which the practice reaches a positive return on its investment. But the soft costs, costs that impact processes and routine tasks, should also be factored into the practice's cost of providing future services. It is only in this manner that a practice can stay ahead: making the effort to perform the analyses necessary to understand the true costs of doing business. Then management can use the results of this powerful data to make necessary changes and improvements.

To the Point

The bottom line is that physician practices should take the steps necessary to analyze their businesses just as other industries do. The medical practice industry, as a whole, still does not apply full analytical and costing techniques to its business. These are increasingly critical steps in maintaining the financial viability of a practice in today's regulatory healthcare environment of ever-changing reimbursement models and an increasingly competitive landscape. If a practice is not aware of its basic costs for providing services and the full practice resources required to so, and if it does not find a way to work at its most efficient and competitive level, it will be very difficult to maintain profitability, retain staff, and attract future business partners.

CHAPTER 8

Measuring and Managing Cash Flows

Edited by Lee Ann Webster, MA, CPA, FACMPE

After completing this chapter, you will be able to:

- Explain the objectives of cash management and the critical role cash management plays in overall resource management.

- Develop a practical approach to managing the medical group's current cash position.

- Describe the sound precepts of an effective internal control system for cash.

- Identify the nature and purpose of the cash flow statement and its uses in the overall financial management of medical group operations.

- Develop a cash flow statement and interpret the principal ideas it conveys about cash flows.

- Design an approach for forecasting future cash flows and developing a cash budget.

- Implement the use of a petty cash fund for a medical group.

- Provide examples of the possible problems and consequences that could evolve from faulty cash management practices.

- Incorporate the use of short-term investments into the cash management process.

One of the most valuable assets a medical group has is cash: Cash provides the means to acquire resources to conduct the practice, satisfy creditors and suppliers of resources, and compensate physicians and staff. Without adequate amounts of cash, the practice would be unable to operate or would experience great hardship and stress. Thus, managing cash becomes a matter of continuous focus for the financial manager. The objectives of cash management can be broken down into three areas:

1. The first objective is to have the right amount of cash on hand at the right time. Obvious problems will arise if there is too little cash to satisfy obligations as they become due. Less obvious are costs that result from having too much cash that is not yielding a return.

2. A second objective is to protect against the misappropriation of cash and other short-term resources. This objective is achieved by establishing and carrying out the proper internal control policies and procedures and by ensuring that adequate safeguards are developed and exercised.

3. A third objective is to provide an accounting of one's stewardship over cash through the proper type of reporting on the major cash flows for given time periods. These reports also provide a basis for planning future cash flows.

Cash management should be viewed as a before-the-fact control system. Unlike profit planning, in which operations can continue for a time if losses occur, when a medical group's cash is exhausted, immediate action must take place. By continually planning for cash needs, the group can be certain that adequate, but not excessive, cash is available when needed.

This chapter is organized around the present, past, and future information and tools needed to manage cash. In the next section, we will examine the data and tools necessary to manage the current cash position. Next we will treat, in some depth, the major reporting vehicle for presenting past cash flow information. After that we will look at ways to help plan for future cash flows and what instruments to use. This section will be followed by some long-term strategies for cash management. The chapter will close with anecdotal material on real events that describe some lapses in cash control and the dire consequences.

MANAGING THE CURRENT CASH POSITION

There are two important questions the financial manager needs to know: How much cash is available? Where is it being held? Ideally, the manager should have an accurate picture of both the amount and the timing of cash flows for the entire practice. As we will see later, the cash budget projects cash inflows and cash outflows by month for the next year. An annual picture of cash flows by month shows seasonal patterns and allows the manager to schedule once-a-year payments as well as other discretionary payments, such as capital expenditures and professional liability insurance premiums, during months that are most beneficial. Also, the cash budget may indicate that cash inflows for a particular month will exceed cash outflows. Thus, for that month, the group should have no cash flow problems. However, in other months, cash outflows may be greater than cash inflows, causing a deficit unless a large balance of cash is maintained. Cash planning for the entire year is accomplished through the cash budget, which is covered in a later section. The day-to-day control of cash requires two major tools: the short-term cash plan and the daily cash report. These two approaches will be covered in the next two sections.

THE SHORT-TERM CASH PLAN

The short-term cash plan is a dynamic tool for short-term cash management. The period covered by the plan and the detail of projection depend on the fluctuations of cash and the precision with which the cash is managed. Generally its length will be at least one month.

For most medical groups, cash flow projections by day for the next week, and then by week for the remainder of the month, provide an adequate approach to managing short-term cash. For example, the short-term cash plan presents four weeks of data showing daily cash flows for week 1 and weekly cash flows for weeks 2, 3, and 4. At the end of each week, the short-term cash plan is "rolled over." A new short-term cash plan will show on a daily basis the expected cash flows for week 2 and show on a weekly basis the expected cash flows for weeks 3, 4, and 5. This arrangement will continually "roll over" each week, thereby keeping the short-term cash plan current.

The advantages of this short-term cash planning can be illustrated in the following example that utilizes data in Exhibits 8.1 and 8.2. The short-term cash forecast, as shown in Exhibit 8.1 for the month of January, would be prepared based on the organization's longer-term cash budget (covered later). The forecast indicates that there will be a cash drain in January, because production was low during December, and therefore, cash collections will be low during January. Also during January, professional liability insurance premiums will be due and a higher level of production is anticipated, thereby resulting in larger cash outflows.

For simplicity, Exhibit 8.1 presents the tentative short-term cash forecast for the first four weeks limited to weekly cash flows. As can be observed, a large cash deficiency appears in the first week of January, primarily due to the payment of the professional liability insurance (included in the $140,000 accounts payable

EXHIBIT 8.1 ▪ **Short-Term Cash Forecast by Week for the Month of January**

	Week 1	Week 2	Week 3	Week 4
Beginning Cash Balance	$100,000	$(63,700)	$(30,500)	$10,300
Cash Inflows				
Electronic Payments				
Blue Cross	20,000	20,000	25,000	25,000
Medicare	12,000	12,000	15,000	15,000
Other	15,000	15,000	12,000	12,000
Total Electronic Payments	47,000	47,000	52,000	52,000
Lockbox Payments	5,000	7,000	7,000	8,000
Patient payments (front desk)	2,000	2,500	2,500	2,500
Credit card payments	2,000	2,000	2,000	2,000
Capitation payment from HMO	—	20,000	—	—
Other	2,000	1,000	1,500	500
Total Cash Inflows	58,000	79,500	65,000	65,000
Cash Outflows				
Net payroll (including physicians)	—	20,000	—	90,000
Payroll taxes	80,000	—	7,000	—
Refunds	700	800	700	800
Accounts payable	140,000	25,000	15,000	10,000
Other	1,000	500	1,500	250
Total Outflows	221,700	46,300	24,200	101,050
Ending Cash Balance	$(63,700)	$(30,500)	$10,300	$(25,750)

amount). A smaller deficiency occurs in weeks 2 and 4. Assuming the financial manager had been using sound cash management practices prior to January, the long-term planning of the cash budget would have forced the accumulation of some funds in anticipation of the January deficiencies. Therefore, let us assume that funds generated in earlier months were invested in marketable securities and that a line of credit was established at the bank. Given this tentative short-term forecast in Exhibit 8.1, the financial manager must revise the forecast to meet the cash needs and provide for a minimum cash balance.

A short-term cash plan is developed from the information now available and is shown in Exhibit 8.2. The cash plan is based on a minimum required cash balance of $25,000. Management decided to sell $40,000 of marketable securities and to borrow $50,000 on the line of credit. They planned to repay the loan in the second and fourth weeks as cash is generated. An alternative approach would have been to spread the payment to the insurance company over several months. The choice also must depend on the relative cost of each. In this illustration, the final short-term cash plan met the group's cash needs and maintained a minimum cash balance of $25,000. It should be noted that the short-term cash plan projected cash flows by week for the next month. Daily projections for weeks 1 and 3 may have indicated the need for additional borrowings if cash payments were scheduled early in the week and cash receipts were expected late in the week.

EXHIBIT 8.2 ■ Short-Term Cash Plan by Week for the Month of January

	Week 1	Week 2	Week 3	Week 4
Beginning Cash Balance	**$100,000**	**$26,300**	**$25,500**	**$66,300**
Cash Inflows				
Electronic Payments				
Blue Cross	20,000	20,000	25,000	25,000
Medicare	12,000	12,000	15,000	15,000
Other	15,000	15,000	12,000	12,000
Total Electronic Payments	47,000	47,000	52,000	52,000
Lockbox payments	5,000	7,000	7,000	8,000
Patient payments (front desk)	2,000	2,500	2,500	2,500
Credit card payments	2,000	2,000	2,000	2,000
Capitation payment from HMO	—	20,000	—	—
Other	2,000	1,000	1,500	500
Sale of investments	40,000	—	—	—
Borrowing	50,000	—	—	—
Total Cash Inflows	148,000	79,500	65,000	65,000
Cash Outflows				
Net payroll (including physicians)	—	20,000	—	90,000
Payroll taxes	80,000	—	7,000	—
Accounts payable	140,000	25,000	15,000	10,000
Refunds	700	800	700	800
Other	1,000	500	1,500	250
Repay borrowing	—	34,000	—	5,000
Total Outflows	221,700	80,300	24,200	106,050
Ending Cash Balance	**$26,300**	**$25,500**	**$66,300**	**$25,250**

THE DAILY CASH REPORT

A vital report for every medical group is the daily cash report. It serves a similar function to that of a fuel gauge on a motor vehicle. This report permits the financial member to monitor the cash position on a current basis and to see that the projection in the short-term cash plan is achieved. Deviations from the short-term cash plan may require corrective action — sometimes immediately. For example, it may be necessary to shift cash from one bank to another, sell or purchase short-term investments, or borrow or repay loans from the line of credit.

The daily cash report is even more important for the group that does not prepare a formal cash budget or a short-term cash plan. Since cash management is carried out informally in those cases, the daily cash report serves as the only tool to plan for cash needs and to monitor the cash position. Exhibit 8.3 illustrates the daily cash report. The key information includes:

- Book and bank balance of each cash account;
- Summary of daily receipts; and
- Summary of daily disbursements.

Some groups may desire only the information on account balances presented at the bottom of Exhibit 8.3. In addition to book (or checkbook) balances, the bank balance may be obtained using Internet or telephone banking. This information serves at least two purposes: (1) determining the float position of each account and (2) determining the adequacy of compensating balances. Float refers to the lag period from when a check is issued to the time when the check clears the issuer's checking account. Compensating balances are additional requirements imposed on borrowers by commercial banks beyond interest charges and require the borrower to maintain a specified demand deposit balance at that bank. Inadequate compensating balances may result in additional service charges, difficulty in obtaining loans, or higher interest rates.

The information in the upper portion of Exhibit 8.3 displays cash collections by pay type and major expenses by category. It is considered good financial management to collect patient payments at the time of service, at least copayment amounts. Note that the illustration provides a line for cash receipts collected at the front desk.

Groups that do not maintain a cash budget or short-term cash plan might include a section on the report providing a cash forecast for the next few days. Financial managers are strongly encouraged to use daily cash reports because they improve cash planning by helping to avert cash crises and allow a more even distribution of cash to physicians. If administrators feel they do not need to plan for cash needs, they are probably maintaining too much cash. Using daily cash forecasts will frequently lead to lower financing cost of operations, stronger credit standing, and more satisfied physicians.

EXHIBIT 8.3 ■ Illustration of Daily Cash Report

Beginning Cash Balance	$_____	
Cash Receipts		
Electronic Payments	$_____	
Blue Cross	_____	
Medicare	_____	
Other	_____	
Total Electronic Payments	_____	
Lockbox payments	_____	
Patient payments (front desk)	_____	
Credit card payments	_____	
Capitation payment from HMO	_____	
Other	_____	
Total Cash Receipts	$_____	
Total receipts and beginning balance	$_____	
Cash Disbursements		
Net payroll (including physicians)	$_____	
Payroll taxes	_____	
Accounts payable	_____	
Employer retirement plan contributions	_____	
Refunds	_____	
Other	_____	
Total Disbursements	$_____	
Ending Daily Cash Balance	$_____	

Bank Account/Number	**Book Balance**	**Bank Balance**
General account	$_____	$_____
Payroll account	_____	_____
Refunds account	_____	_____
Other	_____	_____
Total Ending Cash Balance	$_____	$_____

The administrator may find it useful to keep a month-to-date cash spreadsheet, which details the receipts, disbursements, transfers, and running balance by bank account by day for each month (see Exhibit 8.4). The information in this spreadsheet can be used to provide a proof of cash for use in connection with the bank reconciliation.

EXHIBIT 8.4 ■ Month-to-Date Cash Spreadsheet for Bank Account

| | | | | CASH RECEIPTS | | | |
	Date	Electronic	Lockbox	Credit Card	Clinic	Other	Description
Balance Forward							
Sat	1-Jan						
Sun	2-Jan						
Mon	3-Jan	2,134.76	1,788.22	1,560.22	3,100.00		
Tues	4-Jan	8,977.53	1,020.21	900.00	1,200.00		
Wed	5-Jan	35,000.03	3,901.22	888.22	2,050.00		
Thurs	6-Jan	18,009.22	2,277.53	500.00	4,977.22		
Fri	7-Jan	7,877.24	1,090.43	1,088.88	2,197.90		
Sat	8-Jan						
Sun	9-Jan						
Mon	10-Jan	6,902.12	3,338.97	1,500.00	3,665.00	35,982.11	Capitation HMO
Tues	11-Jan	9,092.71	1,088.66	2,200.00	1,400.22		
Wed	12-Jan	28,799.53	2,398.67	786.44	1,909.50		
Thurs	13-Jan	21,222.34	1,986.46	3,126.33	2,110.30		
Fri	14-Jan	5,877.22	2,238.95	701.00	529.90		
Sat	15-Jan						
Sun	16-Jan						
Mon	17-Jan	4,992.11	1,000.87	210.00	4,201.98		
Tues	18-Jan	9,223.44	2,187.60	890.00	1,602.10		
Wed	19-Jan	37,188.29	1,876.54	3,011.11	1,876.36	3,500.00	Expert Witness Fees
Thurs	20-Jan	23,111.21	2,198.07	1,790.50	2,367.92		
Fri	21-Jan	6,266.59	1,287.45	1,112.55	891.50		
Sat	22-Jan						
Sun	23-Jan						
Mon	24-Jan	6,999.22	977.62	765.00	3,523.67		
Tues	25-Jan	8,902.34	1,238.70	1,890.33	1,785.60		
Wed	26-Jan	39,555.32	2,654.81	3,123.09	3,793.19	79.20	Vendor Refund
Thurs	27-Jan	19,014.23	901.00	888.21	2,054.73		
Fri	28-Jan	8,921.85	3,198.54	791.31	650.34		
Sat	29-Jan						
Sun	30-Jan	5,899.21	2,111.89	810.20	4,590.21		
Mon	31-Jan	12,900.24	1,004.55	1,400.77	1,543.28		
Total		326,866.75	41,766.96	29,934.16	52,020.92	39,561.31	
Total FFS Collections						450,588.79	
Total Cash Receipts						490,150.10	

Checks	Tax Deposits	Other	Description	Book Balance	Bank Balance
				167,205.32	306,230.75
				167,205.32	306,230.75
				167,205.32	306,230.75
	119,325.22			56,463.30	73,456.32
59,222.61				9,338.43	65,230.65
				51,177.90	80,230.21
				76,941.87	83,222.31
				89,196.32	92,123.44
				89,196.32	92,123.44
				89,196.32	92,123.44
				140,584.52	141,622.52
15,204.79				139,161.32	152,802.55
				173,055.46	181,203.55
				201,500.89	206,222.52
		83,555.76	Net Payroll	127,292.20	165,222.50
				127,292.20	165,222.50
				127,292.20	165,222.50
				137,697.16	145,930.25
32,627.96				118,972.34	155,222.93
	36,902.44			129,522.20	135,202.22
				158,989.90	162,555.91
				168,547.99	170,987.56
				168,547.99	170,987.56
				168,547.99	170,987.56
19,345.67				161,467.83	180,203.57
				175,284.80	189,202.57
				224,490.41	236,502.66
				247,348.58	249,631.52
	382.01	3,457.82	Refunds	257,070.79	261,305.99
				257,070.79	261,305.99
				270,482.30	272,381.29
	15,982.52	85,201.55	Net Payroll	186,147.07	230,222.91
126,401.03	172,592.19	172,215.13			

IMPROVING CASH FLOWS

Medical practices can improve their cash flows in a number of ways. Some of these are discussed below.

A Healthy Revenue Cycle

Practice personnel should attempt to collect all copays from patients at the time of service. If practice personnel can compute the amount due after the patient's insurance company pays, the practice should attempt to collect this amount, as well. Practice management should consider a policy requiring self-pay patients to pay at the time of service and be prepared to work out suitable payment plans for patients who cannot pay larger bills at this time. The practice should communicate the fact that these payments are due at the time of service in advance of the patient's appointment. Accepting credit cards makes paying easier for many patients. Also, many health savings plans provide healthcare credit cards for employees to use for their medical bills; these patients can become upset when the practice does not accept these cards, as they must then complete and turn in the paperwork and wait for their reimbursement.

Insurance companies should be billed promptly, with special care taken to ensure that the practice is sending a "clean claim." Denials should be worked promptly. Billing and collection personnel should follow up on unpaid claims from both insurance companies and patients. Effective revenue cycle management will speed up cash flows and spread cash collections more evenly.

Timing of Billing by Suppliers

The practice should strive to time the due dates for its vendor bills to correlate with its cash receipts. For example, a practice that receives a large capitation payment from an HMO during the second week of each month might attempt to arrange for certain vendors' bills to be due after this time. Many suppliers will cooperate in setting more convenient payment dates. Thus, financial managers might request that suppliers invoice the group at dates that fit the group's cash flow schedule.

Payment of Vendors

In general, the best practice is to pay bills at the time that they are due. If a practice pays its bills early, then it loses the cash flow advantages of using the money for the extra time period. If a practice pays its bills late, then it risks a poor credit rating.

Harvey Mackay, author of *Swim with the Sharks without Being Eaten Alive*, offers a contrarian view on the prompt payment of bills. He advocates paying promptly, claiming that the goodwill this creates with vendors is more valuable than the use of the money for the extra time period. Mackay explains, "The way you pay your bills says something about the kind of person you are to deal with. Whether it's the man who painted your house or the firm that delivers your raw stock, you'll always get a better shake if you pay the same day you get the bill."[1]

Thus, managers should weigh the advantage of longer use of funds by waiting until the due date to pay bills against the benefits of maintaining a more favorable relationship with vendors by paying early.

Payment at the End of Discount Periods

When a vendor offers a discount period, the best strategy calls for paying at the end of the discount period. The practice should almost always take advantage of discounts, since missing a discount results in the group paying a higher effective interest rate. For example, if a vendor offers a cash discount of "2/10, net 30," this means that either (1) a 2 percent discount can be taken if paid in 10 days, and if not (2) the full amount is due in 30 days. Failing to take advantage of this discount would cost the medical group 2 percent for use of the supplier's money for an additional 20 days. Since there are 18 20-day periods in a year, the effective annual rate is approximately 36.5 percent.

Arranging Deferred Financing

Through negotiations with suppliers, it is often possible to make major purchases and extend payments over several months. This is particularly true if the practice is a valuable customer or if the vendor has significant competition. Many suppliers will extend payments for 90 to 120 days without additional cost. In other cases, the added interest a supplier may charge is often lower than the group's borrowing cost.

Controlling Claims Payments

Medical groups that pay claims to other providers, such as those in subcapitation arrangements, should establish a schedule for paying claims to those providers, for example, paying these claims once or twice a month on set dates. Having a schedule helps the practices keep cash levels high as long as possible and earn income on short-term investments. The desire to control claims payments to the maximum extent must be balanced by any need for favorable relations with physicians and other providers outside the group.

Arranging for Earlier Receipt of Capitation Fees

The practice should attempt to arrange earlier due dates for capitation payments as part of the group's negotiation with the HMO. The HMO itself is normally paid by employer groups in the first half of the month.

Strategic Timing of Payroll

Another strategy is to set the practice's payroll dates to maximize cash flow. For example, because physician payroll is usually a practice's largest expense, it might make sense to pay this at the end of the month. Support staff salaries are often paid semimonthly or biweekly to accommodate those employees' personal budget needs.

Take care in determining the physicians' regular salary (which they expect to receive no matter what) in relationship to their bonus. If the practice sets the regular physician compensation too high, it risks a cash crunch should the practice fail to realize sufficient profits or cash flow. Use regular salary amounts that are easily obtainable but sufficient to meet the physicians' normal living expenses, leaving the bonus pool for excess monies. The timing of bonuses is crucial. For example, a practice with a lower cash flow during the first quarter will probably not want to pay a physician bonus at that time. Cash basis practices will want to pay a bonus at the end of the year for tax-planning purposes.

Managing the Payment of Employer Retirement Plan Contributions

Federal tax laws currently allow all employers (including cash-basis taxpayers) to deduct contributions paid to qualified retirement plans up to the due date of their income tax return (including extensions). For example, a corporate calendar-year practice could wait until its tax return due date of March 15 of the following year to make its retirement plan contribution (or until September 15 if it gets an extension). This deferral can be especially useful to cash-basis practices in their attempt to minimize income taxes at the end of the year while maintaining sufficient cash for operations at the beginning of the following year. Be careful not to abuse this tool by pushing contributions too far back while failing to accumulate the cash necessary to fund the contributions; this can create significant cash flow problems when the practice is up against its extended due date and does not have sufficient funds to pay its retirement plan contribution.

Keep in mind that this option to defer retirement plan funding until the tax return due date is only available for the *employer* retirement plan contributions. Amounts withheld from employees for 401K deferral contributions or plan loan repayments must be remitted to the plan promptly.

INTERNAL CONTROL OF CASH

In chapter 2, we stated that an internal control process safeguards the assets of the practice; provides for reliable and accurate information; and ensures compliance with organizational objectives, policies, and procedures. Medical groups have reported that one of the most important objectives of a financial information system is to provide proper internal control over cash. An effective internal control system for cash is intended to:

■ Establish custody over cash;

■ Protect cash from theft or fraud;

■ Limit the temptation of otherwise honest employees; and

■ Provide a check on accuracy and reliability of cash records.

The internal control of cash requires a fairly extensive and concentrated series of procedures. The following discussion highlights some of the more popular methods of establishing internal control over cash.

EXHIBIT 8.5 ■ **Segregation of Duties (General Theory)**

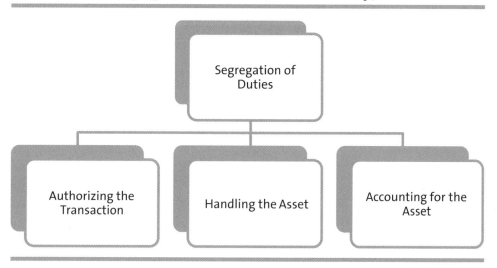

Segregation of Duties

An effective internal control process requires that cash functions be divided among personnel in such a manner that makes embezzlement or theft of cash more difficult. This means that employees with cash functions should not perform incompatible functions, so responsibilities for handling cash, recording transactions, and authorizing transactions should be separated. No one person should have complete authority over the entire sequence of transactions that involve cash: for example, from the purchase of a resource through payment. The general theory regarding segregation of duties is shown in Exhibit 8.5.

For cash, the two primary areas requiring segregation of duties are (1) cash receipts and (2) cash disbursements.

Internal Control over Cash Receipts

Specific individuals in the group should be designated to handle and be responsible for cash. Others should not be permitted to do so. Furthermore, the practice should segregate the functions relating to cash receipts to ensure that the person(s) who handles cash and checks does not post the payments and related adjustments, and still another person performs the bank reconciliation.

Accounting records must be kept by persons who do not handle or have access to cash. Thus, cashiers should not be permitted to record transactions in patient accounts receivable, and accountants responsible for receivables should not physically handle cash receipts or payment.

Finally, still another person should be responsible for reconciling the bank account. This person should not handle cash or post the accounting records.

EXHIBIT 8.6 ■ **Segregation of Duties for Cash Receipts**

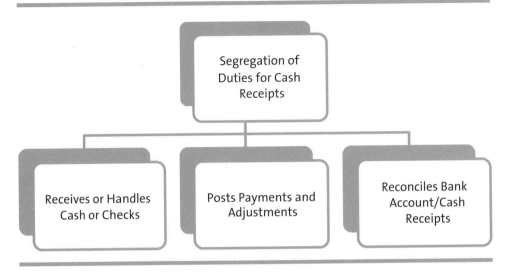

The suggested segregation of duties over cash receipts is shown in Exhibit 8.6. Other tips regarding control over cash receipts include:

- Medical billing software generally allows for assigning staff members access to various functions. Make sure that those employees who receive cash receipts are not allowed access to the payment posting and adjustment functions.
- Maximize use of bank lockboxes and electronic payments to minimize the amount of cash that is physically in the office. This enhances segregation of duties by avoiding office staff access to that cash.
- If your practice receives checks from patients and insurance companies in the mail, consider having two staff members open the mail together.
- One way to expedite the deposit of checks into the practice's bank account is to use a check-scanning machine at the office that transmits the check information to the bank for electronic deposit. To further eliminate the potential for embezzlement or misplacement of the check, have the checkout personnel scan the check in front of patients and give them their receipts at that time.
- All cash receipts should be deposited intact daily. No payments should be made out of undeposited cash receipts. Only the petty cash or change fund should remain on the premises overnight.
- A verifiable record should be made immediately after each cash receipt, such as a remittance advice.

Internal Control over Cash Disbursements

The practice should ensure proper segregation of duties among employees with cash disbursement functions. Exhibit 8.7 shows the suggested segregation of duties for cash disbursements personnel.

EXHIBIT 8.7 ▪ Segregation of Duties for Cash Disbursements

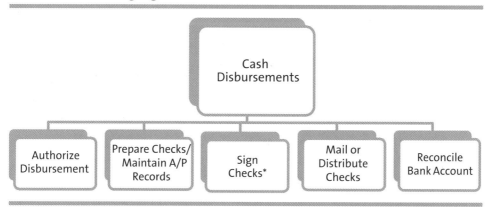

* including use of facsimile signature stamp

The functions of authorizing disbursements, preparing checks and maintaining the accounts payable records, signing checks, and mailing or distributing checks should be performed by different individuals. Yet another person with no other cash disbursement responsibilities should reconcile the bank account. Note that in some smaller practices, the functions of signing checks and authorizing transactions are combined. While it is important for the check signer to review the supporting documentation for all of the checks that he or she signs, it is especially important for check signers who bear the sole responsibility for authorizing transactions.

In some practices, especially smaller groups, the physicians may give check-signing responsibility to a "trusted" employee who also prepares the checks, mails or distributes them, and maintains the accounts payable records. Sometimes this person even reconciles the bank account. Such practices violate the recommended segregation of duties and leave the practice vulnerable to embezzlement, even when such employees have never committed such offenses in the past. A 2010 study by the Association of Certified Fraud Examiners (ACFE) revealed that only 7 percent of employees who committed occupational fraud had been previously convicted of a fraud-related offense.[2] Every criminal commits a first crime; the failure of a practice to institute recommended internal controls could provide the temptation that leads an honest employee to becoming a dishonest employee.

Another common question is why it is necessary for the mailing or delivery of checks to be performed by a separate person. It may seem like common sense to give these documents back to the accounts payable clerk to mail; after all, the accounts payable clerk maintains those records and should seemingly be able to perform this function most effectively. The problem with this scenario is that a signed check is a cash equivalent. A dishonest accounts payable clerk who performs both of these functions might prepare checks payable to bogus vendors or open up personal checking accounts in the name of legitimate vendors and misappropriate checks payable to those vendors. He or she might prepare checks with the intention of changing the payee or amount. These frauds would be much more difficult to perpetrate if the accounts payable clerk does not receive the signed checks to mail and distribute.

So the recommended work flow for cash disbursements would be (1) a supervisor approves invoices for payment, (2) the accounts payable clerk processes the checks and gives them to (3) a physician or administrator for signature, who signs them and gives them to (4) another employee to mail. And (5) another executive, administrator, or financial employee reconciles the bank account.

A caution regarding facsimile signature stamps: Some practices use facsimile signature stamps of legitimate check signers' signatures to sign checks. While this practice may be convenient when the authorized check signer is a busy physician or works in another location, it is a risky practice that can weaken internal control over the case disbursements function. A person who has access to the facsimile signature stamps should have no other function in the cash disbursement process. For example, this person should not be responsible for preparing or mailing accounts payable checks. Even though this individual is technically not an "authorized check signer," this person *does* have the ability to provide an authorized signature on a check. Practices should seriously consider eliminating facsimile signature stamps.

Electronic payments: Most practices must make some of their payments electronically. For example, many tax payments are required to be made in this manner. In addition, some vendors may require that payments be made electronically. In other cases, the terms for timing of payment may be so narrow that payments made sending a paper check through the mail could lead to potential late charges and/or finance charges. The practice should ensure segregation of duties with regard to the electronic payments just as it should for paper checks. Many banks allow for dual controls on automated clearing house (ACH) payments, which allow for one individual to initiate a transaction and another to approve the transaction.

Other controls over cash disbursements: Medical groups should also use the following internal controls over cash disbursement:

- Cash disbursements should be made by check or by bank ACH, unless specifically authorized from petty cash. (See discussions regarding Internet Banking and Petty Cash later in this chapter.)
- The checks should be prenumbered, and the stock of blank checks should be kept under adequate safeguards with access given only to persons authorized to sign checks.
- Void checks should be destroyed. If the group prefers to save these, then it should (1) tear out the signature portion of the check and (2) keep them under the safeguards similar to blank checks.
- No payments should be made without proper authorization and verification of the amounts due. When checks are signed, the signer should have all supporting documentation available for review to ensure that the disbursements are valid and appropriate.

■ Restrict the use of company debit or credit cards. Giving someone a credit or debit card is similar to giving that person access to cash. Consider an expense reimbursement or expense advance situation as an alternative. Remember that when an employee requests a check, practice management has the ability to review the documentation and refuse the request. With the cards, the practice is liable for these disbursements without the right to review the documentation in advance to determine the legitimacy of the business purpose for the disbursement. Furthermore, getting the related copies of invoices and other documentation after the charge is made can sometimes be difficult. Credit and debit cards further increase the risk that personal, unauthorized, or otherwise inappropriate expenses will be incurred by the practice.

Some financial institutions issue credit cards that can be set up to allow only certain classifications of expenditures to be made using the cards. Management generally has the ability to determine which types of expenditures will be allowed. Practices that use credit cards should consider using cards that offer these types of controls.

General Cash Controls

Some recommended general controls are as follows:

■ For the protection of the medical group, the cashier and others who handle cash regularly should be bonded.

■ Cash balances should be verified daily through the daily cash report and review of bank activity over the Internet.

Internal Control Checklist

Medical groups may have audits performed of their financial statements and, in the process, have their system of internal control evaluated, as well. An internal control checklist used by the auditor (see Exhibit 8.8) provides an opportunity to review the areas examined during the evaluation. A "no" response to an item indicates a possible weakness and should be examined for possible modification to improve the internal control procedures.

Bank Reconciliation

A critical part of control over cash is the reconciliation of every bank account. Because it constitutes the verification of two independent accounting systems, it is important that the bank reconciliation be performed by a person who does not have responsibility for cash or maintaining the related accounting records. These reconciliations should generally be performed by an individual at a high level within the organization, although very small groups may have an outside accountant perform this function. Exhibit 8.9 provides a simplified example of a bank reconciliation. Note that this form provides double proof of the correct cash balance.

EXHIBIT 8.8 ■ Internal Control Checklist

Yes	No	Recommended Practices
		Cash fund
		Petty cash or change fund maintained (imprest system)
		A custodian is responsible for this fund
		Fund reimbursement is made directly to the custodian
		Custodian has no access to accounting reports
		Custodian has no access to cash receipts
		Physically secure place for fund storage
		Surprise audits conducted periodically
		Rule prohibiting employee check cashing
		Cash receipts
		All cash receipts deposited daily
		Daily list of mail receipts
		Daily reconciliation of cash collections required
		Cashier personnel separated from accounting functions
		Cashier personnel separated from credit functions
		Cash custodian apart from negotiable instruments
		Bank account properly authorized
		Bank instructed not to cash checks from the clinic to the clinic
		Comparisons made between duplicate deposit slips and detail of accounts receivable
		Comparisons made between duplicate deposit slips and cash book
		Cash disbursements
		Recording, authorizing, and check-signing activities completely separate
		Support required for check signature
		Control exercised if check-signing machine or facsimile signature stamp used
		Limited authorization to sign checks
		No access to cash records or receipts by check signers
		Detailed listing of checks required
		Check listings compared with cash book
		No checks payable to cash allowed
		Checks are prenumbered
		Physical control over unused checks
		Destruction or mutilation of voided checks required
		All disbursements made by check, unless specifically authorized from cash or ACH
		ACH payments require separate initiation and approval
		Control over and prompt accounting for all electronic payments
		Control over and prompt accounting for interbank transfers
		Bank reconciliation
		Reconciliation between bank and books conducted at least monthly
		Cash balances should be verified daily through the daily cash report and review of bank activity over the Internet (or other appropriate means)
		Person responsible for reconciling bank statements is independent from accounting or cashier duties
		Bank statement sent directly to the person responsible for reconciliation
		General
		All employees who handle cash are bonded

EXHIBIT 8.9 ▪ Bank Reconciliation

Balance per books	$ xxx	Balance per bank statement	$ xxx
Add:		*Add:*	
Amounts that have been added by the bank to the account that have not been recorded on the books (e.g., proceeds from a bank loan)	$xxxx	Amounts that have been recorded on the books that have not yet been recorded by the bank (e.g., deposits in transit)	$xxxx
Subtract:	xxx	*Subtract:*	xxx
Amounts that have been deducted by the bank that have not yet been recorded on the books (e.g., bank service charges)		Amounts that have been deducted on the books that have not yet been recorded by the bank (e.g., outstanding checks)	
Corrected balance	$xxxx	**Corrected balance**	$xxxx

In the past, good internal control practices included performing reconciliations on a monthly basis promptly upon receiving bank statements in the mail at the beginning of the month. With the advent of Internet banking, practices can reconcile bank balances at any time during the month. Moreover, today's increased frequency of electronic transactions, including both cash receipts and disbursements, makes more frequent review of bank activity and bank reconciliations a recommended practice.

Internet Banking

Today's fast-paced use of electronic transactions demands that practices use Internet banking. Practices are now receiving funds from many payers electronically, paying many of their taxes electronically, and paying some vendors electronically. As discussed above, practices should be viewing their bank account activity online on an ongoing basis and reconciling their bank balance on an interim basis throughout the month. The increased potential for fraud demands that the practice be vigilant in reviewing this data. Unauthorized or questionable transactions should be reported promptly to the bank, as the time frame for reporting these items and being reimbursed for the related losses may be short. Also, banks may consider a lack of certain internal controls within the practice a sufficient reason for not reimbursing those losses.

In connection with the setup and ongoing use of its Internet banking function, the practice should be vigilant about Internet security. Be very careful about which individuals have access to view bank account information and even more vigilant as to which individuals are given authority to initiate and authorize cash transactions. Have independent individual(s) with information technology expertise review the security of all computers and networks involved in Internet banking.

One advantage of Internet banking is that it can provide physicians with better opportunities for oversight of cash functions. For example, back in the days when the practice received only a paper bank statement in the mail, the person who received this statement had the potential to alter it or remove damaging evidence, such as unauthorized checks, from the envelope. In contrast, altering or removing the data that appear in the practice's online banking activity would be very difficult, and multiple people can view it — not just the person who has the paper bank statement. Furthermore, the physicians' busy schedules seeing patients during office hours often allowed little time for reviewing banking activity. Internet banking allows them to view this activity from home, thus providing additional oversight over cash.

MEASURING CASH FLOWS

In chapters 3 and 5, we discussed two of the three basic financial statements in some detail: the balance sheet and the income statement. In this section, we want to give further attention to the third financial document: the cash flow statement. Under the accrual method of accounting, the balance sheet, which provides the status of the group's assets, liabilities, and owners' equity, and the income statement, which summarizes the results of operations, present only a limited picture of the medical group's financial activities. Comparative balance sheets show the net changes in assets and liabilities but do not reflect the major transactions that brought about these changes. Even though the accrual income statement provides a realistic picture as to the success of practice operations for a given time period, it falls short of showing what effect operations have on the cash balance of the practice and what other transactions were undertaken that did not affect the period's revenues and expenses. Thus, neither statement provides a full indication of the resources provided and the uses to which they were put during the period. The missing link is to have a presentation of what occurred to perhaps the most vital resource of the group — cash. The cash flow statement is directed at presenting this past history for the last accounting period, usually a year. Our discussion of the cash flow statement assumes that the group is following the accrual basis of accounting. A cash flow statement is not required for practices using the cash method of accounting or an OCBOA (other comprehensive basis of accounting). Groups using these other methods may wish to prepare a cash flow statement, particularly if they have large differences between net income and cash flow.

PURPOSES AND USES OF THE CASH FLOW STATEMENT

Even though we have stressed the importance of the income statement as a crucial measurement of progress in business, many individuals feel that cash flow information is equally important in assessing a business's future performance. The usefulness of the cash flow statement is borne out by its portrayal of information about:

- A practice's activities in generating cash through its major operations or "reason for being" and to provide an indication of the likelihood and amount of cash distributions to the owner-physician and for other reinvestment purposes

▪ Its financing activities, including both debt and additional investment by the physicians

▪ Its investing activities, such as the purchase of new equipment or other healthcare practices or entities

The information on the cash flow statement can assist users or readers of the statement in assessing several factors about the practice, such as its financial and operating risks, its financial flexibility, its liquidity position, and the likelihood of profitability. Each of these factors will be discussed next.

Financial Risk

This risk involves the likelihood that the practice's cash flows may become inadequate to cover its debt service requirements (assuming there is debt owed by the group), that is, that cash will be insufficient to cover periodic debt interest and principal payments. Financial risk is a function of the group's financial structure (relative proportions of debt and equity); that is, the lower the portion of debt to equity, the smaller the financial risk. Since debt repayment and interest requirements are satisfied by cash payments, which are provided largely from operational earnings, information about the group's cash flows from operations is useful in assessing its ability to cover the debt service requirements. A greater ability to cover these requirements results in a lower financial risk.

Operating Risk

This involves the likelihood of a practice experiencing unexpected reductions in the demand for its services. If this risk is high, cash flows from operations may become insufficient to provide funds to continue the practice at its normal level. It may become necessary to obtain cash from outside the group or have physician-owners contribute additional funds. The availability, amount, and timing of these needed funds may place a serious burden on the group's financial position and operating capability.

Financial Flexibility

Financial flexibility is related to operating risk and encompasses the ability of a business to weather bad times and respond to new investment opportunities as they come along. For example, the severity of a high level of operating risk can be alleviated if the practice can borrow funds or sell unneeded assets. Also, by having funds readily accessible to invest in a new piece of equipment or a new service line, the group may be able to increase its cash flow from operations fairly quickly. The reporting of the cash flows from operations thus shows the group's sensitivity to situations that may require immediate cash.

Liquidity

Liquidity refers to the makeup of the current assets and the proportion of those assets that are comprised of cash and near-term cash items, such as highly marketable securities. The more liquid a group is, the smaller the chance that it will experience cash flow problems and strains. It will also survive downturns more easily or be able to take advantage of new investment opportunities with available cash. Accurate assessment of a group's liquidity position is important.

Profitability

The cash flow statement helps to show the relationship between accrual net income reported on the income statement and cash flows. Sometimes, a group will show a high level of net income but lack sufficient funds to distribute cash to the physicians or invest in other new options. Identifying the relationships between income and cash flows helps to project meaningful forecasts of earnings and cash flows.

In summary, a cash flow statement provides management and interested outside individuals with information to assess the following:

- Future cash flow potential
- Ability to pay debt service obligations and other liabilities
- Ability to distribute cash to the physicians
- Why earnings and net cash receipts and payments differ
- Investing and financing transactions

Further, the cash flow statement can provide answers to some questions frequently heard among physicians about their group's operations, such as:

- Why are cash distributions to physicians less than the net income for the group?
- Where did the group raise additional cash besides the cash flow from operating the practice?
- How are the new acquisitions (e.g., new group just acquired or new equipment) being financed?
- Is the group borrowing funds to continue the distribution of cash to physicians at a certain level?

ELEMENTS OF THE CASH FLOW STATEMENT

Cash flow statements must categorize cash flows into three discrete types: operating, investing, and financing. In advocating the three-way style, the accounting profession stated that its presentation format emphasizes the relationship among certain components of cash flows that will assist in the analysis of financial performance. By having both cash inflows and cash outflows within each of the three categories, cash flows are perceived as related to each other, such as cash proceeds from borrowing transactions and cash repayments of borrowings shown under the financing category of the statement.

A description of the three categories of activities used in cash flow statements follows. Exhibit 8.10 presents a summary of the major cash inflow and outflow transactions found in the categories within the statement.

Operating Activities

These activities are associated with delivering medical services or products to patients as the normal activity of the practice. The cash effects of these activities are the cash inflows (such as collections from patients or third-party payers) and cash outflows (such as payments for supplies and salaries). Generally, most of these transactions wind up as items on the income statement, although their recognition on that statement may differ in timing from that on the cash flow statement because of the accrual cash-basis dichotomy. (See examples in Exhibit 8.10.)

EXHIBIT 8.10 ■ Statement of Cash Flows — Three Category Classifications of Cash Inflows and Outflows

Cash Inflows	Cash Outflows
Operating activities	
■ Cash from patients	■ Cash purchases of supplies
■ Collection of accounts receivable	■ Payment of accounts payable, payroll, and other services
■ Receipt of interest, rent, dividends, and other cash revenues	■ Payment of interest, rent, and other cash and accrued expenses
Investing activities	
■ Sale of investment securities	■ Purchases of investment securities
■ Sale of property, plant and equipment, and intangible assets	■ Purchases of property, plant and equipment, and intangible assets
■ Collections of notes receivable and other loans	■ Loans made or purchased
Financing activities	
■ Obtaining short-term or long-term loans	■ Repayment of loans
■ Issue of capital stock, mortgages, notes, etc.	■ Repurchase of capital stock and retirement of bonds and other long-term debts
	■ Payment of dividends

Investing Activities

These activities include cash inflows and outflows related to investments, such as purchasing or selling equipment or buying or selling investment securities. (See examples in Exhibit 8.10.)

Financing Activities

These activities pertain to the various aspects of providing financing to the practice, such as obtaining and repaying loans from creditors, receiving additional contributions from physicians as further investment in the practice, and dividends and distributions of retained earnings or capital to physicians and other owners. (See examples in Exhibit 8.10.)

PRESENTATION FORMAT OF THE CASH FLOW STATEMENT

A formal cash flow statement for the East Slope Medical Group is presented in Exhibit 8.11. To support the underlying sources of the cash flow data, East Slope Medical Group's balance sheet and income statement are also presented in Exhibits 8.12 and 8.13.

Note the major breakdown of the cash flow statement into the three basic segments: operating, investing, and financing. Also observe how the combined changes in these three categories explain the net change in the cash balance (decrease of $40,000) during the year 20X1. The beginning balance of cash ($240,000) is added to the net change in cash to produce the ending cash balance ($200,000), which ties out to the cash balance on the balance sheet.

In preparing the operating activities section of the cash flow statement, two choices are available: the direct method and the indirect method. The direct method shows the major types of operating cash receipts, such as "cash received from patients," and cash payments, such as "cash paid for supplies, salaries, and other services of the practice," to arrive at a net amount of cash provided by operating activities. The indirect method computes the same amount of net cash provided by operating activities but accomplishes it by a circuitous route. The starting point is net income shown on the accrual-based income statement to which several types of other adjustments (summarized in Exhibit 8.14) are added or deducted. These adjustments include add-backs for noncash expenses such as depreciation, additions or deductions for changes in specific current asset and current liability accounts, and add-backs or deductions for gains and losses incurred from the disposition of long-term assets. While somewhat confusing, the indirect method does present items that explain the differences between accrual income and cash flows from operating activities that are not included in the body of the cash flow statement under the direct method. It is also generally less time consuming for the accountants to prepare, since the numbers come primarily for the income statement and the changes in the balance sheet. Most cash flow statements found in general practice follow the indirect approach.

EXHIBIT 8.11 ▪ **East Slope Medical Group's Cash Flow Statement**

	20X1	20X0
Cash Flows from Operating Activities		
Net income (loss)	$37,000	$3,000
Depreciation	120,000	70,000
Unrealized gain on marketable security	(15,000)	—
(Gain) on disposal of equipment	(20,000)	—
Unrealized gains and losses on investments	—	—
Deferred income taxes	15,000	(10,000)
Changes in assets and liabilities:		
(Increase) decrease in accounts receivable	(50,000)	42,000
(Increase) in accounts receivable (other)	1,000	(1,000)
(Increase) decrease in prepaid expenses	(2,000)	4,000
Increase (decrease) in accounts payable	4,000	(12,000)
Increase (decrease) in payroll, benefits, and taxes payable	9,000	12,000
Increase (decrease) in claims payable	3,000	(4,000)
Increase (decrease) in claims payable IBNR	1,000	(2,000)
Increase (decrease) in income taxes payable	1,000	(12,000)
Net cash flows from operating activities	104,000	90,000
Cash Flows from Investing Activities		
Purchase of marketable securities	(100,000)	—
Purchase of leasehold improvements	(10,000)	(25,000)
Sale of equipment	20,000	—
Purchase of land for future clinic site	—	—
Purchase of equipment	(345,000)	(23,000)
Net cash flows from investing activities	(435,000)	(48,000)
Cash Flows from Financing Activities		
Net increase (decrease) in notes payable	(95,000)	(25,000)
Net increase in long-term debt	326,000	(55,000)
Proceeds from issuance of common stock	60,000	—
Net cash flows from financing activities	291,000	(80,000)
Increase (decrease) in Cash	(40,000)	(38,000)
Cash at Beginning of Year	240,000	278,000
Cash at End of Year	$200,000	$240,000

EXHIBIT 8.12 ▪ East Slope Medical Group's Balance Sheet

	20X1	20X0
Assets		
Current Assets:		
Cash	$200,000	$240,000
Marketable securities	115,000	—
Patient accounts receivable, net of allowance for doubtful accounts of $50,000 in 20X1 and $47,000 in 20X0	640,000	590,000
Accounts receivable — other	2,000	3,000
Deferred tax debits — current	—	—
Prepaid expenses	12,000	10,000
Total current assets	969,000	843,000
Investment:		
Land held for future clinic site	150,000	150,000
Property and equipment, at cost:		
Leasehold improvements	75,000	65,000
Equipment	625,000	575,000
	700,000	640,000
Less: Accumulated Depreciation and Amortization	325,000	500,000
Property and equipment, net	375,000	140,000
Other Assets:		
Goodwill	15,000	15,000
Total Assets	$1,509,000	$1,148,000
Liabilities and Stockholders' Equity		
Current Liabilities:		
Notes payable	$—	$95,000
Current maturities of long-term debt	66,000	—
Accounts payable	60,000	56,000
Accrued payroll, benefits, and taxes	210,000	201,000
Claims payable	16,000	13,000
Claims payable — incurred but not received	3,000	2,000
Income taxes payable	2,000	1,000
Deferred taxes	15,000	5,000
Total current liabilities	372,000	373,000
Long-Term Liabilities:		
Long-term debt, less current maturities	260,000	—
Deferred taxes	15,000	10,000
Total long-term liabilities	275,000	10,000
Total liabilities	647,000	383,000
Stockholders' Equity:		
Common stock, $1 par, authorized 200,000 shares: issued and outstanding 100,000 shares	100,000	90,000
Contributed capital in excess of par	325,000	275,000
Retained earnings	437,000	400,000
Total stockholders' equity	862,000	765,000
Total liabilities and stockholders' equity	$1,509,000	$1,148,000

EXHIBIT 8.13 ■ East Slope Medical Group's Income Statement

	20X1	20X0
Revenues		
Patient service revenue (net of contractual allowances and discounts)	$7,100,000	$6,590,000
Provision for bad debts	(100,000)	(90,000)
Net fee-for-service revenue	7,000,000	6,500,000
Capitation revenue, net	200,000	220,000
Other	110,000	90,000
Total medical revenue	7,310,000	6,810,000
Operating Cost		
Support Staff Costs:		
Staff salaries	1,680,000	1,600,000
Payroll taxes	160,000	153,000
Employee benefits	260,000	230,000
Total support staff cost	2,100,000	1,983,000
General Operating Cost		
Information technology	190,000	200,000
Drug supply	250,000	252,000
Medical and surgical supply	170,000	175,000
Depreciation	120,000	70,000
Professional liability insurance	90,000	85,000
Other insurance premiums	11,000	10,500
Building and occupancy	620,000	610,000
Administrative supplies and services	103,000	105,000
Professional and consulting fees	70,000	75,000
Clinical laboratory	260,000	240,000
Radiology and imaging	90,000	80,000
Promotion and marketing	32,000	30,000
Total general operating cost	2,006,000	1,932,500
Total operating cost	4,106,000	3,915,500
Total Medical Revenue after Operating Cost	3,204,000	2,894,500
Less: NPP Cost	690,000	600,000
Total Medical Revenue after Operating and NPP Cost	2,514,000	2,294,500
Less: Physician Cost	2,350,000	2,200,000
Net Income (Loss) after Provider-Related Expenses	164,000	94,500
Other Income (Expense):		
Interest expense (net)	(150,000)	(90,000)
Unrealized gain on marketable securities	15,000	—
Gain on disposal of equipment	20,000	—
Interest expense (net)	(115,000)	(90,000)
Income before Provision for Income Taxes	49,000	4,500
Provision for (reduction of) Income Taxes	12,000	1,500
Net Income (Loss)	37,000	3,000
Retained Earnings, Beginning of Year	400,000	397,000
Retained Earnings, End of Year	$437,000	$400,000

EXHIBIT 8.14 ▪ Calculating Operating Cash Flow from Net Income (Indirect Method)

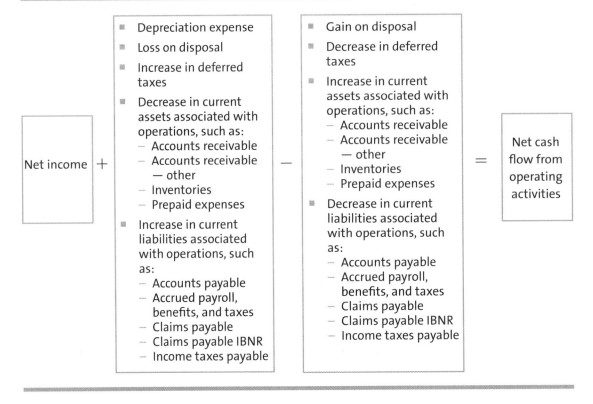

The following interpretative inferences about the contents of the cash flow statement for the East Slope Medical Group for 20X1 in Exhibit 8.11 should be noted:

▪ The net income ($37,000) on the income statement for the year ended December 31, 20X1, is the first item shown under the Operating Activities section that is prepared following the indirect method. Notice that this amount is less than the net cash provided from operating activities ($104,000). This is primarily due to the noncash expense for depreciation of $120,000 being added back to net income to increase the cash flow from operations. The $50,000 increase in the accounts receivable balance had a negative impact on the net cash provided from operating activities. The practice's total medical revenue for 20X1 increased by $500,000, a greater than 7 percent increase over the level achieved in 20X0. But part of the increase in revenue was not collected at the end of 20X1, as evidenced by the increase in accounts receivable. This revelation about the disparity between accrual net income and cash provided by operations shows one of the valued information elements that the cash flow statement brings out and might be used as a way to explain (in part) why cash distributions to physicians might be less than the corresponding net income.

- Other adjustments to net income in the Operating Activities section of the cash flow statement show the offsetting interplay between the changes in various current asset and current liability accounts, such as the increase in accounts receivable discussed above, which decreased cash flow from operations, and the increases in accounts payable and accrued payroll, benefits, and taxes, which have the effect of increasing cash flows from operations.

- Under cash flows from investing activities, we note that the practice purchased marketable securities for $100,000 and equipment with a cost of $345,000. The equipment acquisition was apparently financed by the issuance of a long-term note payable (net of current-year repayments) of $326,000, as indicated under cash flows from financing activities. Note also that short-term notes payable were retired (totaling $95,000) during the period. Also, note that the practice received $60,000 from a new physician shareholder in exchange for the issuance of stock.

- The ending cash balance of $200,000 represents a decrease from the balance of cash at the beginning of the period, which was $240,000. By reviewing the statement of cash flows, we can see the combination of operational and financing cash flows that brought about the change in this balance.

Do not confuse the cash flow statement with an income statement prepared using the cash basis. The latter statement might be referred to as a statement of cash receipts and disbursements. This statement only reflects cash receipts from patients and other payers for the rendering of medical services, which are considered as revenues for the period under the cash basis and shows only cash payments for expenditures classified as expenses to produce the revenue. The cash flow statement shows not only cash flow from operations but also cash inflows and outflows for other transactions not shown on the statement of cash receipts and disbursements, such as proceeds and repayments of loans, acquisitions of equipment, and other long-term investments. Thus, the statement of cash receipts and disbursements is a limited view of cash movements during an accounting period and is not equivalent to a cash flow statement.

FORECASTING AND PLANNING FUTURE CASH FLOWS

Earlier, we introduced the short-term cash plan that predicts cash flows for the immediate future of the group's operations — that is, for several weeks or days within the next month. Its objective is to identify potential cash shortages and excesses so that the financial manager can take appropriate action to manage the current cash position. Now let's turn to planning for a full year.

The Cash Budget

A logical extension of the short-term planning thrust is the cash budget, which schedules the timing of cash flows by month for the coming year. The cash budget represents the major instrument for planning the use of cash during the next operating year. As a planning instrument, it is the result of a deliberate and careful process of scrutinizing the scope and timing of the operations for the following year and measuring the effects of these events on the cash balances needed for carrying out the total group plan. A cash budget is more than a mere prediction of what cash flows will be; it is also a forecast of cash needs. The cash budget assists in planning future cash flows in these ways:

- Since the final cash budget is the result of a series of trial drafts of cash forecasts, each trial raises questions about whether the operating plans are too ambitious for the cash that will be generated in the next year. If so, some revisions may then be made to the operating plans.
- The cash budget will show when and if a short-term loan is needed and when it can be repaid.
- The cash budget identifies the month that is best for scheduling discretionary or unusual payments, such as bonuses, once-a-year debt service, and annual professional liability insurance premiums.
- The cash budget can anticipate the development of a continuing cash surplus that calls for a review of investment possibilities, a reduction of debt, or an additional distribution to the physician owners.

Clearly, these examples show that the cash budget is a useful tool for internal planning. It can assist management in highlighting key decisions related to cash for the coming year. Also, once adopted, the cash budget may be used as a control benchmark that, when compared with actual cash flows, will indicate the accuracy of cash flow predictions and the need for revising projections for future months.

Another important function of the cash budget is its use in negotiating a loan or line of credit from banks and other lending institutions. A key component of the loan application is the cash budget. Lenders are favorably impressed by cash planning, especially when it is at a level of detail that shows the overall cash picture, along with why the loan is needed and when the loan is likely to be repaid. During periods of tight credit, even preferred borrowers will increasingly be asked to provide cash projections. To volunteer this information in advance is a hallmark of strong overall planning, a sign of good management, and an indication of an intent and ability to repay the loan requested. Hence, the cash budget is a positive factor in loan negotiations.

The cash budget, like other financial plans, is no better than the sources of data on which is it based. For this reason, we will indicate the data and sources of information needed to construct a cash budget in the next section.

Cash Budget Data and Sources

To build a cash budget for a medical group, the following data are necessary:

- Beginning cash balance
- Projected cash receipts from patients and third-party payers (also miscellaneous income)
- Projected cash operating expenses

- Projected cash expenditures for capital acquisitions and long-term investments
- Projected cash receipts from other sources (e.g., sale of investments)
- Required cash borrowing and debt repayment
- Ending cash balance

These data may be arranged in any format that is useful to the group's management. The format shown in Exhibit 8.15 emphasizes the importance of operations to the cash position. It also highlights, in sequence, the impact of nonoperating sources of cash, nonoperating uses of cash, and cash borrowings on the ending cash balance. The next section introduces the supporting schedules for this cash budget, along with a discussion about the related data sources.

EXHIBIT 8.15 ■ Cash Budget

Upper Mountain Medical Group
Cash Budget for the Year Ended 12/31/20XX

Supporting Schedule Exhibit Number		January	February	March
8.16	Cash collections from patients	$173,000	$201,000	$218,500
8.17	Less cash operating expenses	236,015	170,515	174,515
	Cash increase (decrease) from operations	($63,015)	$30,485	$43,985
	Add beginning balance	14,000	10,000	12,470
	Ending cash balance before nonoperating and financial transactions	($49,015)	$40,485	$56,455
	Add: cash from nonoperating sources			
8.19	Sale of short-term investments	35,000	0	0
	Subtotal	($14,015)	$40,485	$56,455
	Less: cash payments for nonoperating items			
8.20	Payment on installment debt for land	2,000	2,000	2,000
8.20	Repayment of short-term debt	0	26,015	0
8.18	Assets in capital budget	0	0	10,000
8.19	Purchase of short-term investments	0	0	33,000
	Subtotal	$2,000	$28,015	$45,000
	Ending cash balance before borrowing	($16,015)	$12,470	$11,455
8.20	Add: borrowing to maintain minimum cash balance	26,015	0	0
	Ending cash balance	$10,000	$12,470	$11,455

The Beginning Cash Balance

This balance is the actual amount shown in the accounting records for the beginning cash balance. If the cash budget is prepared before the end of the current year, the beginning cash balance must be estimated.

Projected Cash Receipts from Patients and Third Party Payers

The key element in the preparation of any budget is the projected volume of service to be provided. This level affects both the cash budget and the profit plan in two ways:

1. The amount of cash to be collected from patients is a direct result of billings for the services performed.

2. The amounts of variable operating expenses (such as supplies) and step-fixed operating expenses (such as many medical support salaries) relate to the level of activity. This factor also has an impact on the relationships among cost, volume of service, and profits. These relationships will be examined in chapter 11.

Several approaches can be used to project the level of services and future revenue. These also will be discussed further in chapter 11. Each of these methods starts with a projection of the volume of services to be provided to patients. For the FFS portion of revenue projection, gross charges are determined by applying the proposed fee schedule to this projected volume of services. Estimated adjustments must be deducted from gross charges to arrive at billings to patients and third-party payers.

A practical approach to projecting volume of activity involves asking physician and ancillary department heads to forecast the volume of service they expect to provide during the next year. As a starting point, each physician is provided with the actual amount of service (number of patients seen or procedures performed) by month and in total for the year. The physician then indicates the percentage change, above or below last year, for each month and for the year as a whole.

The amount of estimated cash collections by month are determined by applying historical collection patterns to the billings of patients. To illustrate, assume the historical collection pattern is:

- 30 percent collected in the month after billings
- 50 percent collected in the first month after billings
- 10 percent collected in the second month after billings
- 5 percent collected in the third month after billings
- 5 percent uncollectible

If January billings are $200,000, $60,000 for those billings will be collected during January; $100,000 in February; $20,000 in March; and $10,000 in April. In addition, $10,000 will not be collected. Cash collected in January will include

EXHIBIT 8.16 ◾ Budgeted Cash Collections from Patients

Upper Mountain Medical Group for the Year Ended 12/31/20XX

Estimated patient billings related to budget year		Estimated cash collections by months in the budget year*			
		January	February	March	etc.
October	$200,000	$10,000	$—	$—	$—
November	180,000	18,000	9,000	—	—
December	170,000	85,000	17,000	8,500	—
January	200,000	60,000	100,000	20,000	10,000
February	250,000	—	75,000	125,000	25,000
March	250,000	—	—	75,000	125,000
	etc.				
Cash Collections		$173,000	$201,000	$228,500	$ etc.

*The assumed collection percentages are as follows:

- 30% collected in the month of billing
- 50% collected in the first month after billing
- 10% in the second month after billing
- 5% in the third month after billing
- 5% uncollectible

5 percent of October billings, 10 percent of November billings, 50 percent of December billings, and 30 percent of January billings. Exhibit 8.16 illustrates the determination of estimated cash collections by month from estimated patient billings. January billings are $200,000, while collections are $173,000. Billings in February and March are $250,000, while cash collections are $201,000 and $228,500, respectively.

Projected Cash Operating Expenses

Data for the operating expenses in the cash budget can come from three sources:

- First, last year's cash expense data, by month, adjusted for any anticipated changes such as the level of staffing, rates of compensation, and price changes.
- Second, a consolidation of cash expenses prepared by responsibility centers that relates to their planned level of activity.
- Third, a monthly profit plan on a cash basis.

EXHIBIT 8.17 ■ Budgeted Cash Operating Expenses

Upper Mountain Medical Group
for the Year Ended 12/31/20XX

	January	February	March	etc.
Human resources expenses				
Physicians' salaries	$77,560	$77,560	$77,560	
Nurses' salaries	21,420	21,420	21,420	
Ancillary department salaries	15,225	15,225	15,225	
Administrative and staff salaries	8,550	8,550	8,550	
Medical support salaries	9,200	9,200	9,200	
Housekeeping and security salaries	1,560	1,560	1,560	
	$133,515	$133,515	$133,515	
Physical resource expense				
Supplies (detail oriented)	$11,500	$11,500	$11,500	
Occupancy and use — building	9,000	9,000	9,000	
Occupancy and use — utilities	5,000	4,000	4,000	
Maintenance and repairs	2,500	2,500	2,500	
	$28,000	$27,000	$27,000	
Purchased service and general and administrative expenses				
Data processing	$5,000	$5,000	$5,000	
Professional accounting services	0	0	3,000	
Professional liability insurance	65,000	0	0	
General and administrative	$4,500	5,000	6,000	
	$74,500	$10,000	$14,000	
Total cash operating expenses	$236,015	$170,515	$174,515	

Exhibit 8.17 shows a supporting schedule of cash operating expenses by month. Totals from this schedule are included in the cash budget presented in Exhibit 8.15. If responsibility centers are identified, their managers should project the amount of operating expenses necessary to support their center's agreed-upon level of activities for the next year. After these projections are obtained and approved, they must be translated into cash outlays by month. If the responsibility centers were involved in preparing profit plans, however, the first step in quantifying operating expenses for the following year is already completed.

Projected Cash Expenditures for Capital Assets and Investments

Capital budgeting relates to prioritizing and evaluating proposals for the acquisition of fixed assets and other long-term investments. The decision rules and the capital budgeting process will be covered in chapter 14. The preferred decision rule and techniques require all changes in cash flows caused by a capital asset proposal to be scheduled by future time periods. There are at least three possible impacts these cash flows may have on the cash budget:

1. There is usually an initial investment of cash.

2. The net cash inflow generated by the new asset will take the form of increased revenue, decreased operating costs, or a combination of the two.

3. There may be additional cash receipts from sources, such as borrowings or investments by physician stockholders, used to finance the new asset.

In Exhibit 8.15, the $10,000 planned expenditure for the purchase of capital assets was purposely delayed to March when larger cash collections from patients were projected. If the asset had been acquired in January, additional borrowings would have been required. A February acquisition would have required postponement of a portion of the loan repayment to March. Trial cash budgets allow the manager to assess when it is best to acquire a new capital asset in view of other cash flows.

Exhibit 8.18 shows the approved $10,000 outlay that has met all the criteria established by the medical group for acquiring capital assets. In this illustration, there are no acquisitions of long-term investments such as securities or land held for future use. They would be included in this supporting schedule because they require analyses similar to those of operating capital assets.

Projected Cash Receipts from Other Sources

Cash from operations will likely be the medical group's major source of cash. Other sources of cash aside from borrowing might include:

■ Sale of investments, including real property no longer used in operations;

■ Sale of furniture, fixtures, and equipment no longer used in operations; and

■ Cash invested by owners.

EXHIBIT 8.18 ■ Planned Expenditures for Capital Assets

Upper Mountain Medical Group for the Year Ended 12/31/20XX			
	January	February	March	etc.
Planned purchase of capital assets			
Compact automobile	$0	0	$6,000
Waiting room furniture	0	0	4,000
	$0	$0	$10,000
Planned purchase of investments			
Land held for future use	$0	$0	$0
Totals	$0	$0	$10,000

EXHIBIT 8.19 ▪ Planned Other Sources and Uses of Cash

Upper Mountain Medical Group for the Year Ended 12/31/20XX

	January	February	March	etc.
Planned other sources				
Sale of short-term investments	$35,000	0	$0	
Sale of real property	0	0	0	
Investments by owners	0	0	0	
Totals	$35,000	$0	$0	
Planned other uses				
Purchase of short-term investments	$0	$0	$33,000	
Payment of dividends	0	0	0	
Totals	$0	$0	$33,000	

The major uses of cash include:

▪ Acquisition of capital assets and long-term investments;

▪ Acquisition of short-term investments, such as marketable securities;

▪ Payment of cash dividends; and

▪ Other cash distributions to owners besides compensation.

One reason for segregating other sources and uses of cash from both operating cash flows and transactions related to borrowing is because of their more discretionary nature. Usually, the administration exercises judgment as to which months to include these cash flows.

In Exhibit 8.19, the only source illustrated involves the disposition of short-term investments in January in the amount of $35,000, followed by their virtual replacement in March. A possible alternative available to the financial manager would have been to further increase short-term borrowing in January instead. Perhaps by using these short-term investments as security for the loan, its cost could have been reduced, and the transaction costs on the sale and later repurchase of the short-term investments could have been avoided.

Borrowing Cash and Debt Repayment

Borrowing for periods of a year or less is called short term. Banks may require such loans to be "cleaned up" once a year before any further short-term credit is granted. When cash is borrowed on a short-term basis, it should provide financing for seasonal needs. If not repaid out of operations within a year, it must be replaced by a more permanent source. Term or installment loans range from one to five years and sometimes as long as 10. They are commonly used to finance equipment acquisitions that should generate additional cash flows above the required debt service. Long-term loans, in excess of five to 10 years, are usually related to financing improved real property that will generate sufficient cash flows beyond insurance, repairs, taxes, and so on to cover their debt service.

Leases are a hybrid type of debt financing. They vary from month-to-month arrangements at one extreme to an installment purchase at the other. As with other borrowing, the cash flows generated by the leased asset should sustain the lease payments called for by the agreement.

A common reason for businesses to encounter severe financial problems is inattention to the loan terms. For example, a five-year loan is used to finance an asset having a 10-year payback period. In this instance, the trial cash budget, if realistically prepared, should provide a warning signal to management. With increased debt service, a chronic cash drain will appear, indicating a need for either longer term financing or reduced planned expansion.

The use of a short-term loan is needed in Exhibit 8.20 because the payment of the professional liability insurance for the medical group causes a severe cash drain in January. The cash budget also shows that this loan can be repaid in February according to the projected other cash needs and sources. Although it could be easily argued that this loan should be for a longer period, because it is financing insurance that will benefit the entire year, it makes sense to pay it off in February and save interest. The loan has also been "cleaned up," which sets the stage for another loan should it be needed later in the year.

The other loan repayment included in Exhibit 8.20 is the result of an investment decision in a prior period. The medical group is paying for this land at the agreed-upon rate of $2,000 per month.

EXHIBIT 8.20 ■ Planned Borrowing and Debt Repayment

Upper Mountain Medical Group for the Year Ended 12/31/20XX

	January	February	March	etc.
Planned borrowing				
Short-term loan	$26,015	$0	$0	
Total	$26,015	$0	$0	
Planned debt repayment				
Short-term loan	$0	$26,015	$0	
Installment debt for land	2,000	2,000	2,000	
Totals	$2,000	$28,015	$2,000	

Ending Cash Balance

Turning back to Exhibit 8.15, one can see that "ending cash balance" is used within captions at three points in the cash budget. The first shows the amount of cash that would result from adding planned cash flows from operations to the beginning cash balance. This number helps the financial manager decide on the month in which to include discretionary sources and/or uses of cash. In a similar manner, the line captioned "ending cash balance before borrowings," shows what amount, if any, must be borrowed to maintain a minimum balance. The final ending cash balance is the projected position of cash at the end of the month after taking all planned cash transactions as well as the beginning cash balance into account. This figure would be used in the projected balance sheet if one were prepared.

Keeping the Cash Budget Up-to-Date

The cash budget should be maintained a year in advance by adding three more months at the end of each completed quarter. Within the quarter, a monthly short-term cash forecast is prepared using the best current data available. As mentioned earlier, the short-term forecast is broken down by weeks to facilitate cash management of the current position. If the cash budget varies widely from actual data, it will be necessary to revise the budget completely at the end of the quarter.

Summary

At various points in this section, we noted the interrelationship between the operating plan (profit plan) and the cash budget. Amounts derived from the profit plan, such as receipts from patients and cash operating expenses, are key elements in the cash budget. Acquisition of, or changes in, the assets and their finance (resource plans) are also necessary to complete the budget.

It is not surprising that the cash budget is often called a residual budget because it is the result of all other financial plans; however, this should not lead anyone to the conclusion that the cash budget is no more than a carry-over total. It is much more, particularly in the trial cash budget stage. At that point, it identifies the temporary excesses or surpluses of cash that call for investment or borrowing plans. It diagnoses chronic cash drains in advance, which will call for a change in the scope of plans and/or additional permanent financing. It also provides guidance for shifting discretionary cash receipts or payments to an appropriate month.

Exhibit 8.21 shows the importance of the cash budget in coordinating both operating plans and resource plans. Finally, it is a strong managerial tool for negotiating needed financing.

THE IMPREST PETTY CASH SYSTEM

Almost every organization finds it necessary to pay small amounts of cash for a great many items, such as minor office supplies, postage, employees' local travel, and small expense payments. Generally, it is impractical to require that

EXHIBIT 8.21 ■ **Cash Budget Coordination**

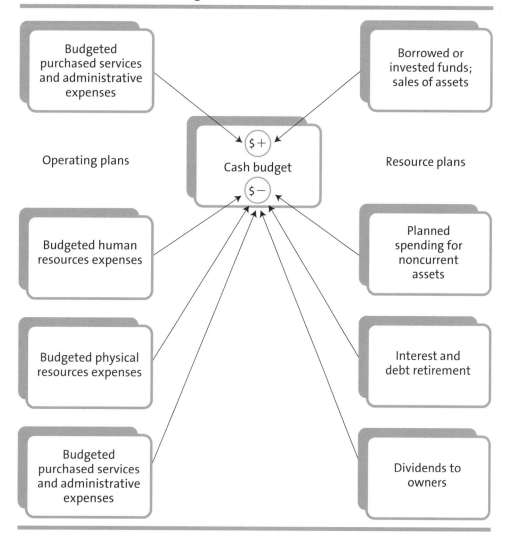

such disbursements be made by check, yet some control over them is important. A common method of obtaining reasonable control, simplicity of operations, and general adherence to the rule of payment by check is the imprest system for petty cash disbursements.

This is how this system usually works:

■ A trusted employee is designated as the petty cash custodian and given a small amount of currency as a fund from which to make small payments.

■ As disbursements are made, the petty cash custodian obtains signed receipts from each individual to whom cash is paid. If possible, evidence of the disbursement should be attached to the petty cash receipt.

- ▪ When the supply of cash runs low, the custodian presents to the financial manager (or individual designated as the check writer) a request for reimbursement supported by the petty cash receipts and other evidence that has been obtained for all disbursements. A check made payable to "Cash" or "Petty Cash" is drawn and given to the custodian to replenish the fund.

- ▪ Care should be taken to monitor the size of the petty cash fund. If it is excessive, the fund balance should be lowered. Similarly, if it is insufficient, the balance should be increased.

Under the imprest system, the petty cash custodian is responsible at all times for the amount of the fund either as cash or in the form of signed vouchers. These vouchers provide the evidence required by the disbursing individual to issue a reimbursement check. Two additional procedures are recommended to obtain more control over the petty cash fund:

1. Surprise cash counts of the fund should be made from time to time by the financial manager to determine whether the fund is being accounted for satisfactorily.

2. Petty cash vouchers should be canceled or mutilated after they have been submitted for reimbursement so that they cannot be used to secure a second and improper reimbursement.

CASH IRREGULARITIES AND THEFTS

Since cash is such a volatile asset, internal control over it must be strong, continuous, and all encompassing. The major approaches to ensuring that controls are effective were covered in a previous section of this chapter. The importance of cash controls probably cannot be conveyed more vividly than by the recounting of medical group managers' "war stories" involving some kind of theft, misappropriation, or shortcoming of procedures. In this section, we would like to mention some of these anecdotes.

- ▪ Physicians in one medical group used the petty cash fund largely to cash their personal checks. Frequently, there was no currency in the fund to provide for the small expenditures that occasionally arose or for change when patients were paying for service at the time of their visit. Also, this same medical group permitted physicians to borrow monies from the fund when they were "short," and long periods of time prevailed before the amounts were repaid.

- ▪ During a surprise cash audit of the petty cash fund at one medical group, the administrator found the intermingling of nongroup monies with the group's fund. In this case, the custodian was a seller of cosmetic products and had mixed in some of those funds with the petty cash amount, apparently using the petty cash fund as a "change bank" for her cosmetic business.

- ▪ A medical group did no short-term or long-term cash planning. Thus, the administrator had little or no idea what the group's cash needs were or what the timing of certain required expenditures was. During one week when payroll checks were to be issued, the administrator discovered that there were insufficient funds in the checking account to pay the staff members.

■ A consultant who performed many operational reviews of medical groups' activities frequently found that some groups do not reconcile bank accounts on a regular basis; in fact, on several occasions, there had been no bank reconciliations made for several years.

MANAGING SHORT-TERM INVESTMENTS

Assets that are closely related to cash are the short-term investments that medical groups enter into for short periods of time. In previous sections, we made frequent references to acquiring and disposing of these investments. Let's take a closer look at how they might be managed in conjunction with cash management.

When the cash position is being built up to meet a large planned expenditure later in the year, the cash in excess of normal needs should be invested for a return. These temporary excesses in the cash account can be transferred to the group's savings account or into other short-term investments and then returned to cash when needed later.

We will not evaluate the desirability or preference for certain types of short-term investments. The most frequently mentioned types of investments that groups select are savings accounts, certificates of deposit, U.S. Treasury bills and notes, money market mutual funds, and commercial paper.

Some of these investment instruments may need explanation:

■ Savings accounts are comprised of time deposits and passbook savings accounts with banks. They earn a fixed rate of interest.

■ Certificates of deposit are marketable receipts for funds that have been deposited in a bank for a fixed period of time and earn a fixed rate of interest. Certificates are offered by banks in a variety of denominations and range in maturity from one month to several years.

■ U.S. Treasury bills are perhaps the most popular short-term investment vehicle. A Treasury bill is a direct obligation of the U.S. government sold on a regular basis by the U.S. Treasury in denominations of $10,000 and upward to $1 million. Maturities are one month, three months, six months, and one year. Interest rates vary depending on the short-term money market conditions.

■ Money market mutual funds, sometimes called liquid-asset funds, sell their shares to raise cash, and by pooling the funds of large numbers of small savers, they build their liquid-asset portfolios. Investors can start their accounts with as little as $1,000 and use these as an investment outlet for small amounts of excess cash. Withdrawals can be made quickly from these accounts using checks drawn on the account balance.

■   Commercial paper represents unsecured, short-term negotiable promissory notes issued by large, well-established companies that need funds for a short time period. Denominations are usually in fairly large sums ($100,000) and thus, would probably be sought by only very large medical groups as an investment medium.

The primary characteristics of these investment options are their short-term maturity dates and the ability for the investors to convert back into cash with a minimum of effort and with less risk of losing their original investment amount. Thus, financial managers must be careful in selecting short-term investments, as safety of principal is the paramount concern.

To incorporate any short-term investments into the cash management process, it is important that these investments are monitored and the amounts of their current values are developed when these investment balances are needed for planning purposes. Thus, each investment should be listed on a schedule that includes this information:

■   Current market value

■   Purchase and maturity date (if applicable)

■   Income to date

■   Yield percentage

Also, the total investment balances for the current and previous months should be made available. This information can be used in preparing short-term cash forecasts if investments are to be liquidated within the month. If they are not, their proceeds should be included in the cash budget for the month in which they are liquidated.

To the Point

■   The objectives of cash management are:
  - Having the right amount of cash on hand at the right time;
  - Protecting against the misappropriation of cash and other short-term resources; and
  - Providing an accounting of one's stewardship over cash through the proper reporting of the major cash flows experienced by the group for definite time periods.

■   The short-term cash plan is a tool to manage cash in a short period of about a month or so and usually includes cash flow projections by day and by week.

- A group can improve the timing of its cash flows by:
  - Presenting the patient with a bill at the time of service;
  - Having suppliers time their billings to follow peak collection periods;
  - Arranging deferred payments for major purchases;
  - Controlling the timing of claims payments; and
  - Arranging for earlier payments of the HMO's capitation to the medical group.

- The daily cash report is a key report that permits the financial manager to monitor the group's cash position on a current basis and to see that the projections in the short-term cash plan are actually achieved.

- The purposes of an effective internal control system for cash are:
  - Establish custody over cash;
  - Protect cash from theft or fraud;
  - Limit the temptation of otherwise honest employees; and
  - Provide a check on accuracy and reliability of cash records.

- Specific internal control procedures promote effective controls.

- The cash flow statement is the third major financial statement, and it provides a history of cash flows experienced by a medical group during the last accounting period, usually for one year. Such information includes:
  - A practice's activities in generating cash through its major operations and providing an indication of the likelihood of cash distributions and cash availability for new investments;
  - Its financing activities, both debt and additional investment by physicians; and
  - Its investing activities, such as the purchase of new equipment and other healthcare entities.

- Information in the cash flow statement can help users assess several factors about the practice regarding financial risk, operating risk, financial flexibility, liquidity, and the relationship between accrual net income reported on the income statement and cash flows. In addition, it provides information about the ability of the practice to distribute cash to the physicians.

- The cash budget is an important document that schedules the timing of the cash flows by month for the coming year. It is the major instrument for planning the use of cash during the next operating year.

■ To build a cash budget for a medical group, these data are needed: projections of cash receipts from patients and third-party payers, projections of cash operating expenses, projections of cash expenditures for capital acquisitions, required cash borrowing, and debt repayment amounts.

■ Short-term investments that provide a liquid form of investment with a "safe" return are attractive vehicles to park excess cash for short time periods when these funds will be required for later use within the group. Investment instruments that fit the criteria of short-maturity and safety of principal are savings accounts, certificates of deposit, U.S. Treasury bills, money market mutual funds, and commercial paper.

REFERENCES

1. Mackay, H. 1988. *Swim with the Sharks without Being Eaten Alive*. New York: William Morrow and Company, Inc.

2. Association of Certified Fraud Examiners. 2010. *Report to the Nations on Occupational Fraud and Abuse: 2010 Global Fraud Study,* Austin, Texas: ACFE.

CHAPTER 9

Improving Your Financial Position by Increasing Collections and Reducing Outstanding Accounts Receivable

Edited by Sara M. Larch, MSHA, FACMPE

After completing this chapter, you will be able to:

- Explain how a medical service becomes an insurance claim or patient statement.

- Describe how A/R are created from medical services and the hydraulics that create them.

- Identify key elements of the front end of billing that are critical for collections and A/R.

- Utilize several techniques to analyze and manage insurance and patient receivables and collections.

- Describe key strategies aimed at increasing cash collections and reducing outstanding A/R.

- Summarize the approaches to considering centralizing, outsourcing, and other hybrid arrangements for back-end billing or key functions.

As the person responsible for finance and financial management, you have likely spent time focused on assets, liabilities, revenues, and expenses. Your usual lexicon includes the balance sheet, income statement, statement of cash flows, and statement of equities. This chapter takes you from those big picture financial statements and drills down into the hydraulics of the revenue cycle and specifically focuses on strategies that increase collections and reduce accounts receivable (A/R).

Your success depends on the financial position of your medical group. Your medical group's financial position is significantly affected by each of the revenue cycle key functions. As a leader, you must make revenue cycle everyone's responsibility, starting with the front end of the practice. Doing things right at the beginning reduces errors (denials) and eliminates rework (outstanding A/R). This chapter will help you analyze your charge and collection trends and turn that information into actionable improvements. It will also provide a look at your billing operation's use of vendors and other ways to maximize your collection performance and keep your A/R at best-practice rates.

The medical group's balance sheet tracks cash and current assets. Your cash includes net patient revenue (collections). The value of the A/R is included as part of current assets if you are utilizing an accrual method of accounting. The income statement will include collections (or net patient revenue), whether the medical group uses a cash or accrual method of accounting. In order to improve a medical group's financial position, it needs to collect revenue quickly and accurately, avoid claim denials and delays in payment, and ultimately keep the outstanding A/R as low as possible.

In order to analyze and manage collection performance and accounts receivables, medical group leaders need a good knowledge of the entire revenue cycle process. Perhaps you can remember a civics class in grade school on "how a bill becomes a law." Let's look at how a medical service becomes a paid bill in Exhibit 9.1.[1]

As you can see, this process includes multiple entities (employer, employees, payers, banks, medical practices, etc. For those insured via their employer, it begins when the employee selects his or her insurance plan during open enrollment. Revenue cycle performance can be impacted by a number of external

EXHIBIT 9.1 ■ How a Medical Service Becomes a Paid Bill

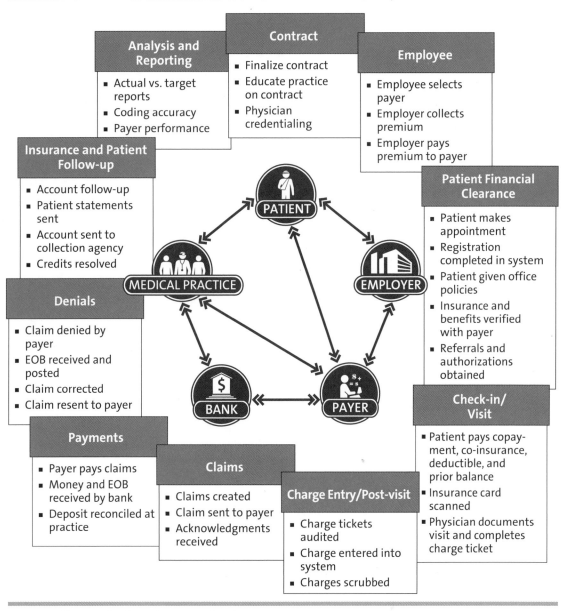

© 2009 Walker, Woodcock, Larch. Reprinted with permission.

forces including changes in payment or reimbursement methods (e.g., bundled payments), patients choosing high-deductible health plans, new delivery models (e.g., patient centered medical home), and, of course, regulatory changes.

To drill further into the revenue cycle, let's look at Exhibit 9.2, which shows the critical billing and collection tasks and how accounts receivables are created.

EXHIBIT 9.2 ■ How Accounts Receivable Are Created

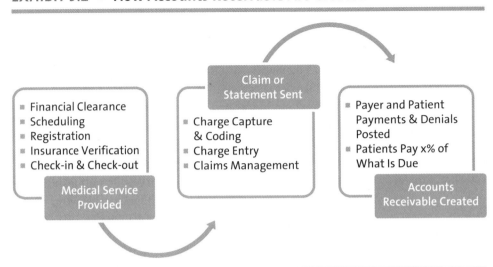

Completing every step efficiently and accurately will determine whether the insurance claim is paid or denied and whether the patients pay their balance due. Doing things right the first time will reduce claim denials and increase the percentage of clean claims that get paid. The next section of this chapter will provide an overview of the critical billing tasks that take place along the way to collecting cash.

FOCUS ON THE FRONT END OF THE REVENUE CYCLE

Medical groups must focus on the front end of their revenue cycle, which begins when a patient calls for an appointment. Appointment scheduling techniques can be applied to increase patient volume, which will increase the medical group's potential revenue. During the initial phone call to schedule the appointment or admission, the medical group's staff will collect all required information. The information and practice policies communicated to the patient set the stage for their future relationship with the medical group. Determining a patient's financial status prior to the date of service has become a critical part of the front end of the revenue cycle. Financial clearance includes verifying insurance with the payer, determining whether a referral or authorization is required, and identifying whether the patient owes money from a prior encounter.

When the patient arrives, the medical group will again confirm any insurance coverage, scan insurance card(s), and ask the patient to pay his or her copay, prior balance, or deductible. Patients not prepared to pay their balance due or those with very high account balances should meet with a financial counselor or the medical group's manager.

Better-performing medical groups have utilized a formal Patient Financial Policy for many years. This policy is given to all new patients and provided annually to all patients. The Patient Financial Policy has been approved by the medical group's governance process and is available in writing to physicians, staff, and, of course, patients. Tom Hajny states, "In too many practices, communication of the financial expectations and asking for payment at time of service is seen as injurious to customer service and an impediment to the patient receiving quick access to clinical staff."[2] Experience has shown that patients usually have less anxiety when they understand the medical group's financial expectations.

During the patient's visit, physicians and other providers document the services provided either on paper or, increasingly, via EHR. The physician's note is the documentation that supports which CPT and ICD-9 code is selected and entered into the group's practice management system (PMS). Only what the physician has documented can be billed to the payer or the patient. In addition to the documentation, which comes in many formats, the medical group will also use a form to communicate to the billing staff what services were performed and what should be billed. This form is often called an encounter form but may also be considered a superbill, charge ticket, or fee slip. Those medical groups with a fully implemented EHR will send CPT/ICD codes directly to the practice management systems without any additional paperwork or staff handoffs. Determining what CPT and ICD codes to use is often a shared responsibility between the physician and the staff. Some medical groups utilize certified coders with many years of experience, but the physician has the ultimate responsibility.

In this chapter, we will not devote time to the important topic of coding except to point out that every professional fee-billing operation needs coding and billing resources available to the physicians, coders, and billing staff. Today, many of these resources are available in online formats for single or multiusers. See Exhibit 9.3 for a list of recommended resources to support coding and reimbursement.

Medical groups need to keep their fee schedule current. They need to make sure their fees are always at or higher than all payers' contracted allowed amounts. The medical group's fee schedule also needs to have a relationship to the

EXHIBIT 9.3 ■ Recommended List of Resources to Support Coding and Reimbursement

Most of these publications are updated at least annually:

- CPT manual
- ICD-9 and 10 manuals
- HCPCS manual
- Medical dictionary
- Medicare and Medicaid bulletins
- Payer newsletters
- Medical specialty publications

practice's cost of providing that CPT service. One way to improve the medical group's financial position is to make sure that the fees charged will cover the costs of the service provided (and a little profit to cover bad debt).

One way to reduce claim denials is to utilize claims scrubbing software to identify which claims are "clean" and ready to go to the payer. When claims are processed with this software, medical groups are able to identify errors or omissions on their claims much faster and earlier in the process. Instead of sending out the "dirty" claim and waiting for it to be denied, the medical group staff can correct the claim and send it out right the first time!

The remaining portion of this chapter will focus on ways to manage, analyze, and reduce outstanding A/R with a focus on increasing cash collections at the same time. We will look at insurance A/R and patient A/R. Insurance claims are pending (no response), paid, or denied. Patient statements are either pending (no response) or paid. The balances due from all insurance claims and patient statements are part of the medical group's total A/R until they are paid. In a perfect world, all claims would be clean of errors and submitted quickly, and the medical group would receive payments starting in 14 days, with the majority of payments received in 45 days. The next four sections will go deeper into payment posting and variances, denial management, insurance follow-up, and patient collection follow-up.

POSTING PAYMENTS AND CONTRACTUALS

At the same time that the insurance payment is posted (electronically or manually), staff will post the contractual allowance (the variance between the group's fee and the contracted payer's allowed amount). If the contractual allowance is posted incorrectly, the A/R will be either overstated or understated. Managers should perform regular payment audits to ensure that staff members are not automatically writing off money that is collectible.

The medical group needs to evaluate the accuracy of the payment against the expected amount defined in the payer's contract. Most medical groups can load payer fee schedules into their PMS. They can then analyze the payments received against the payer's fee schedule to create a payment exception report to follow up on.

When the Claim Is Denied

When medical groups provided a service in the '70s and '80s, they sent a bill to the third-party payer and were paid. In the past 20 to 30 years, the payer's claim process has changed dramatically. As new payer models and payment methodologies were implemented, payers added administrative hurdles to the claim process. The payers' computer systems have become more sophisticated, allowing payers to increase the algorithms used to evaluate a group's claims and increase the denial rate. The higher the claim denial rate, the larger the A/R will be. In a 2011 report, MGMA reported that the median MGMA cost survey participant had 4.5 percent of initial claims denied, and the better-performing practices had 3 percent of claims denied.[3]

Denial management is the study of medical claim denials and how these denials can be prevented. The majority of claim denials are due to a process or performance failure within the group. Common reasons for denials include:

- Insurance verification: Patient's insurance is not valid on date of service
- Incorrect payer: Incorrect insurance
- Registration: Information is incomplete or incorrect
- Charge entry: CPT or ICD codes are invalid
- Lack of referrals or preauthorizations
- Medical necessity: ICD-9 does not support CPT billed
- Documentation: Additional information from the physician/provider is requested
- Duplicate: Payer's system shows that a claim is a duplicate and has either been paid or denied

Denial reports will include the major reasons for the denials and the frequency and dollar value of those denied claims. It is important to also compile detailed data on the claim that was denied to enable the practice to identify the originating cause of the denial. Exhibit 9.4 presents a sample denial report.

Reviewing denial data will point out opportunities for improvement in the medical group. Identifying the originating cause of the denial and improving the process so the denials stop happening will reduce claim denials and the cost to rework, will reduce the time to be paid, and will reduce the A/R.

In addition to understanding the originating cause of the denials and making changes (often on the front end) to reduce errors in the future, the medical

EXHIBIT 9.4 ▪ Sample Denial Report

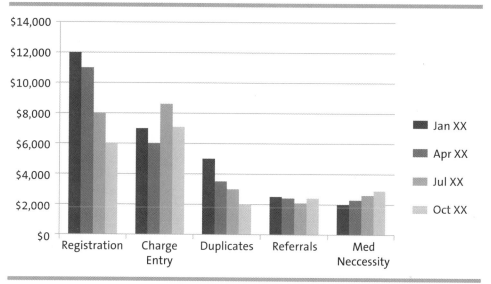

group needs a well-organized denial appeal process. Insurance companies know that a certain percentage of their claims will be denied in error. Being efficient about how to appeal will make it more likely that all denied claims are resubmitted and adjudicated by the payer. Payers have defined claim-filing limits and appeal-filing limits. Appeal-filing limits begin from the date of the explanation of benefits (EOB) and range from 30 days to six months.

Since the medical group has a limited amount of time to submit their appeal, groups are reorganizing their appeal follow-up staff. Dedicated staff members are assigned to work the appeals. These dedicated staff will organize the work according to appeal-filing-limit timing and the dollar value of denials needing rework. The appeals process can be more efficient when also organized by denial reason. For example, if x percent of claims were denied due to lack of referral and all the referrals are located in the same place in the group, working all of those at the same time can be more efficient. The medical group should create template appeal letters for the most frequent denial reasons. There are Web resources and books available that can help a group quickly create a series of letters. Many practice management systems offer appeal modules. It is suggested that the medical group's legal counsel review the letters for compliance with any state or federal collection or insurance regulations.

ACCOUNTS RECEIVABLE — INSURANCE FOLLOW-UP

Unpaid claims should be followed up within 45 to 60 days. Medical groups who maximize their electronic capabilities should be receiving claims status electronically. Others are checking claim status online, and the least efficient will call the payer to inquire about outstanding claims. Medical groups identify insurance collections as a key strategy to reaching their revenue goals. But few groups truly define their collection policy other than to state that older accounts with larger balances should be a priority.

Medical groups with better insurance-collections performance focus on staff training and performance management. Performance management includes traditional revenue cycle metrics such as days in A/R or net collection rate, as well as functional or task measures that ensure cash collections will be the outcome.

Examples of functional or task measures include:

■ Notes on accounts at certain time intervals. Practice should run a "no activity" report, which will identify those claims pending for 45 or 60 days with no payment or denial activity. The staff should contact the payer to verify the claim was received and to determine the reason why no action has been taken.

■ Payment posting current (or collectors could be wasting their time)

■ Credit balances resolved in 60 days

■ Denials due to past appeal-filing limits

■ Systems in place to identify improper, inaccurate, and underpaid remittances

- Performance standards for collectors
- Performance of A/R by provider and payer reviewed

Account follow-up is usually organized in one of four ways: (1) by payer, (2) alphabetically by patient name, (3) by physician/specialty/department, or (4) a hybrid of the other methods. Large groups tend to organize by payer first and then by specialty or physician. Smaller groups will find it hard to organize by payer. With fewer staff, if one staff member is out of the office, there may be no one there to handle a Medicare billing issue.

Insurance collection strategies are usually organized around the major payers. Creating a relationship with a payer's provider relations representative can reap revenue benefits for a medical group. Staffers following up on accounts by payer quickly become very knowledgeable about that payer's billing and coding rules. Scheduling weekly phone calls with provider representatives can ensure an ongoing two-way communication on claim issues. Payers now offer more online and electronic claim status access, which every practice should take advantage of.

Some portion of a medical group's outstanding A/R will need to be written off as bad debt. When all efforts to collect have been exhausted, the account needs to be adjusted utilizing an appropriate write-off code. Each medical group should determine how old is "too old." Monitoring the medical group's performance for days in A/R and percentage of A/R greater than 90 days and greater than 120 days against external benchmarks will help evaluate if A/R write-offs are needed. Exhibit 9.5 compares A/R aging in MGMA better-performing medical groups to all MGMA cost survey participants.

EXHIBIT 9.5 ▪ Percentage of A/R over 90 and 120 Days

	Better Performing	Others	All
Percentage of Total A/R > 90 Days	13.13%	28.09%	22.85%
Percentage of Total A/R > 120 Days	9.00%	22.72%	17.78%

Source: "Multispecialty, All Owners," *Performance and Practices of Successful Medical Groups: 2011 Report Based on 2010 Data.* 2011. Medical Group Management Association.

ACCOUNTS RECEIVABLE — PATIENT FOLLOW-UP

Patient collections are the responsibility of the front-end and back-end operation and part of A/R follow-up. When copayments and deductibles are not collected at the time of service, these balances become part of the total A/R. It is much easier to collect at the time of service then it is to collect after the fact. There are no true obstacles to collecting from a patient at the time of service, only policy or process failures. Patients are more likely to pay when they are at the office and even more likely to pay prior to their visit. At that moment, patients are highly motivated to pay. Once they leave the office, other financial bills become the patient's priority. The patient collection efforts will be more successful if communication to the patient has been conducted. Providing the medical group's financial policy to all patients will be helpful.

Increasing healthcare costs and difficult economic times are causing many patients to consider high-deductible health plans. Add to that trend the continuing increases in the uninsured, and the medical group's future success may depend on how well it collects patient balances. Because of this increased focus on patient collections, medical groups all over the United States are focused on improving the quality of the patient statements they send out. Better-performing practices will turn to the Patient Friendly Billing project for recommendations. This project began in 2001 with patient focus groups, and it has outlined the key success factors in ensuring the billing process is "patient friendly."

The Patient Friendly Billing project is committed to helping create patient bills that are:

- Clear: All financial communications are easy to understand and written in clear language. Patients should be able to quickly determine what they need to do with the communication.
- Correct: The bills or statements should not include estimates for liabilities, incomplete information, or errors.
- Concise: The bills should contain just the right amount of detail necessary to communicate the message.
- Patient Friendly: The needs of patients and family members should be paramount when designing administrative processes and communications.[4]

Improving the patient statement will improve patient satisfaction and ultimately patient collection performance. As the medical group's Web site evolves, consider offering patients the option to submit billing questions via e-mail, to receive e-statements to eliminate the cost of printing, and to mail and pay their bills online in the future. A couple additional tips about patient statements are listed below:

- Are zero balances printed? If they are, the practice management system can suppress the printing and save the cost of forms.
- Are credit balance statements mailed? These statements are normally used as a review mechanism for possible refunds or a location of incorrectly posted payments. Two alternatives seem possible: Either the statements could be sorted and directed to the attention of one person, or the group could prepare a separate list of credit balance accounts.
- How are special collection messages handled? Proper use of color and wording will increase collection.

The use of a collection agency or other outsourced vendor can improve the group's patient collection accounts. Using staff to call and follow up on patient collections takes them away from duties that cannot be easily outsourced, such as charge entry, payment posting, or insurance follow-up. Most medical groups use telephone calls or collection letters to encourage patients to pay before transferring any account to a collection agency. Patients owing the practice money have certain legal rights via the Fair Debt Collection Practices Act (FDCPA).[5] The FDCPA prohibits debt collectors from using abusive, unfair, or deceptive practices to collect payment. It defines parameters that collection staff need to follow, such as hours of the day when you can contact a patient regarding collections. Medical group staff also need to be knowledgeable about their state collection law. Armed with the appropriate laws and regulations, a practice can be confident about pursuing their patients for balances due.

ANALYZING ACCOUNTS RECEIVABLE

Medical group terminology may vary some from the financial world and from the hospital side of our industry. It is important when analyzing A/R that key terms be defined:

Receivables in the financial world: The term "receivables" includes all money claims against individuals, organizations, or other debtors. They arise from various kinds of transactions, the most common in healthcare being the amount owed the provider of medical services on a credit basis. Credit may be granted on open accounts or on the basis of a formal instrument of credit such as a promissory note. Notes are generally used for credit periods of more than 60 days, as in sales of equipment on the installment plan and for relatively large transactions.

Receivables in a medical group: In medical groups, the principal receivables are patient receivables on open accounts, called accounts receivable (A/R). Other receivables include interest receivable; loans to group officers, physicians, and employees; and loans to affiliated entities. In this chapter, we will focus on receivables arising from rendered patient services since they are the major type of receivable that most groups have in their practice.

Practice management systems: All medical groups utilize some type of practice management system (PMS) to support the revenue cycle — from appointment scheduling and billing to A/R management. Small medical groups have been able to take advantage of the increasing number of Web-based practice management vendors offering ever-increasing functionality on a per-physician or per-transaction cost basis. The implementation of EHR with connectivity or single sourcing with a PMS is providing efficiency from the point when the medical service is provided to the point when the patient's account is paid and closed. The PMS is an important tool to manage and control a medical group's accounts receivables. The vendors with higher performance provide functionality that supports a systematic and efficient approach to all steps in the revenue cycle and an impressive set of reports that will analyze and forecast collections.

BILLING TERMS

Gross charges versus gross patient revenue: Both refer to the amount the physician billed for the medical service provided.

Collections versus net patient revenue: Both refer to the amount paid to the physician by the insurance company and/or patient. When the medical group utilizes an accrual basis of accounting, the net patient revenue will be forecasted using historical collection performance against gross patient revenues billed. When the medical group utilizes a cash basis of accounting, the collections are actual cash received.

Why are we focusing on managing A/R and collections? A/R is usually the largest and thus most important asset held by a medical group. Assume a medical group has gross charges (gross patient revenue) of $60,000 per month that are outstanding for an average of 90 days. This creates a necessary but noninterest-earning asset of $180,000. If the time to collect can be reduced by three days, $6,000 can be freed for other uses. On the other hand, a slowdown in collections would cause an increase of three days in the collection period and require an additional investment of $6,000 to maintain the same level of business. Thus, it is extremely important from a cash management perspective to control A/R.

Today's PMS offer an amazing array of collection and A/R reports. Better-performing practices establish appropriate collection procedures and have reports to monitor performance. Action taken to collect accounts and the results attained are recorded in the PMS and then utilized to create electronic work files when further follow-up is warranted. If A/R is written off, another set of reports will track reasons for the write-off, with both monthly and year-to-date summaries.

While statistics about the status of accounts and third-party payers are important, there is no substitute for devoting staff attention to slow accounts because it is people who pay bills. In the next section, we will address several approaches for analyzing A/R.

In this chapter, we are excluding analysis of capitated or other prepaid revenues. When analyzing performance of a medical group, including prepayment revenues in the data can produce potentially misleading trends about managing receivables because these revenues are not outstanding in the sense that revenues from FFS patients are outstanding.

Evaluating the performance of the billing and collection effort requires a look at valid performance measures. Clearly, last month's cash collections tell the medical group how they are doing compared to the budget and answer the question, "Is there enough money to fund payroll this month?" But that is not all the medical group wants to measure. In fact, last month's cash collection total is already an historical trend and not an indicator of future revenue performance.

There are a number of traditional A/R measures that medical groups should track on a regular basis:

- **Net Collection Rate:** The net collection rate lets you know how much money you collected of the money you *could* collect.
  - Calculation: Net collections (collections less refunds) divided by net charges (gross charges less contractual adjustments)
- **Days in A/R:** This turns the dollar value of the current A/R into the number of days of gross charges.
  - Calculation: Total A/R (net of credit balances) divided by the average daily charge (gross charges divided by 365)
- **% of A/R > 90 days:** How much of your A/R has been pending for more than 90 days?
  - Calculation: A/R older than 90 days (aged from date of charge entry) divided by the total outstanding A/R
- **Claim Denial Rate:** This determines the percentage of claims denied upon submission.
  - Calculation: Number of claims denied divided by total claims submitted

NET CHARGES AND CASH COLLECTION ANALYTICS

Trend the net charges (gross charges – contractual adjustments) and cash collections over 12 months. The gap between the two lines will indicate how well the practice is performing. Good performance would cause the two lines to stay close together. Exhibit 9.6 shows that the two lines stay parallel except in June and July. When a medical group sees the performance change, it can

EXHIBIT 9.6 ■ **Net Charges and Collections Chart**

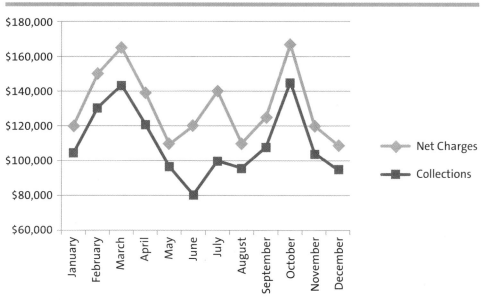

begin to evaluate the causes for the collections delay. These causes could be a disruption in the charge capture or claims processes or a payer's denial rate has increased for a specific reason.

Define what "great performance" means to the medical group. The right reports will clarify the revenue opportunities or, at a minimum, create the need for more research to understand what is going on. Reimbursement performance reports can include more than one indicator. Often, no single indicator tells the entire story.

For example, Exhibit 9.7 shows outstanding A/R at the end of each quarter for a 24-month period. Looking at this one performance measure, total A/R, a practice manager might assume that volumes or charges have also increased in the last two quarters.

Then, he or she looked at Exhibit 9.8, which clearly shows gross charges flattening and decreasing. Thus, A/R increasing looks like a bigger concern.

In Exhibit 9.9, gross charges are shown with outstanding A/R in one chart. This chart is an excellent example of analyzing two revenue measures together. Both measures are trending in a negative direction from better-performing practices. When analyzed together, it is clear there is a cause that has nothing to do with charge volume.

Exhibits 9.10 and 9.11 list the indicators[6] a medical group practice should report on regularly.

The medical group's manager will track many indicators on a daily and weekly basis in areas such as workload productivity, credit balances, claims suspended on edit lists, and so on. There is only one indicator the medical group must monitor each day, and that is cash collected. Better-performing medical groups widely communicate the amount of cash collected each day. This makes it clear that cash is always a focus (no money, no mission) and is an early warning signal of potential down trends in the month.

EXHIBIT 9.7 ▪ Total A/R (in 000s)

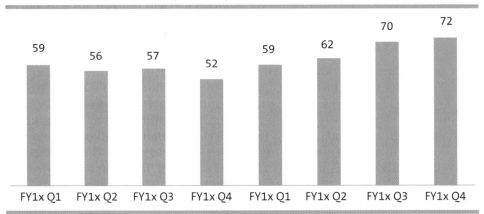

EXHIBIT 9.8 ■ Charges (in 000s)

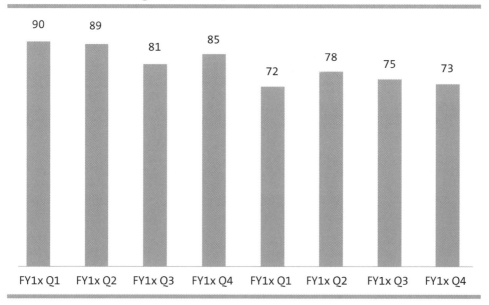

An example of an initial key indicator dashboard can be found in Exhibit 9.12. Start with the indicators that make sense for your medical group, improve and measure performance over time, and add indicators as needed as you move forward.

Next, the medical group should be calculating the same performance measures for each major payer. Even when a group's total performance is very good, there

EXHIBIT 9.9 ■ Charges and A/R Chart

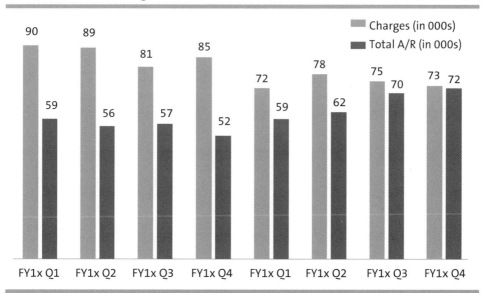

EXHIBIT 9.10 ■ Key Financial Performance Indicators

Revenue Cycle	Total accounts receivable per physician
	Percentage of total accounts receivable 120+ days old
	Days in accounts receivable
	Adjusted fee-for-service collection percentage
Financial	Total medical revenue per physician
	Total operating cost per physician
	Total medical revenue after operating cost per physician
Efficiency	Total operating cost as a percentage of total medical revenue

EXHIBIT 9.11 ■ Multi-indicators to Measure in a Single Report/Graph — Sample

Quarterly Charges & Total A/R

Percentage A/R >120 days and Collections as Percentage of Net Revenue

Lag Day to Post Charges & Days in A/R

Claim Denials by Major Payer & Major Denial Reason

Gross Collection Rate & Net Collection Rate & Percentage Payer Mix Managed Care

may be revenue improvement opportunities within one payer. Evaluating payer performance must include an evaluation of the payer's administrative processes or obstacles.

The medical group's contract negotiators need pricing strategies that relate to the current Medicare fee schedule, develop specific fee floors by product type (indemnity, PPO, HMO), and/or are ready to agree to lower rates for proven volume shifts. Before a medical group practice begins negotiating a new contract or a renewal, it should take time to analyze current business as a percentage of Medicare and compare volume by payer (see Exhibit 9.13 for a sample report). What is the lowest fee that the medical group can afford to agree to? This analysis will help a group frame their pricing boundaries.

EXHIBIT 9.12 ■ Sample Dashboard Indicator

Key Performance Indicator	Dec XX	Dec XX	Qtr 1	Qtr 2	Qtr 3	Qtr 4	Target
AR Days	55	52	49	45			35
% AR > 90 Days	25%	24%	21%	18%			10%
Net Collection Rate	85%	90%	92%	93%			98%
Denial Rate	28%	22%	19%	18%			7%

EXHIBIT 9.13 ▪ Top Payers' Charges and Percentage of Medicare

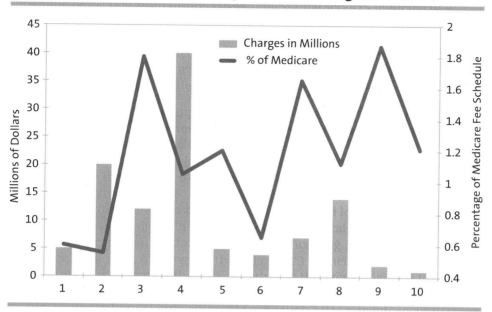

There are a number of recommended ways to categorize and prioritize A/R follow-up. Running a report by dollars outstanding or by payer appeal timelines often provides the best way to organize A/R follow-up staff. The medical group's PMS will provide a number of A/R reports that are very helpful in managing and monitoring the outstanding A/R. Looking at your A/R from several different perspectives may identify new A/R opportunities. Exhibit 9.14 provides a list of several ways to prioritize the accounts receivable.

Experienced administrators and financial managers know that a great deal of time can be spent collecting accounts that do not make sizable reductions in A/R or notable increases in monthly collection totals. For a better payoff, a

EXHIBIT 9.14 ▪ Prioritizing Your Outstanding Accounts Receivable

- ▪ Sort by balance due (highest to lowest)
- ▪ Create dollar buckets appropriate for your specialty ($3,000+; $2,000–$2,999; $1,000–$1,999; $500–$999; $100–$499; $50–$99; $10–$49)
- ▪ Sort by account type, payer type/plan
- ▪ Sort by date claim submitted or date of service
- ▪ Sort by age of account
  - – Create age buckets (120+ days, 91–120, 61–90, 31–60, current)
- ▪ Sort insurance receivables and guarantor receivables separately

careful analysis of A/R, collection activities, debtors, and third-party payers can be useful in zeroing in on major problems. Through careful investigation, the financial manager will be able to determine which analyses are appropriate for a medical group.

Third-party analyses assist the financial manager in identifying areas that need attention, particularly those related to third-party payers, such as:

- Identification of insurance companies that become collection problems;
- Identification of reasons given by the third party for not paying; and
- Development of a third-party payer fact sheet.

DEFINING GOALS AND ACHIEVING THEM

Organizing, forecasting, planning, communicating, and measuring staff effectiveness by results are all management's responsibility. Defining staff performance expectations will tell the staff how to prioritize their time each day.

Some examples of staff performance indicators for medical group A/R functions are:

- Monthly outstanding accounts
- Percentage of bad debt to gross charges and to net charges
- Number of complaints voiced to administration
- Gross collection rate
- Average monthly collections
- Average time span from charge to claim that is out to the payer
- Number of claims per week
- Gross and net collection ratio by financial class or payer

APPROACHES TO CONSIDER: OUTSOURCING, INSOURCING, AND OTHER HYBRID ARRANGEMENTS

If a medical group is wondering if it should outsource or insource its billing, the first question to answer is why it is asking the question. Most often, the question has been prompted by a concern that the medical group's billing performance is just not good enough, or perhaps one of the physicians "heard" that outsourcing or insourcing is the best way to go.

Before a medical group considers a decision to change billing structure, it needs to ask why they want to change. Is the revenue cycle performance below industry benchmarks? If not, then experts would suggest that no change is the best decision. One thing everyone can agree on is that a major change in any part of a medical group's billing operation will result in a short- to mid-term cash impact. If the change is implemented poorly, the group could have a much longer-term impact. Thus, a medical group should not even consider outsourcing or insourcing if performance is at or above industry standards. If there are specific functional areas that need to be improved, outsourcing that area only might improve performance. For example, some medical groups have outsourced their self-pay collections after sending only one statement and waiting only 30 days because they don't have the staff in the medical group to effectively work those accounts. Those are the kinds of decisions a medical group might want to consider before looking at outsourcing the entire billing operation.

So how does a medical group decide which billing model is best for the group? First, it is important to realize that there is no "best" way, or all medical groups would be doing it the same way. Instead, there is "best for your medical practice, today and for the next few years." Now, let's move on to discuss differences in these approaches and how a medical group might decide what is "best" for it.

Some experienced medical group managers believe that "no one collects our money like we do." But there can be compelling reasons why a medical group should outsource.

Outsourcing: Contracting with an External Vendor for Billing

Will outsourcing reduce the billing costs?

Some medical groups believe that outsourcing can reduce their cost of billing. Unfortunately, there are a few vendors who quote really low prices (in conference exhibit halls, during a presentation, etc.). Then when the medical group does its due diligence, it determines that the vendor's definition of "billing" and the medical group's definition of "billing" are not the same. It is extremely important to agree on the scope of services that will be delivered before pricing is analyzed. Examples of billing functions that are sometimes optional, and thus will be cost added to the quoted base price, can include: charge capture, payer credentialing, physician coding and compliance, payer contract analysis, collection agency, and so on. A medical group needs to understand what it is currently spending on billing (for everything including IT) and then try to price out each functional area. When the scope of billing services is similar, the costs of billing are pretty comparable with the following exceptions.

- ▪ Since payment posting and charge entry are high-production areas, it is possible for a larger staff operation to get some efficiencies.

- ▪ Self-pay collections, claims processing, and patient statement mailing are usually cheaper at higher volumes; an outsourced vendor may have enough volume across all clients to keep these functions at a lower per-unit cost.

- ▪ Large billing vendors often have made significant investments in technology that will allow staff to maximize efficiency and reduce errors.

Will outsourcing reduce the time spent on billing?

Some medical group leaders consider outsourcing because they believe it will reduce the time they spend dealing with billing and billing issues. That is not true! When the billing is outsourced, it is critical that the medical group leaders stay involved, evaluate the billing company's performance on a regular basis, and create a working relationship with a specific individual. During the sales and implementation phases, the outsourced billing vendor may involve several people to help get the group set up and ready to get that first claim out the door. Ask the vendor to identify the representative for your group's account — the person who will be interacting with the group on a regular basis. It cannot be more than one person. Obviously, there may be more than one person who provides services (usually someone else does reports, etc.), but the medical group needs to know who will be its advocate and troubleshooter as needed. Who will the medical group leader call or meet with if billing performance is not as good as you expected? Managing an outsourced billing contract takes a lot of work; failing to understand that and commit the appropriate resources can be a major reason why the outsourced model doesn't deliver the expected results.

Remember that geography is a powerful thing. When a medical group outsources billing, the front desk staff and the physicians feel like they just don't have a relationship with that group of people. Most often, the billing team is located in another part of town or as technology has advanced, even out of town. Geography is a powerful negative force in human interaction. Make sure that if the group outsources, you do everything in your power to create regularly scheduled face-to-face interactions and frequent online meetings that will ensure that everyone feels like they are on the same team.

Negotiate a great contract

Be really explicit about the scope of services in the vendor contract. It is sad to walk into a physician practice that has its billing outsourced, and no one can answer questions about who is handling physician coding problems or the status of credentialing or why monthly reports are not available until the end of the next month. It must be clear for every billing function (in detail) who is handling each step in the billing process (the medical group or the vendor?). Here is an example:

A vendor's contract states that they are responsible for charge entry. Physicians want to know if all of their charges have been billed. Who is responsible for that? Charge capture is not mentioned in the scope of services, thus that falls to the medical group. The outsourced billing vendor is going to be responsible only for entering the charges given to them — not for making sure that all charges were sent to them. Can you see how specific this relationship needs to be? It isn't any easier when you insource your billing; you still have to make sure that both charge capture and charge entry are happening, but at least you don't have the argument of who is accountable for it.

Is it more likely for some specialties to outsource more often than others?

"Notably, those referral-based specialties such as neonatology, radiology, anesthesiology, pathology and those physicians specializing as hospitalists rely on registration conducted elsewhere. . . . Many of these specialties have found outsourcing to be a compelling option."[7]

Insourcing: Moving Billing Back to the Medical Group

Most of us know what it takes to run our own billing operation within our medical group. But if a medical group manager accepts a new position or acquires a new medical group, he or she may inherit a billing operation that is in transition. The issues related to bringing billing in house (insourcing) are every bit a challenge! A few highlights to consider:

- ■ **PMS:** If the medical group has a new PMS that includes a billing and A/R module, then it will implement those modules while hiring the billing staff. It takes a lot of resources to do both concurrently.

- ■ **Staffing:** The most important key to excellent billing performance is hiring an experienced and talented billing expert to manage this new operation. In some cases, that person will also be the practice administrator, and in other cases, the group will hire a new billing manager to take responsibility for the new staff and day-to-day operations. As more physician medical groups are affiliating with health systems, the billing expert might work for the health system and report up through the hospital revenue cycle department. Regardless, the human resources effort in staff selection and training is enormous and not without some glitches along the way, usually.

- ■ **Space, Hardware, and Maintenance:** If this is a new operation in the medical group or health system, the required space to support this new team and the required fixed assets and computer hardware are significant upfront investments. There are a number of one-time costs that will take place throughout the first year.

- ■ **Communication:** Two of the biggest positives of having billing within the medical group are the opportunity for excellent communication with physicians and front desk staff. Don't forget to take advantage of this opportunity for frequent face-to-face interactions. Regularly scheduled meetings to discuss performance and opportunities for improvement are an enhancement to any revenue cycle process.

Consider Hybrid Models to Maximize Collections

Depending on the size of the internal collection staff, partnering with one or more outside vendors can be an important link in the chain of a strong collection program. The smaller the staff, the more the medical group needs to depend on an outside vendor to play an active role in increasing total cash flow. Historically, medical groups have used professional collection agencies. Today, medical groups increasingly use a variety of outside vendors to support and supplement their revenue cycle. The choice of an outside vendor and how well it performs can make a considerable difference in overall collection results and patient relations.

Use of outside vendors

Before an account is released to an outside vendor, the medical group needs to attempt to collect the amount due. At some point, it becomes fruitless to continue to spend time and money trying to collect overdue accounts internally. As patients continue to select high-deductible health plans and other new payer models, it is imperative that accounts be worked consistently. If the medical group does not have sufficient or experienced staff to stay current on A/R, it must release the accounts to an outside vendor to be worked in a timely fashion. Continuing to hold on to accounts receivable for 90 or 180 days when no one is available to work the accounts will result in reduced collection performance.

Before finalizing a relationship with an outside vendor for collection services, two important questions need to be asked:

1. Are the vendor's fees reasonable when contrasted with internal collection costs?

2. Is the probability of collection greater with the vendor than it is with the internal staff?

Other topics to consider:

3. How does the vendor interact with the medical group's patients? Collection activities, however polite and courteous, often raise patient anxiety. Involvement of an outside vendor, which may have staff better equipped to handle these situations, can help protect the image of the medical group.

4. Who can the medical group call for a reference check on the outside vendor? Follow-up with the references is essential. The vendor's current customers should be able to answer about the start-up transition, how soon the medical group received cash, and the ongoing cost of doing business with the vendor.

5. Consider using more than one outside vendor. Usually a vendor has a specialty niche that it is known for. Some handle "early out" or precollections. Others utilize attorneys for large, complex accounts.

Some medical groups are tempted to write off an account rather than refer it to an outside vendor for collection. Two things happen if groups go in that direction. First, it is likely that the patient community will hear of the medical group's tendency to write off debts. This type of reputation can cause even more nonpayment by patients, thus increasing collection costs considerably. Second, writing off collectible balances is not fair to paying patients. In the long run, the medical group's cost of practice must be paid by someone. An indirect result may be increased charges for all patients. In today's competitive and transparent environment, holding down costs must be a prime consideration.

What will it cost?

The newer outside vendors that offer collections services (early out, precollections, etc.) use a variety of fee and commission structures. They also have a variety of recovery rates. Look for outside vendors with strong recovery rates who charge a low flat fee per account. When you assign accounts to an outside vendor earlier in the collection process (at 45–60 days), their fee will be lower than traditional collection agencies — sometimes less than half what a medical group might be used to paying collection agencies. Traditional collection agencies usually accept accounts for collection on a contingency basis (i.e., no collection, no charge). They charge a commission only on funds actually collected. Collection agencies charge contingent fee commissions ranging from 25 to 40 percent. Accounts previously handled by other agencies that require legal action or accounts transferred to out-of-town agencies may put the fee at a higher percentage.

Attorneys for Collection

Who gets the better collection results — collection vendors or attorneys? If volume only is judged, the answer is collection vendors. However, some medical specialties use attorneys for collection services on large or complex accounts. Assuming contingency fees for collection activity are competitively priced, there are some benefits to using attorneys:

- Greater impact on patients when a letter is received from an attorney rather than a collection vendor
- Patient perspective that this matter is more serious and a legal suit might occur
- Attorney ability to file suit quicker and for less cost
- Attorney ability to spread legal costs over numerous accounts
- Attorney ability to deal with other attorneys in accident cases

Many collection vendors offer legal services, too, so all options should be explored.

To the Point

As the person responsible for finance and financial management, your focus has been on assets, liabilities, revenues, and expenses. Accounts receivable are a key driver in collection performance and stating the medical group's financial position. In order to analyze and manage collection performance and A/R, medical group leaders need an excellent knowledge of the entire revenue cycle process. In this chapter, we have discussed both internal and external forces that impact revenue cycle performance. A/R and cash collection performance will not be maximized if the medical group has inadequate staffing or uneven work flow or if staff members do not follow procedures. In order to decrease A/R and increase cash collections, the financial manager must focus on solving particular problems that are hampering performance, such as clearing up a backlog of billing, adding staff to needed areas, collecting at the time of service, getting action from third parties, or decreasing the time an account is held before collection starts. Reducing A/R and increasing cash collections will improve the financial position of every medical group.

REFERENCES

1. Walker Keegan, D., Woodcock, E., and Larch, S. 2009. *The Physician Billing Process: 12 Potholes to Avoid in the Road to Getting Paid*, p. xxvi. Englewood, CO: Medical Group Management Association.

2. Hajny, T. G. 2003. "Patient Flow and the Revenue Cycle," *Journal of Medical Practice Management* (Nov/Dec): 135–36.

3. Medical Group Management Association. 2011. *Performance and Practices of Successful Medical Groups: 2011 Report Based on 2010 Data*. Englewood, CO: Medical Group Management Association.

4. Healthcare Financial Management Association. 2012. Patient Friendly Billing, Chicago, IL, Retrieved from www.hfma.org/hfma-initiatives/patient-friendly-billing/patient-friendly-billing--purpose-and-philosophy.

5. Fair Debt Collection Practices Act Web site. Retrieved from www.ftc.gov/bcp/edu/pubs/consumer/credit/cre27.pdf. Accessed May 15, 2012.

6. Walker Keegan, D., Woodcock, E., and Larch, S. 2009. *The Physician Billing Process: 12 Potholes to Avoid in the Road to Getting Paid*, p. xxvi. Englewood, CO: Medical Group Management Association.

7. Larch, S. 2011, January 12. "Out-Source or In-Source Your Medical Billing: How Do You Decide?" *Getting Paid: Leading Ideas and Opinions on Medical Billing and Practice Management*. Retrieved from http://www.kareo.com/gettingpaid/2011/01/out-source-or-in-source-your-medical-billing-how-do-you-decide.

PART II

Using Financial Management Information to Manage Operations

CHAPTER 10

Managed Care Issues

Edited by Daniel D. Mefford, CPA, MBA, FACMPE

After completing this chapter you will be able to:

- Explain the major concepts of managed care.

- Identify the main managed care participants in the marketplace.

- Outline a medical practice's motivation to contract for managed care.

- Differentiate between the types of risk in managed care contracts.

- Identify core components of a typical managed care contract.

- Link cost control mechanisms to a medical practice's managed care activities.

- Explain the importance of continued professional development in the emerging arena of managed healthcare.

- Access self-development tools to follow managed care's evolution.

Despite an abundance of media information, the subject of managed care remains an enigma for many people. In this chapter, we will provide a basic definition of managed care and compare managed care with traditional fee-for-service (FFS) healthcare delivery. To further enrich the general concept of managed care, we introduce the major financial stakeholders in a managed healthcare delivery marketplace. The introduction and proliferation of managed care led to many cultural changes in how patient care is provided and to the inception of new integrated provider mechanisms. We will name and provide basic definitions of these innovative organization forms.

When entering a managed care contract, one of the key areas a medical group practice will have to assess relates to how much risk it is able and willing to accept. To help assist in this task, we present a three-tiered model on the various risk levels. The discussion of various risk arrangements in this section will include remarks on how organizations can effectively manage cost in a managed care environment.

Due to the centrality of managed care contracting in thriving medical group practices, a major segment of this chapter is dedicated to the explanation of a list of commonly used elements in managed care contracts. Negotiation skills and relationship-building abilities are essential in determining a financial manager's aptitude toward sustaining successful managed care activities. After a contract is negotiated, the question of how to manage the contract becomes most important. Included are highlights of some of the more innovative methods organizations are using to manage these agreements.

This chapter is intended to provide some basic working knowledge of managed care issues. However, the authors strongly suggest a deeper examination into the various managed care subject matters as a major component of any financial manager's continuing education effort. Thus, we close the chapter with suggested resources to stay abreast of managed care developments and an attempt to predict future developments in the ever-changing managed care marketplace.

WHAT IS MANAGED CARE?

Since the modern era of healthcare delivery took shape in the United States, reimbursement for any medical service performed was generally on a FFS basis and paid for in arrears. Within this framework, patients or their insurers paid for healthcare services only after or at the time such services were rendered. Under most FFS, indemnity health insurance plans, physicians practiced medicine with considerable latitude in clinical treatment alternatives; meanwhile, consumers had similar latitude to choose which physicians they would seek treatments from in meeting their healthcare needs. Significant changes in the healthcare delivery system and movement away from the traditional FFS system began to occur in the 1980s. At that time, a great number of providers explored the group practice concept, and health plans started to negotiate directly with these larger group-practice organizations. Resulting contractual arrangements obligated affiliated physicians to accept and treat certain patients at a predetermined reimbursement level. The health reform debate of the early 1990s further opened the wedge for managed healthcare delivery in the United States, as the debate raised considerable alarm regarding the long-term economic impacts of the prevailing fragmented and increasingly expensive healthcare delivery system on American society as a whole.

Under the traditional FFS financial system, providers, including both hospitals and physicians, were reimbursed for their services on the basis of either their clinical gross charges or their actual costs of rendering medical services, depending on the individual payer. This payment system tended to promote inefficiency and has been a major factor, along with advances in technology and new drugs, in creating the rapid inflation experienced by the healthcare industry in the United States throughout the latter stages of the twentieth century. In a spiral-like fashion, the more providers charged and the higher the costs for delivering healthcare services, the greater their medical revenues. Obviously the traditional FFS system presented providers with a disincentive to contain much of the costs associated with healthcare delivery.

The disposition and growth of managed care delivery systems are a direct result of ostensible problems with the increasing amount of money spent on healthcare services nationwide and the inflation in the cost of those services. The sweeping movement to the organizational form of managed care known as health maintenance organizations (HMOs) was seen as an alternative to the inflationary and greatly fragmented FFS system. HMOs and other managed care organizations (MCOs) adopted the concept of managed healthcare delivery as a system in which the provider of care is incentivized to establish mechanisms to contain costs, control utilization, and deliver services in the most appropriate settings. Market by market, managed healthcare delivery systems have become the most powerful force for reshaping the healthcare landscape in the United States today.

The many methodologies that the managed care marketplace has adopted center on three key factors: (1) controlling the utilization of medical services, (2) shifting financial risk to the provider, and (3) reducing the use of resources in rendering treatments to patients. Methods to curtail utilization and reduce costs have been developed and refined over the last 30 years and seem to be primarily directed at changing the culture of medical practice at all service delivery access points. Among these cultural changes are the following:

- Mandating outpatient surgery for many operations
- Same-day admission surgery
- Step-down units, which provide care at a lower intensity than inpatient care sites
- Nonduplication of services
- Drug formularies
- Nursing homes as an alternative to long-term hospitalization
- Home healthcare as a more prevalent means of providing quality care
- Hospices
- Nurse triage call centers and other measures aimed at directing consumers to the appropriate level of medical care
- Inpatient critical pathways
- Patient education focusing on wellness and prevention
- Care coordination strategies like case managers and hospitalist programs

To explore other concepts of managed healthcare delivery in deeper detail, let's examine the following definitions taken from the mainstream healthcare literature.

Managed care is an attempt at a coordinated approach to deliver a full continuum of healthcare services through a system designed to measurably meet the objectives of delivering appropriate care by the appropriate provider at the appropriate venue at the appropriate time and utilizing appropriate resources such as staffing and technology.[1]

The concept of managed care embodies a direct relationship and interdependence between the provision of and payment for healthcare. Central to understanding managed care is the population orientation and the organization of care-providing groups or networks that take responsibility and usually share financial risk with the insurer for a population's medical care and health maintenance.[2]

Managed healthcare delivery does not necessarily imply the incorporation of an HMO. HMOs are only one organizational form that managed care may take. There are various managed care organizational models that offer a range of health plans. The specific dynamics of each managed care market account for differences in the popularity and growth of such models. A local ownership presence also appears to contribute in the development and acceptance of some models over others. In addition to HMOs, the most prevalent MCO models today are preferred provider organizations (PPOs), point-of-service (POS) plans, and exclusive provider organizations (EPOs).

The various organizational structures managed care can assume typically involve concepts and processes aimed at affecting the amount of money spent on healthcare services by changing the behavior of the two parties who have the most significant direct influence over healthcare services utilization — patients and providers. MCOs attempt to achieve this objective through the use of several control mechanisms that characterize the organization of service delivery. The following list provides the reader with a baseline understanding of these core concepts and processes. A more detailed discussion of many of these concepts and processes is included throughout the remainder of the chapter.

Primary care physician (PCP): A general practice physician, usually a family practitioner, internist, pediatrician, or occasionally an obstetrician/gynecologist who has specific enrollees (patients) assigned to him or her by a health plan for routine medical care. The PCP serves as the primary and first contact in many managed care organizational models and operates as the gatekeeper. This role includes providing primary healthcare services and authorizing referrals to specialists and testing facilities when necessary.

Capitation: Provider organizations receive a fixed, previously negotiated periodic payment per member covered by the health plan in exchange for delivering specified healthcare services to the members for a specified length of time, regardless of how many or how few services are actually required or rendered. Usually, these payments are adjusted for enrollee age and sex, but they generally do not consider the amount of individual patient care provided. The term "per member per month" (PMPM) is the commonplace calculation unit for such capitation payments.

Utilization review: Utilization review encompasses the comprehensive set of strategies and techniques used by healthcare professionals, insurance companies, and the government to evaluate the necessity, appropriateness, and efficiency of healthcare services. The utilization review process may take the shape of prospective, concurrent, or statistical review, and can include chart reviews or the requirement for advance permission prior to surgery. Superior utilization management systems monitor for underutilization as well as for overutilization. Depending on the managed care network, peer review groups, public agencies, or utilization review committees may perform the utilization review procedures. For example, Medicare and Medicaid generally require that hospitals have a standing utilization review committee.

Financial risk: In the traditional FFS setting, a provider organization generally has a direct clinical and financial relationship with the patient, or the patient may have an insurance company that will reimburse the patient or provider for expenses incurred as a result of medical service delivery. Within this context, the charge for any medical service is determined by the functional fee schedule of the medical practice at the time service was rendered. The fee schedule is somewhat price sensitive to the marketplace yet generally covers all practice expenses plus the desired levels of physician compensation and any retained earnings or profits. Obviously, a medical practice will set a fee schedule that meets its financial needs (detailed information on constructing an appropriate fee schedule was discussed in chapter 7). The financial risk of the medical group involves the possibility that all or some of the revenue amount may not be collected and the uncertainty over when such revenue will be recouped. The reward in the traditional FFS arrangement is that the revenue amounts from payers are likely to exceed the actual cost of services if charges are adequate and expenses are reasonably controlled.

In contrast, often under managed care arrangements, providers receive payments prospectively. The basic financial risk of a medical group entering into these contracts is that the group must manage the total delivery of healthcare services within the scope of its contract so that the total cost of services provided to health plan members is less than the revenue received. The reward for assuming this type of financial risk is timelier and, hopefully, increased cash flows based on more predictable patient volumes and better service-volume management. Specific risk arrangements will be discussed later in this chapter.

THE MANAGED CARE MARKETPLACE

In recent times, medical groups often associate managed care contracting with simply becoming participants in the locale's various health plans and then either building the group through projected increases in patient volumes or simply maintaining an existing volume in an effort to keep patients from migrating to another competitor. Yet, there is an abundance of contractual relationships between payers and providers to facilitate the delivery of healthcare services in a managed care environment. Savvy healthcare financial managers will seek to recognize the complex dynamics and key opportunities associated with each of these economic relationships while building or sustaining a thriving medical practice. As financial managers approach different factual situations, they should critically examine the relationships that exist between and among the various market participants. The most straightforward arrangement, although generally unusual in today's business climate, is a direct financial relationship between the patient and the provider. Healthcare is provided as a directly billable service to the patient who is the only responsible party to compensate the provider for the services rendered. Financial managers should recognize that many patients elect not to claim their insurance coverage for certain medical services and that MCOs routinely do not cover all possible services in their benefit packages, thus creating the need for competent processes to handle this manner of transaction. Direct contracting for the provision of healthcare services between large employer groups and physician organizations or other provider enterprises, such as integrated delivery systems, presents a variant of this arrangement.

By design, however, the majority of managed healthcare delivery systems customarily involve the coordination of multiple contracted stakeholders. To understand the most dominant forms of managed care in today's healthcare marketplace, it is helpful to think of the interrelationships of the three main market participants:

1. Healthcare purchasers (patients, employers, or even providers)
2. Insurers and MCOs (government based, commercial)

3. Providers (individual physicians, medical group practices, integrated delivery systems [IDSs], physician hospital organizations [PHOs], independent practice associations (IPAs), management services organizations [MSOs], physician practice management companies [PPMCs], ambulatory surgery centers [ASCs], etc.)

The government and commercial insurance companies, along with hospitals, physician groups, consumer cooperatives, and individual patients, all compose the purchaser element of the managed care marketplace. Purchasers of medical services in today's healthcare marketplace are now usually organized and demand lower costs and improved care compared to individual patients directly interacting with providers under typical FFS arrangements. Because of economic pressures, organized purchasers can apply in the negotiation process for care, this factor alone has driven much of the sweeping change in the healthcare system. For example, large employers are becoming exceedingly influential purchasers because they are involved in determining what constitutes reasonable and appropriate health insurance costs. In addition to their negotiation power in relation to health plans, employers also hold significant market influence with organized public interest groups in different arenas articulating healthcare policy matters.

Providers are at the core of the managed healthcare delivery systems as they have the most influence on the actual processes and outcomes of patient care. Providers include physicians, hospitals, and midlevel providers such as nurse practitioners and physician assistants and other individual and institutional providers that are directly involved in the delivery of healthcare services. As a result of the proliferation of managed healthcare delivery, many providers have made the transformation into numerous new and important business structures, as discussed in greater detail in the next section.

Finally, many MCOs and other insuring entities, responding to their own business objectives and potentially significant economic pressures from the market, have developed into huge conglomerates that imaginatively attempt to integrate the economic realities of health insurance with the productive assets of healthcare service delivery. In their weaker expressions, MCOs aggressively bargain with provider enterprises for lower (discounted) reimbursement fees. However, in their most robust form, MCOs attempt to completely shift the financial risk of providing services from the insurer to the provider so that the provider will have "incentives" to manage care efficiently. This occurs despite the fact that both types of organizations are in completely different business lines.

Arrangements between the provider entity and the insuring party or MCO are generally guided by a negotiated contract for a specified period of time. The spectrum of these agreements reaches from very simple discounted FFS arrangements carrying minimal financial risk to complex risk contracting more commonly known as capitation. Managed care contracts may contain many conditions and provisions that can potentially threaten the long-term financial stability of a medical practice if not examined and researched by experienced personnel. The authors recommend that financial managers seek such expert guidance prior to finalizing and executing agreements with MCOs. Issues specific to managed care contracting are approached in greater detail in a later section.

The Rise of Integrated Provider Mechanisms

Since the introduction of managed care, a number of new, integrated provider organizations were fashioned for the principal purpose of bringing previously fragmented providers together to deliver healthcare services, all for reasons related to the growth of managed care. Integrated provider organizations regularly develop medical service delivery strategies that use various managed care procedures and methods, such as case management and clinical pathways, and generally rely on discounted FFS, global, or individual capitation agreements to compensate affiliated providers for their services.[3] In many situations, integrated provider organizations will serve as the primary conduit between a payer organization, such as a health plan, and individual physicians.

Integrated provider organizations are usually designed as separate legal entities for a set purpose, customarily to jointly market their constituents' services to enhance their competitive positions in a managed care market and/or to provide management and administrative services in support of medical service delivery strategies and programs.[4] Regional differences and market maturity factors have generally led to the popularization of some integrated organizational forms in favor of other integrated provider arrangements.

A definitive summary of these integrated provider mechanisms is beyond the scope of this chapter. Furthermore, the functionality or name of an organization in one community may be vastly different from what an organization with a similar name does in another metropolitan area. However, the following list provides the more prevalent examples of these integrated provider organizations:

Integrated delivery systems (IDS) are networks of organizations that provide or coordinate and arrange for the provision of a continuum of healthcare services to consumers and are willing to be held clinically and fiscally responsible for the outcomes and the health status of the population served.[5] Generally consisting of hospitals, physician groups, health plans, home health agencies, hospices, skilled nursing facilities, and other provider entities, these networks may be built through "virtual" integration processes encompassing contractual arrangements and strategic alliances as well as through direct ownership.[6] There are many models of integrated delivery systems including those developed around former multihospital systems (e.g., Intermountain Healthcare in Utah), those created around physician groups (e.g., Mayo Clinic in Minnesota, Arizona, and Florida), those built around insurance companies and hospital systems (e.g., Cigna-Lovelace Clinic in Texas), and other hybrid models representing various combinations of provider organizations (e.g., Allina in Minnesota and Kaiser-Permanente, which delivers healthcare in many states).[7]

Physician-hospital organizations (PHOs) are cooperative ventures that bring physicians and hospital providers together in a separate, vertically integrated business enterprise. PHO as a business entity does not deliver healthcare services but generally coordinates the provision of services through the PHO's contributing physician and hospital providers. The PHO's foremost business function is to better market the health services of the PHO's individual and institutional providers through the development of a single unified healthcare product.[8]

Independent practice associations (IPAs) are networks that bring together otherwise separate physician practices in a united manner to deliver healthcare services in a managed care environment. In an IPA enterprise, individual physicians or provider groups typically establish ownership and/or contractual relationships with the network organization. Under the terms and provisions of those arrangements, the individual physicians or medical groups typically agree to provide healthcare services to health plan beneficiaries under network-sponsored managed care contracts. As with PHOs, IPA networks do not actually deliver healthcare services directly to the consumer but are organized to coordinate or arrange for the provision of healthcare services to consumers by the providers participating in the network.[9]

Management services organizations (MSOs) are business enterprises that may be jointly owned and sponsored by physicians, hospitals, or other capital partners to provide management and administrative support services to physicians in a managed care market. Physicians, hospitals, or other parties may also solely own these management support organizations. MSOs customarily do not provide healthcare services to consumers. Rather, they are generally created to provide an assortment of practice support services such as sophisticated utilization control mechanisms and other elements of the managed care "infrastructure" that must be acquired and employed by providers under managed care. Some MSOs go beyond a simple "service bureau" function by purchasing the assets of affiliated physicians and entering into long-term management agreements with the "captive" provider network. Some MSOs have also broadened their ownership base and character by engaging outside investors to help capitalize the growth and development of the practice management infrastructure for affiliated providers.[10]

Physician practice management companies (PPMCs) are usually publicly held or entrepreneurially directed enterprises that acquire total or partial ownership interests in physician organizations. PPMCs are generally regarded as a particular type of MSO; however, the motivations, goals, strategies, and structures arising from their unequivocal ownership character — development of growth and profits for their investors, not for participating providers — differentiate them from other MSO models in important ways. Like other MSO models, PPMCs customarily do not provide healthcare services directly to consumers. PPMCs characteristically provide an assortment of practice support services, such as billing and collections, managed care contract negotiations, physician practice management, network development, utilization and quality management, information systems and data management, claims payment, and marketing development, to compete effectively in a managed care environment.

Ambulatory surgery centers (ASCs) are specifically licensed business ventures that operate exclusively for the purpose of furnishing a range of surgical services on a same-day outpatient basis. Physicians or hospitals may jointly own such entities, or other parties may also own solely these free-standing surgical centers. Many ASCs provide administrative support services to affiliated physicians and mid-level providers but generally do not employ physicians because of the corporate practice of medicine statutes that exist in many states.

On March 23, 2010, the Affordable Care Act (ACA) was signed into law. This law formalized a federally mandated approach to managed care by providing a series of healthcare policy changes. One part of that act was to create an additional managed care entity called Accountable Care Organizations. While initially ACA envisioned this organization to be a group of primary care physicians who could accept financial risk on a group of Medicare beneficiaries, the non-Medicare managed care market has begun to develop its own means of defining organizations capable of providing accountable care. In many cases, some form of shared financial risk with the provider community, in the form of risk pools and/or bonus pools, is being developed as of this writing. While there have been legal challenges to the constitutionality of the ACA, the law may well redefine how providers "manage" patient care in the future.

MOTIVATION TO CONTRACT FOR MANAGED CARE

An analysis of the underlying reasons why and with what parameters a medical group would consider contracting with the MCOs in their market can be an insightful exercise for the group before considering any health plan's specific programs. Connected with this analysis is the necessity for the group's management team to revisit their overall goals and objectives. By focusing on the strategic direction of the organization, the medical group will be able to ascertain whether entry into managed care corresponds with or runs contrary to the expressed directions that the organization desires to pursue.

While the scrutiny of a medical group's individual goals and objectives will be unique for each group and each market, there are certain common goals with which many medical groups ascribe that can serve as a checklist to compare motivations for entering the managed care environment. These motivations are summarized below in question form. Each group should be introspective and consider the following questions: Do we want to . . .

- Maintain our market share? Will we risk losing patients on the whole if we do not "lock in" programs like HMOs? Are we currently experiencing declining patient registrations? Do employers in our community consider traditional indemnity programs (like Blue Cross) too expensive? Is the population declining in our area?
- Increase our share of the market? Do we have an opportunity to preempt other providers by being the "first" to accept full-risk arrangements? Could our medical group become an exclusive or preferred provider for a major MCO, employer, or union? Is the population growing in our area? Is there an opportunity to expand the medical practice in our geographic base?

▪ Change our patient mix? Have we had difficulty attracting particular age groups or individuals within our service area because we currently do not contract with their insuring parties? Do we offer a service that is underutilized?

▪ Decrease our collection period? Have we had problems collecting from current patients? Is our accounts receivable volume too large? Is our cost of collection activities excessive?

▪ Retain our FFS reimbursement system, perhaps through a PPO arrangement? Is the medical group prepared to assume the insurance risk for patient care under capitation arrangements? Are MCOs attracting patients away from our group at an increasing rate? Have we had an unfavorable experience with an MCO?

▪ Follow the leader? Have the medical group's competitors become involved in these programs? Have colleagues from other geographic areas encouraged our participation? Have physicians who normally refer patients to us enrolled in these programs?

▪ Risk a negative impact on physician compensation levels as a result of managed care participation? Will the medical group have to develop and implement new physician compensation systems? Would the medical group slowly splinter and potentially dissolve if decreasing medical revenue amounts yield lower physician compensation?

Another introspective exercise deals with assessing the overall impact if the group decides to enter into a managed care contract. Again, this analysis can uncover potential changes in the business and clinical routines of the practice that may be contrary to the ultimate desires of the physicians and governing group of the organization, or they may reveal modifications to those customs with which all can cope.

The movement toward managed care systems has made a profound impact on the standards by which providers conduct their practices. The following list of five principal areas where the impact is most significant elaborates on the writing of Aaron and Breindel.[11] The areas affected are:

▪ Access to managed care networks
▪ Practice size and structure
▪ Price competition
▪ Product differentiation
▪ Information systems

Access to Managed Care Networks

Access to managed care networks refers to the avenues through which a medical group offers its services. In order to contain costs, managed care systems restrict to varying degrees the patient's choice of provider to those physicians who have a contractual relationship with the managed care plan. Thus, in many markets, providers might be somewhat restricted to distributing their services primarily through individual managed care plans, and patients might not necessarily have access, at the same economic level, to all desired providers. Because of these potential circumstances, the establishment of ongoing, productive relationships with managed care plans is important to the successful operation and growth of a group practice.

Practice Size and Structure

Large group practices seem better positioned to compete successfully in the managed care market because of their bargaining power with individual managed care plans. Larger practices often have this edge because of their productivity potential and their enhanced ability to support sophisticated utilization review and control mechanisms (which are attractive to managed care plans). Also, larger group practices tend to have more means to build and support a superior degree of professional administration and financial management, including employee specialization and talent. Such management talent coupled with an enterprise-wide, systematic approach to allocating the appropriate time to negotiating and performing due diligence typically facilitates the most attractive managed care agreements. Finally, a large practice can support a wider range of medical services — a feature that managed care plans can promote in their marketing to potential subscribers.

Price Competition

Price has become one of the principal determinants that managed care plans use to make decisions on the medical practices they include in their networks. The increasing importance of price competition impacts financial managers because of the dire need for an effective and accurate cost accounting system.

The effects of price competition for practice services are principally understood in the context of the group's cost accounting system. Financial managers need to be able to quickly determine the exact cost of at least 10 the most frequently delivered services by the practice so the organization can effectively negotiate managed care contracts. Without this knowledge and expertise, there is the potential for the group to either price itself out of the market or price its services so low that the medical practice becomes unprofitable.

Product Differentiation

Product differentiation means that a group practice has the ability to distinguish its services from those of its competitors. In the past, medical group services were relatively undifferentiated, but in a managed care environment, product differentiation can be a useful growth strategy. Groups that are able to differentiate their types of services will be in a better position to negotiate with managed care plans than groups that compete on price exclusively. If a physician group's services are truly unique, or if the group can quantify superior quality and patient satisfaction, it may be possible to convince the MCO that the plan's product will be enhanced by using the group's team of physicians. In so doing, the managed care plan can be likewise differentiated from other competing plans and will attract more subscribers. There are several ways that medical groups can differentiate their practice. Patient satisfaction surveys, hospitalist programs to coordinate inpatient care, urgent care centers, call centers, and demand management activities are some of the more prevalent examples. Another differentiating technique is based on the reputation of superior quality or extremely specialized expertise. The Mayo Clinic, now operating in Minnesota, Arizona, and Florida, presents a great illustration of this approach because of their long-standing reputation of quality care and superior service.

Information Systems

Medical groups need sophisticated and powerful information systems capable of compiling and using extensive amounts of clinical, financial, and operational data. The financial risk associated with providing medical services in a managed care environment can only be managed effectively through the use of sophisticated information systems that are able to track detailed patient histories, the scope of treatment provided, and the underlying costs for each patient-care episode. Other core tasks of an effective information system include additional cost accounting functions, patient eligibility, referral tracking, monitoring actual costs per referred specialist, diagnosis management (e.g., identifying the top 10 ICD-9 or CPT codes used in the practice), claims adjudication, total chronic care cost analysis, and the calculation and examination of incurred but not reported (IBNR) subaccounts.

As stated previously, one of the primary thrusts of successfully administering managed care contracts rests on the physician organization's utilization review and control processes and disease management functions, all enabled or hindered by the medical group's information systems. To be successful in these activities, utilization review and disease management programs require comprehensive and timely information about the procedures, treatments, and other clinical details of the services provided. Generally, medical groups that have information systems with the capability to capture this type of utilization information in an expedient and interpretative manner are more attractive to potential contracting partners than those groups that make little effort in this area. Information systems were discussed in more detail in chapter 4.

ASSUMING RISK

The traditional FFS environment represents, assuming appropriate collection processes, a minimal amount of financial risk to the medical group for providing their services. In other words, providers under an FFS system mainly face the financial risk of not pricing clinical episodes of care in line with market demand. However, the managed care environment introduces many different levels of financial risk for medical groups to consider. The nature of this complexity and the notion of transferring the risk associated with pricing future, unresolved states of medical demand to provider entities requires savvy decision making on the part of providers. The authors recommend the use of actuarial consultants and other professional resources when attempting to sort through the various risk arrangements MCOs bring to the negotiating table.

Within managed care models, there are generally three levels of financial risk that can be assumed by a medical group. Representing a low level of financial risk is the concept of "risk sharing" where medical groups get paid discounted FFS equivalent rates for services provided to subscribers of a health plan. The possible loss from this risk level generally results from the medical group potentially realizing only a limited increase in patient influx from a managed care plan and/or no significant acceleration of (i.e., advance) payments for services. The group must decide if it is willing to trade discounting its charges for potential volume, or in some cases, to maintain and protect an existing patient base. Groups may find it helpful to design several flexible budgets to aid this type of decision making so that the decision process is based on the actual variance in the practices' historical expense data related to claims submission and time to payment as opposed to merely accepting the deal. Flexible budgets are discussed in more depth in chapter 11.

Related to the risk sharing or the "managed care lite" model is a contractual agreement based on some percentage, usually above 100 percent, of the RBRVS RVU reimbursement allowable plus the potential for a bonus based on measures of successful performance. For example, if the medical group meets certain utilization targets established mutually by the group and the contracted health plan, additional rewards, bonuses, or surpluses may be allocated to the group. The only additional risk to the medical practice is to not "earn" the reward (assuming the contractual RVU reimbursement rates cover all practice overhead and physician compensation).

At an intermediate degree of financial risk, the MCO's contract provisions might involve the establishment of a withhold fund or risk pool. Created by diverting a portion of the group's reimbursement amounts (20 to 25 percent) — generally related to the projected level of subscriber utilization of medical services — into an account controlled by the MCO, these amounts may be returned to the medical group pending the actual utilization of medical services below a specified level for a given time period, then the group and the managed care entity will share in an agreed-upon percentage of the risk pool funds. If patient utilization rates are above the specified level, the group will share little or no amount from the pool of funds and, thus, potentially stands to collect less than its customary discounted FFS amount. In some contracts, the group may even be at risk for a portion of the deficit arising from an established budget.

A third level of risk, and the most detrimental if not managed appropriately, exists when a medical group is paid a predetermined capitation (per capita) rate regardless of the utilization of medical services. As previously discussed, capitated payment systems involve arrangements between an MCO and providers under which the providers are paid an actuarially calculated per-person payment to deliver a specific menu of services to a defined population over a given period of time, regardless of the actual demand for services by individual patients. In this scenario, most, if not all, of the financial risk of providing protection from future, costly professional services rendered to a health plan's members, before those events become certain, is shifted to the medical group. In other words, medical groups contract to offer certain medical services to health plan enrollees that they may not be able to entirely supply themselves, and for which they have to assume financial responsibility for the demand of these services in the future and their price.

To allow access to the most appropriate specialists for their patient population, medical groups with full professional risk may enter into additional contracts on an FFS or subcontracted basis with specialty groups to perform these services. In essence, the same levels of risk assumed by the primary capitation contractor may then be levied on a select number of specialists as subspecialty capitation agreements. Carve-outs are another measure that primary capitation contracting medical groups use to help curtail potential losses from more costly medical services. During the negotiating process, medical groups might decide to exclude or "carve out" certain higher-risk services (e.g., mental health, pharmacy, cardiology, oncology, orthopedics, etc.) in their contract with the MCO rather than accepting that risk directly and then repackaging it to other providers. The authors generally caution that only the most sophisticated provider organizations should enter into capitation arrangements inclusive of pharmacy risk. The substantial information systems required to identify inappropriate utilization and the high costs associated with inventorying new drugs and direct-to-consumer advertising, which entails more provider time to research and explain the efficacy of certain drugs, have all but made pharmacy risk the domain of mature and sophisticated provider organizations.

Contracting for carve-out capitation describes the situation in which an MCO contracts with various specialty providers to deliver designated specialty care required by enrollee populations. Tantamount to carve-out capitation, contracting only for chronic care capitation presents highly focused medical groups with some exciting opportunities if the organization has appropriately developed and positioned its people, processes, planning, and technology. In this circumstance, specialty providers contract with an MCO to deliver designated specialty care required by a subset of enrollees identified as having chronic conditions (e.g., AIDS, congestive heart failure, asthma). In both cases, reimbursement is based on a capitated rate with the specialty providers. A carve-out or chronic care capitation rate is generally a single price for an entire episode of acute or post-acute services including surgery, facility, ancillary providers, and consulting physicians. To develop this single payment, a detailed analysis of the cost incurred by each provider in the continuum is broken down by CPT code for assessment by the health plan and the contracting medical group. Once assessed, the medical group must decide if the potential financial benefits outweigh the risk exposure of the group. The main benefits of accepting carve-out or chronic care capitation include its potential for more accurate and predictable expenditure projections for costly medical services and more closely aligning the incentives of specialty providers with those of the payer.

In a manner similar to accepting physician services capitation or specialty carve-out risk, medical groups accepting global capitation contracts are obviously exposed to the greatest amount of financial risk due to the scope of medical services, both inpatient and outpatient, covered under the terms of the contract. Global capitation refers to the payment made to a provider entity in exchange for arranging for all covered services by an enrolled population. If actual utilization rates and expenses exceed those anticipated in the development of the contracted global capitation rate, the "true" cost of medical services will exceed the capitation revenue received, and the medical group will be the only party responsible for the loss. Medical groups without exceedingly strong capital reserves should consider this possibility very seriously when evaluating any variety of global capitation agreements.

MANAGED CARE STRATEGY DEVELOPMENT

In the previous sections we defined the basic concepts of managed care, compared these with an FFS market orientation, and described some of the possible risk arrangements medical groups might encounter in the marketplace. Before we introduce the typical components of a managed care contract, directing one's attention to how a medical group develops a managed care strategy plays a paramount role in a contract's development. Determining the medical group's overall managed care strategy will greatly aid the evaluation of present and future contracts and will give the group a platform of information from which to identify its best alternative to a negotiated agreement or "BATNA" positions. Not all inclusive, but still considered a substantial baseline from which to frame decisions involving managed care strategies and participation objectives, the medical group's management and negotiating team should be clear on the following criteria:

- Establishment of acceptable risk limits and reimbursement methods
- Understanding of minimum data and information system requirements, such as financial systems, marketing systems, medical management systems, and so on to successfully administer managed care agreements
- Identification of key members of the medical group and designating them as principal representatives of the practice to discuss and negotiate an affiliation with managed care entities
- Selection of the minimum and maximum parameters related to administrative requirements such as capital expenditures, administrative costs, staffing, and so on that will be useful in evaluating various types of managed care contracts
- Understanding of the typical risk arrangements offered in the organization's geographic service area (i.e., how the different contracts operate and the general financial considerations at stake)
- Determination of time frames for all financial accountings and fund settlements

The chosen criteria should address all elements of managed care contracting that are important interfaces with any aspect of the medical group. Again, it is important that these determinations be made before reviewing and negotiating the actual agreement with the health plan's representatives. The criteria should also convey a timetable for actions to be taken so that the assigned negotiation team can develop a judicious approach to the search for the most suitable MCOs with which to affiliate.

NEGOTIATING MANAGED CARE CONTRACTS

Negotiating a successful managed care contract requires first and foremost that medical groups have invested an adequate amount of time and resources in preparation for the process of actually composing the deal as discussed in the previous section. Items such as understanding the local and national managed care environment, identifying the group's ideal contracting positions and next best alternatives on sensitive issues, determining the full costs associated with each unit of service the medical group renders, and assembling a skillful team of negotiators who look out for the best interests of the medical group all contribute significantly in the development of an attractive agreement.

Before any face-to-face negotiations take place between the medical group and the health plan, the medical group should select its negotiation team. Generally, the team should be composed of the group administrator and/or financial manager, the information systems manager, the medical director, the utilization manager or nursing supervisor, the group's attorney, and any other important outside professionals such as accountants, consultants, or actuaries that the group may desire present. The best advice that this team can receive is to be prepared to deal with all aspects of managed care contracting and to have thoroughly discussed the group's desired positions and deal breakers on all-important issues of the contract. The group's negotiators must keep in mind that the contract, although it may be only for a year or so, is likely to evolve into a long-term relationship. Its provisions will have a profound impact on the overall operations and financial viability of the medical practice.

When entering into the contracting process, the medical group will likely be presented with a standard participation agreement. Physicians and the contract team must understand that this initial contract prepared by the managed care entity will be favorable to that entity's interests at the expense of the medical group. Some agreements may be more biased than others, so negotiating a fair agreement may be difficult under any circumstances. In most cases, though, an agreement can be modified to provide more equitable terms between the parties. Most contracts then need to be tailored to the objectives and desired ends of the medical group. Negotiators should prepare for the following issues:

- Even though the initial contract offered by the managed care entity is favorable, the entity will entertain some changes to this document. The group must not assume that the "standard form agreement" presented cannot be changed. If the entity is inflexible, this will most likely not bode well for a successful future relationship. On the other hand, if the insurer is open to changing its standard agreement, most medical groups will not have the bargaining presence or position (either in numbers or position in the marketplace) to fashion a wholesale revision of the original contract. In general, the group must accept the premise that the contract provisions will remain as proposed unless it can present a convincing case for changing them.

■ Before negotiations begin, the medical group should have determined whether it has the capacity to render the desired services and the parameters of "give and take" they may have in adjusting this capacity estimate. Also, the group team should have an understanding, agreed to by the governing body and a majority of the physicians, as to the price range that will be acceptable to the group.

■ The medical group should have investigated the MCO. While a full-scale investigation is not practical, the medical group should undertake an inquiry about the entity's operations and style of conducting business, its financial soundness, and its compliance with state law. At the very minimum, the MCO's latest financial statements should be reviewed. Contacting the state's department of insurance can also provide information about the financial operations of the entity. In addition, references from other providers and administrators from those organizations that are, or were, part of the managed care system should be obtained.

■ The medical group should identify those provisions that must be changed in order to accommodate the needs and goals of the medical group. The strategy for approaching the discussion of making these changes should be developed prior to any meetings. And the team should have not only carefully considered its position on these areas decided but also determined a "fall back" position.

MANAGED CARE CONTRACT PROVISIONS AND APPLICABLE COST CONTROL MECHANISMS

The development and negotiation of satisfactory managed care contracts are rapidly becoming two of the most tactical decisions made by the medical group. Group management must therefore become thoroughly familiar with all aspects of sound contracting procedure and terminology to meet its objectives and long-term aspirations.

Every contract presented to a medical group, whether from an HMO, PPO, POS, or other health plan, or directly from an employer, will contain certain similar provisions and conditions. While the specifics of each agreement section will vary by payer, all medical group contracts with the various permutations of managed care entities will address many of the same subjects and will generally spell out the rights, responsibilities, and due process of each party involved. The following sections introduce and define typical contractual terms and provisions. Each subsection includes information on cost control issues. These include:

■ Type of contract: individual or group

■ Services the medical group must render to plan members

- ▩ Geographic service area
- ▩ Reimbursement rates and payment calculations
- ▩ Payment method and billing procedures
- ▩ Provider network inclusive of all participants
- ▩ Risk pools and bonuses
- ▩ Utilization review and care coordination requirements
- ▩ Provider profiling
- ▩ Referral restrictions
- ▩ Professional liability insurance issues
- ▩ Reporting requirements for each party
- ▩ Renewal and termination of the contract
- ▩ Exclusivity and assignment clauses
- ▩ Other provisions

Individual versus Group Contract

With an individual contract, the MCO contracts with a group of physicians on an individual physician basis. Each physician is credentialed separately and signs the contract with the MCO as an independent party. However, group contracts are the preferred format by many organizations. In this situation, the MCO contracts with the entire group of physicians as a single business entity, which allows for one signature, usually by the practice administrator or another senior management staff member serving as the officially authorized representative for the group, should the agreement need amendment, renewal, or termination. With a group contract, the doctors are listed as providers in the contract but do not have to individually sign the agreement. The principal advantage of a group contract is that it creates a single contracting voice and strategy for the medical group throughout both the negotiation process and the effective contract period, provided the authorized representatives have the full support of the medical director and other important physicians when acting on the medical group's behalf. Additionally, if a physician leaves the medical group during the contract period, the contract generally does not terminate. Should a new physician join the practice during the contract period, that individual's name is simply added to the existing contract, typically without any signature, consent, or other execution measure by the new physician. However, most health plans will require credentialing of the new physician under any circumstances.

Services the Medical Group Must Render to Plan Members

This basic provision should first list a detailed account of the services the medical group will provide under the contract, called a responsibility matrix. The responsibility matrix delineates who is responsible for delivering care and the degree of care assumed by the provider group. It is important when the group agrees to provide a stated range of medical services that they understand what the reimbursement rates are for each of those services so any capitation payments can be appropriately split between specialty and primary care. Without a clear definition of the medical services the group's physicians will provide and which services will be provided by others in the network, the group may hold itself open for additional liability if the managed care entity makes poor choices in the assignment of care responsibility. To help track the full cost of medical services appropriately, the medical groups should insist on a definition of the services to be rendered by CPT code and the place of service. This level of specificity will allow the medical group to track all expenses based on claims data and makes clear to both contracting partners which specific treatments and medical services will be covered by the health plan.

A second aspect of this provision relates to specifying whether the medical group must provide care to only a designated number of patients or be available to all patients who visit the practice. The medical group could lose control of its patient panel if it does not have the right to notify the managed care entity that it no longer has the capacity to accept new patients. The third element of the services provision pertains to the functional meaning of the phrase "to provide care of the highest quality" if this condition is in the contract. A clause that requires the medical group to provide services under a different standard of care than otherwise stipulated by state law or local standards can open the group up to additional malpractice risks. Physicians should only be held to that level of professional service that is in accordance with local standards or set by law.

Geographic Service Area

Medical groups should give critical consideration to accurately and completely identifying the service area in which the medical group must provide or arrange for medical services. This is particularly important in capitation contracts where the medical group must make arrangements for care in a variety of different counties. Having patients in a metropolitan area or community not serviced by the medical group can lead to excessive treatment and referral expenses, especially if the plan members tend to use urgent care services at a higher-than-average rate.

Reimbursement Rates and Payment Calculations

The price paid for medical services rendered under the managed care agreement is one of the greatest concerns to a medical group. In general, there are two types of fees and payments for services with variations fashioned to suit the parties involved: discounted FFS or capitation arrangements.

Discounted FFS basis: Under this reimbursement methodology, a discount is applied to the physician's charges, with the contract stating whether the discount applies to the customary charge schedule of the physician group or to a standardized charge that may be based on a community-related charge schedule. It also should specify the method for determining maximum charges so that the managed care entity may not impose unilaterally the maximum charge limit. In other instances, the discounted FFS reimbursement amount will be based on a fixed rate for the service rendered. Here, the medical group should compare these fixed charges to the charge schedule currently in effect with the group to determine its aggregate impact. Often, the discounted FFS payment is based on either the *Federal Register* resource-based relative value scale (RBRVS) or St. Anthony Publishing's *Relative Values for Physicians*. In this scenario, the payments do not necessarily follow the full amount as determined by those scales but represent some percentage thereof.

Capitation: A more sophisticated approach to managing medical service demand, as previously discussed, capitation reimbursement methodologies require that the medical group provide a stated range of services for a fixed price per month. Because the per-capita reimbursement rate does not vary given the scope, intensity, or frequency of the services rendered, the financial risks assumed by the medical group are much greater in capitation agreements than in discounted FFS arrangements. In addition, capitation arrangements may lead to further financial risk if the scope of services covered under the contract requires the medical group to refer patients outside of the practice. The group will be required to pay for the services rendered by other medical specialties. To the extent that the referral physician is not under an appropriate risk-bearing contract with the medical group holding the agreement with the MCO, the medical group will pay the referral physician on a FFS basis out of the fixed capitation payment it receives. This represents an enormous potential risk for the medical group.

To mitigate some of this potential risk, medical groups should develop and employ sophisticated IBNR accounting methodologies to assess and understand the complete scope of costs associated with delivering each and every contracted service to the enrolled population. The objective of IBNR accounts is to project and quantify future financial liabilities. These future liabilities are potential medical expenses for authorized referrals that the system has not captured, and for which claims have not yet been received. The financial insolvency of some medical groups has resulted from underfunding or not utilizing IBNR accounts. Generally, IBNR amounts should be "booked" at the individual patient level but monitored at the aggregate level to assess the group's proficiency in this area. One note of caution to the reader, however: Over-allocating funds to various IBNR accounts can prove just as severe as under-allocating since these funds can't be used to support ongoing expenses or investment activities. Maintaining adequate cash flows is extremely important for medical groups, so these accounts should be monitored closely. Lines of credit from reliable lending institutions provide medical groups another measure to smooth out cash flows and protect against unforeseen circumstances that lead to higher-than-expected costs per plan member.

The manner in which the capitation amount is expressed in the agreement needs careful consideration. The group should insist on payment amounts adjusted for age and sex considerations in the membership. Such payment adjustments should be determined or verified by an independent actuary prior to contract executive. This age/sex breakout is vital because the medical group assumes the additional actuarial risk that the age and sex of the health plan enrollees will match the projections of the managed care entity throughout the agreement term when accepting a payment expressed as a single PMPM figure.

Obviously, when a capitation arrangement is the methodology selected by the MCO and medical group, the calculation of the actual reimbursement rates is a key ingredient of the contract for both parties. The steps that a medical group should take to develop this rate will be described in some detail in a later section of this chapter.

Payment Method and Billing Procedures

The timing of payments to the medical group is also an important aspect of the agreement. As stated previously, one of the prime benefits of a managed care contract for a medical group is the certainty and projected increased speed of payments for the service providers delivering to health plan members. Frequently, contracts will contain maximum flexibility concerning time of payment by the purchaser. Medical groups should resist leaving the payment terms open. For services based on a discounted FFS basis, the managed care entity should agree to provide payment shortly after the statement is received. For capitated agreements, contracting experts recommend that the PMPM fees should be paid based on the number of members assigned to the physicians as of the 15th of the month in which services may be rendered, rather than the contracting standard — the first day of each month. Health plan beneficiaries do not magically change employment or select new health plans or new primary care physicians on the first of every month; thus, there's never a "true" snapshot. The mid-month payment alternative affords a more rational and fair way to facilitate the leveling of membership counts over the length of the contract. Should an assigned member leave after the 15th, the provider retains the whole month's PMPM amount; if the member becomes eligible after the 15th, the health plan keeps the premium, but the situation is much more likely to result in a wash that way. As a further refinement in the payment process, medical groups may seek a reconciliation of the estimated membership to actual head counts as of the 15th of the following month, and the payment amount would be adjusted appropriately.

Good negotiators will also seek to include a provision to apply an interest charge or penalty to delinquent payments; otherwise, the MCO will have little incentive for making timely payments, and the only recourse the medical group ultimately may have will be to sever the relationship. Recently though, many states, and now the federal government, have attempted to pass legislation requiring the prompt payment of outstanding amounts by health plans with varying degrees of effectiveness.

Another important aspect of capitation payments is determining for which patients the medical group is clinically obligated to provide healthcare services. Often overlooked is this specific designation of who is on the member list and who is to be added or deleted. All patients who present themselves for care at the medical group should be accurately identified so that the appropriate services can be provided to plan subscribers and so that payment arrangements (including collection of copayments or deductibles) can be made before the patient leaves the office. Without a current member list, the medical group will lose the opportunity to make other payment arrangements for patients who are no longer covered under the managed care agreement. Old or inaccurate eligibility lists can lead to rendering care to individuals who have no coverage at all and have to be billed after the services are provided. Bad debts can rise dramatically in these instances. Also, there should be provisions that limit the MCO to retroactively add or delete patients from its list of subscribers. Usually, judicious and efficient preregistration processes avoid such potential billing problems.

Medical groups should determine what billing requirements must be met to allow for accurate processing and payment of claims. Usually defined as a "clean claim," medical groups often underestimate the complex systems and brainstorming required to ensure accuracy of claims processing and payment in managed care arrangements. Frequently, agreements are vague in this area, and this could lead to a delay in having the claims satisfied. Thus, specific billing instructions and conditions should be carefully delineated within the contract's language.

Provider Network

The composition of the group physicians, other outside groups or specialists, and other servicing entities, such as hospitals and laboratories, that when combined form the total pool of care providers, needs to be identified in this area of the agreement. In a managed care network, PCPs generally operate as gatekeepers, and each enrollee is required to choose a PCP who coordinates the individual's care. In the provider network, there must be sufficient PCPs to allow reasonable access to a physician for routine and urgent visits.

In addition, most managed care networks include contracted physicians in as many specialties as possible. Normally, in provider arrangements, the health plan itself will hold contracts in rare specialties so that the network can be approved by the state regulatory agency to cover a wide spectrum of healthcare needs, but the network is expected to be able to deliver services in all routine specialties.

Risk Pools and Bonuses

As discussed earlier, a risk pool allows the managed care entity to retain a certain percentage of the payment due to the medical group, which will be remitted to the group only if certain financial and patient care projections are met. The contract should state the amount to be withheld and the basis upon which this fund will be remitted to the group or retained by the managed care entity. In many instances, this provision will be vaguely expressed in the agreement. The medical group also must determine whether the risk pool remission is based on the performance of the group's practice alone, on physicians in the same specialty, or on all network physicians in general. Another factor the medical group must ascertain is if the risk pool remissions would be affected by hospital and/or pharmacy costs. The broader the financial risk is spread among healthcare providers, the more an individual medical group will be at risk for actions that are beyond its control.

The magnitude of the risk pool depends on the behavior of the providers during the period of time when the risk pool was active. Correlating physician compensation with payments out of risk pool payments is an effective means to influence provider behavior. The time allotted for remitting withheld amounts should be specified in the contract. It is desirable to require that these fund transfers be made within 30 to 60 days after the conclusion of the operating year of the plan. Without this requirement, the medical group is allowing the managed care entity to have an interest-free loan at the expense of the group. Some groups negotiate interest accrual on surpluses during the contract term, but this could be a two-way street in the event of deficits.

A corollary concept to risk pools is a bonus pool. This takes the form of contract provisions promising benefits to physicians based on the overall operation of the managed care plan for the year. Frequently, this incentive is touted as the major benefit for participation. In a sense, the objective is sound in that, as the managed care entity succeeds, the physicians and the group also profit. However, in many agreements, determining the nature and calculation of the bonus pool is difficult because of the vagueness of the terms and the lack of specificity in the derivation of the bonus amount. The contract should call for frequent and verifiable data from the MCO.

Utilization Review

Also, as discussed earlier, a utilization review describes the set of techniques used by healthcare professionals, insurance companies, and the government to evaluate the necessity, appropriateness, and efficiency of care. At its core, the utilization review process seeks to eliminate the duplication of medical services and inappropriate utilization. In most contracts, the physician and/or medical group is required to participate in a utilization review program and quality assurance activities and to abide by the terms, conditions, and operations of such programs. Even participation is a necessity. The medical group must not blindly agree to the utilization review measures and quality assurance activities suggested by the managed care entity. In many instances, the managed care agreement will require participation but not provide details on how such programs will be implemented. There should be some agreement and detailed illustrations of the procedures the medical group will be obligated to follow, and of the physicians' responsibilities to comply with the intentions of the program. Much of this information is embedded in the "physician manual" that is considered part of the contract.

It is important that the group's physicians be involved in the approval process of any utilization review activities outlined in the contract, and that the physician manual and any other supporting documentation referred to in the contract also be reviewed in advance of contract execution. Furthermore, medical groups should seek a contract clause that enables the group to observe the utilization review programs and quality assurance activities currently undertaken by other contracted physicians to ensure that they are consistent with the standards of care rendered by the group.

Provider Profiling

As an alternative to or in conjunction with utilization review, some large insurers now present clinical and coordination of care profiling data to providers who contract with them. Developing a provider profiling system requires the incorporation of many assumptions. Therefore, the medical group should ask the following questions, both to gain sufficient understanding of the data and to protect its own interests as much as possible:

- What is being profiled?
- What assumptions were included in the profiling analysis?
- Do they fit the physicians' practice style?
- Will the insurance share complete data with the physicians? (Medical groups should insist on this.)
- Against whom or what was the physician profiled? (Medical groups should insist on being compared to similar practices in the same geographic region.)
- What are the objectives of the insurance profiling system?
- How will this data be used?
- What can individual physicians do to make sure that their compensation will not decrease?
- What is the insurance company's position, both official and perceived, on saving money at the cost of decreasing quality of care?
- What mechanisms are open to the medical group to dispute the data?

(Provider profiling is discussed in more detail in chapter 12.)

Referral Restrictions

As mentioned earlier, the managed care contract will indicate the makeup of the provider team for plan subscribers. In addition, a provision must also state under what conditions patients may be referred to a member of the network and the procedures to effect such referrals. From a quality and coordination of care viewpoint, physicians in the medical group must be satisfied that referral providers meet their standards. In certain groups, a physician/facility referral panel may be established to evaluate the quality of care provided by network members, with the results of their evaluations being part of the process used to make referrals by group physicians. Without some assurance on referral quality, the group may be increasing its professional liability risk with an inappropriate referral that they may be obligated to make because of required treatment protocols.

Regardless of the contractual arrangements on referral restrictions, excessive referral patterns eventually will result in dissatisfaction and contractual rate increases. As a protection, the medical group may employ a number of procedural changes within their operations to curtail excessive referral costs. These are:

- Assign each patient to a primary care physician who is the required gatekeeper for access to other services.
- Require written authorization for referrals within and outside of the medical group.
- Restrict the requested range of services and limit the number of visits to an appropriate number, given the apparent diagnosis.
- Require that all tests be done within the medical group, if possible.
- Limit the time during which a consult must be completed, including arranging appointments.
- Prohibit the use of secondary referrals (that is, the first specialist cannot refer to a second specialist without the approval of the medical director).
- Require a written report from the specialist on the final status and history of the referred case (often this must be received before payment is made).

Professional Liability Insurance Issues

A standard contract provision involves the participating physicians having adequate malpractice liability insurance for the care they render. A physician who has limited or no insurance invites malpractice suits and exposes the entire medical group and managed care entity to being parties of these legal encounters. Medical groups should be expected to provide this insurance.

The managed care agreement, however, should not give the managed care entity too much discretion in determining the professional liability insurance carrier or the amount of coverage required. Also, MCOs should not be allowed to require an increase in the amount of professional liability insurance carried by the medical group or be permitted to name itself as an additional insured on the policy of the medical group. While adding the managed care organization as an additional insured is sometimes possible, pursuing such a measure is usually not a desirable option. The "hold harmless" discussion that follows provides additional useful tips that the medical group should carefully consider regarding "indemnification" of the payer by the provider.

Reporting Requirements

Managing plan operations centers around the use of appropriate data about the care rendered to plan members. Thus, the contract should spell out the types of data and reports the medical group must submit to the managed care entity and the timing for submitting such information. The content, timing, and frequency of the reports are critical and may be enforced with meaningful penalty clauses. However, the medical group should avoid giving the managed care entity full access to the financial records of the group. Similarly, certain information about health plan results is useful to the management of the medical group, and these information components should be provided by the managed care entity on an agreed-upon regular schedule. For example, it is important to review the financial stability of the health plan at least on a quarterly basis. This information will help the medical group's management review the results of the contract and assist them in deciding on a renewal of the agreement.

Renewal and Termination Clauses

Managed care agreements have a specified term during which they will be in effect. Generally, the shorter the time period, the less risk a group assumes. One-year terms are appropriate for most managed care arrangements. These agreements will often automatically be renewed unless action is taken by one of the parties to do otherwise prior to the renewal date. Management should closely note the renewal notification date so that the agreement will not automatically renew without their knowledge.

The contract also should state the conditions and reasons why either party may terminate the agreement prior to the indicated expiration date. The conditions for termination should be fairly specific and not leave interpretations up to either party's personal judgment. For example, a standard reason for the medical group to terminate the contract would be if the managed care entity failed to meet its responsibilities and obligations stipulated in the agreement. Specific references should be made to the group's right to terminate if the managed care entity fails to make prompt payments to the medical group.

Once either party has decided on termination, a provision should address the relationship in three aspects:

1. **Handling patients' medical records.** The agreement probably will contain clauses that specify under what circumstances and by what means the attending medical group should transfer a patient's records to a provider. Because of the extensive work that photocopying this information entails, the agreement should indicate that the medical group should bear no cost for this effort or that it be provided a reasonable payment for this service.

2. **Treatment of patients hospitalized at termination date.** In this case, the group should agree to a continuation of payments under the terms equal to or exceeding the original contract.

3. **Fate of existing patients.** Obviously, the medical group will want to terminate its relationship with these patients under the managed care plan as soon as possible. On the other hand, the managed care entity will want to continue this relationship for particular patients until the anniversary date of the employer-sponsored plan under which the individual patients received coverage. At the very least, the agreement should provide that the managed care entity will not assign new patients to the medical group from a particular employer; that it will reassign all patients as quickly as possible; and that, in any event, the obligation to continue treatment for any particular patient will cease upon the first anniversary date that occurs for that patient's group policy.

Exclusivity and Assignment Clauses

Exclusive arrangements can be beneficial for the medical group when the MCO is exclusive to them for providing care to all the MCO's patients in the area. However, caution should be exercised in allowing for a mutual exclusivity provision where the medical group cannot contract with another MCO.

Assignment: If the medical group or MCO wants to assign their contract to another entity, the language should allow for approval or consent by both parties. In the event of a merger of two HMOs, for example, the medical group should include language that allows for the reimbursement rates to proceed at the higher of the merged companies.

Other Provisions

In addition to the specific areas covered above, there are several other topics that deserve some comment when considering the overall managed care contract. Each of these topics will be briefly mentioned below.

Hold harmless provisions: These clauses require the medical group to reimburse the managed care entity for any costs, expenses, and liabilities incurred by the entity because of any actions or alleged actions by the medical group. Known as "liabilities assumed by contract," they jeopardize the coverage of the medical group's professional liability insurance. When a group agrees to this type of provision, it often does so without the benefit of reimbursement coverage from its professional liability policy, thereby requiring the group to underwrite these expenses itself. Generally, medical groups should stay away from this particular provision due to the potentially high expenses that the group could incur. However, if the group finds itself in the unpleasant position where it faces accepting such a provision or risking the potential dissolution of the practice, expert advice needs to be sought from the group's legal counsel prior to acceptance.

Compliance with rules, regulations, and procedures: Often, managed care agreements contain general statements that the medical group agrees to abide by all rules, regulations, and procedures established by the managed care entity now or in the future. Groups should avoid this open-ended provision because it obligates them to unforeseen actions and contingencies. The preferred approach is to require that these matters be submitted to the medical group for review before they become part of the contract. If so, appropriate documents should be attached to the contract as exhibits.

Confidentiality and access to records: If the contract specifies that the medical group must keep confidential certain information designated by the managed care entity, the group management should exercise caution. These provisions should delineate a procedure to identify information to be kept confidential. An ambiguous clause creates a risk that an inadvertent discloser will be construed as a breach of contract.

These agreements may contain permission for the managed care entity and third parties to access the medical care records of plan subscribers. The medical group should not agree to such release of information unless procedures required by state law are followed. If this contract provision is agreed to without a reference to state law requirements, the medical group will be placed in an untenable position of choosing to break the contractual obligation to disclose the information, or to breach the patient's right to privacy. Finally, the physician/group should avoid agreeing to a release of information that allows the costs of photocopying to be borne by the medical group.

Handling of disputes: The question of how to handle disputes that arise between the contractual parties needs to be addressed in the agreement. Should an independent party be designated to intervene to settle certain types of disagreements? If arbitration is included, is that the best method for settling any disputes that occur? The pros and cons of mediation, arbitration, and court action should be reviewed with the medical group's attorney. Any action should be held as close to the group's home location as possible and under the laws of the state in which the group is located.

Group termination of patients' membership: When would it be in the best interests of the medical group to initiate action to terminate a subscriber to the plan? It seems appropriate that the agreement should prescribe the conditions for the group to act in this manner. For example, the group should be allowed to discontinue patients' membership and coverage if they (a) do not pay their copayments and deductibles, (b) abuse the plan or group services, (c) do not follow medical advice, or (d) disturb or otherwise endanger group staff or patients.

Contract changes: This element was alluded to earlier but bears reiteration. Although not permitting the changing of contract provisions without prior approval of the involved parties is fundamental to contract law, a clause should be included to state this requirement per se. Alterations to the agreement should not be undertaken by either of the parties without obtaining the other party's prior consent to the change. Of importance in this regard is the ability of the managed care entity to lower the premium charged to the patient. This action should also involve the approval of the medical group. The notification period for changing the reimbursement should tie to the termination notice. In other words, if the HMO gives notice to reduce your payments in 30 days, the medical group should be allowed to terminate the contract within 30 days. This is now a standard and can be effectively negotiated with the MCO.

Finally, medical groups must be certain that managed care agreements accurately reflect their levels of understanding and are clearly delineated on the following leverage points:

- The risk the provider entity assumes
- The actual reimbursement rates and calculation methods
- Any referral obligations that would require other physicians or hospitals to provide services to beneficiaries covered under the arrangement with the contracted medical group

This completes our overview of essential contract provisions that constitute a satisfactory and sound managed care contract from the standpoint of the medical group. The authors strongly recommend the incorporation of experienced healthcare attorneys in the negotiation process to assist medical groups in their quest to participate only in those contracts that present fair and reasonable provisions and opportunities.

Other Cost-Control Measures in Managed Care

As noted above, cost management issues were addressed as part of each of the previous sections. However, other cost-control measures exist that financial managers should take the time to investigate and make part of their standard "toolbox" in a managed care environment. We will briefly outline these areas next.

Clinical practice guidelines: Practice guidelines are defined as "systematically developed statements to assist practitioner and patient decisions about appropriate healthcare for specific clinical circumstances."[12]

Although seen by many as yet another impingement of physician's autonomy, practice guidelines can be a valuable tool for cost containment. Their underlying motivation is to curtail variation and to reduce cost in patient care. Large variation in how patients are treated for the same disease status suggests that some physicians may not be fully aware of the specific effect of their treatments. Good practice guidelines are founded on evidence-based research, which means that there is sufficient clinical data to support the benefits of prescribed guidelines. However, opinions on the efficacy of the guidelines are varied. Implementation should definitely not be solely based on projected cost savings but needs to be carefully considered with the clinical staff of the practice.

Outcomes review: If the practice has a sufficient information management system, outcomes review can help decrease expenses. Careful analysis of how the treatment compares with the reported outcome (derived from patient satisfaction information from healthcare utilization data resulting from patients who received a particular treatment) can lead to surprising results that may help to allocate resources more effectively.

Continuing medical education on managed care topics: Continuing medical education (CME) is a standard piece of the professional development of the practice's physicians. As much as possible, physicians should be encouraged to attend managed care seminars and workshops to ensure that the clinical leaders of the practice fully understand the implications that managed care contracting may have on their practices' financial success, practice patterns, and clinical outcomes. However, internal education sessions (e.g., short presentations at regular staff meetings) can significantly add to the staff members' awareness of how to make the medical practice most profitable. Administrators should try to convince their leadership to attend professional education programs on a regular basis to increase their effectiveness in advising the medical group's management on managed care issues.

Regular contact with purchasers: It may seem obvious, but many group practices neglect to maintain contact with their assigned provider representative or contracting person of the MCO. Getting paid as agreed to in the contract may require careful monitoring and regular follow-up by the group's financial manager or other designated party.

ESTABLISHING A CAPITATION RATE

An essential part of evaluating the impact of capitation on the contracting medial group is to analyze carefully the projected costs of providing the healthcare services covered within the terms of the proposed contract. This type of cost analysis helps to establish for the medical group the desirability of accepting capitation amounts in exchange for the delivery of certain medical services to a health plans' enrollees with unresolved states of medical service demand. Cost analysis can also be used to evaluate the capitation proposal of an umbrella organization with which the medical group contracts, such as an MSO or IPA. Cost analysis covers certain parameters of operation — including the anticipated utilization of healthcare services based on prior experience and the fees associated with pricing clinically integrated episodes of care — within which the medical group must operate if the capitated arrangement is to be successful.

By engaging the cost analysis approach, the medical group must determine to its satisfaction that it can operate within the revenue limitations established by the health plan's cost assumptions. In other words, the medical group must conclude from the cost analysis that the capitation amounts will lead to sustainable practice growth and support desired levels of physician compensation over the duration of the agreement for the contract to be executed. Making this decision requires input from an actuary or competent financial consultant who can assist the medical group with a meticulous analysis of its existing practice patterns. The advisor(s) should inform the medical practice regarding the operational experience of other medical groups contracting with the same MCO and recommend any changes that must take place in the group's delivery processes, systems, and mechanisms to make the capitated arrangement successful.

There are at least two methods used to determine costs of services rendered by the medical group and by referrals outside the medical group. These methods are commonly referred to as (1) FFS or actuarial method and (2) cost or budgetary method. A combination of the two methods may also be used. A brief description of each method follows.

FFS Method

The FFS method projects the cost of the medical services that the medical group or referral physicians potentially could render to health plan enrollees on the basis of FFS equivalent charges of those providers for all covered services. The variables used include the anticipated frequency of medical services rendered per health plan member per year and FFS charge equivalents for those services, which are derived from the medical group's or other providers' fee schedules. If the medical group lacks good cost data or if the proposed capitation rate estimate is small in scope, this method should provide a capitation rate estimate that approaches the contribution revenue of similar FFS arrangements. To negotiate substantial capitated reimbursement arrangements, it is essential that the medical group have available monthly and year-to-date summaries of FFS charge equivalents for medical care services rendered to the MCO's members.

There are many types of data sources and key areas for data analysis that are critical in the development of FFS cost assumptions for the delivery of medical services under more sizable capitation contracts. These include Blue Cross/Blue Shield, Medicare Cost Reports, HMO Industry Profiles, and many other local and industry-based statistics resources. A preliminary step to the collection of data is the development of an outline of covered services by the MCO with separate categories for each area for which capitation cost factors are to be projected.

Determining the appropriate capitation rate for a medical service category depends on a combination of two variables: (1) frequency of utilization per member per year and (2) average cost per unit of service. A capitation cost factor, or cost PMPM, is the product of the annual frequency and average FFS charge divided by 12. Such factors must be developed for each of the service categories covered in the MCO's benefit summary. Once determined, these factors are used to develop a capitation cost schedule that can then be compared to the capitation rates offered in proposed contracts by MCOs.

Cost or Budgetary Method

There are several approaches to projecting costs in the process of developing capitation rates under this second general method. They range from a marginal or incremental cost approach to a full cost approach.

To use an incremental cost approach, the medical group must analyze its "true" incremental costs of providing services to a large number of health plan members (e.g., per 10,000 members) based on staffing requirements, supply and equipment costs, and additional facilities expenses. If the medical group's FFS revenues are sufficiently covering the costs of operation including anticipated growth and providing a desired level of profit, then something less than 100 percent of the FFS equivalent charges will be adequate to cover the incremental costs of rendering services to the MCO's members.

Another cost approach, sometimes called the budgetary method, projects the costs of medical service delivery by analyzing the anticipated demand for services and translating this demand into terms such as the number of FTE physicians or other providers required per 1,000 health plan members. Separate measures of demand are established for each provider type and specialty covered in the contract proposal. The demand measures define the staffing requirements for physicians and other healthcare personnel or facilities for the MCO's membership. The staffing requirements can be combined with an average cost per physician (including base compensation, fringe benefits, malpractice insurance premiums, education allowances, etc.) to determine the cost of physician services per 1,000 members. Additional provisions may need to be included in this analysis for the medical group's staff supporting other clinical services, such as laboratory and X-ray services. The costs for some of these factors may be determined by using a procedure analogous to the FFS-equivalent charges approach discussed above.

The key element underlying the budgetary method is the productivity level of healthcare personnel (particularly physicians) and the utilization patterns of health plan members. For example, an assumed utilization rate of three primary care physician office visits per plan member per year and an assumed provider productivity rate of 4,000 office visits per primary care physician translate into the need for one primary care physician per 1,333 prepaid members (4,000/3). This need is equivalent to .75 physicians per 1,000 members (1,000/1,333). This figure may be further split among different specialties such as family practice, pediatrics, obstetrics/gynecology, and internal medicine physicians. Depending on the medical group's delivery system for surgical specialties, productivity estimates should also consider the allocation of time to hospital as well as clinic settings.

If the capitated arrangement is slated to comprise more than 25 percent of the medical group's total patient population, a more detailed cost study should be considered for arriving at an appropriate capitation payment. This study should be designed to accurately determine the medical group's expenses associated with the delivery of healthcare services to both the FFS and capitated populations — and indeed each section of the capitated population (i.e., commercial, Medicare, and Medicaid). For an absolutely thorough cost analysis, capitation rates could be better defined in terms of these actual expenses. Such a cost study should allocate expenses on a departmental basis between the capitated patients by market sector and the FFS patient population. The allocation might be done according to the FFS equivalent of medical services rendered or according to the number of units of services rendered using a standardized relative value study. Once costs have been allocated to each department within the medical practice, the fully loaded cost PMPM can be determined for capitated patients according to the prospective budget of the medical group.

For medical groups that are evaluating capitated contract opportunities, projecting the unit costs of procedures is critical, especially when renegotiating capitation payments and the amounts of copayments required for specific procedures. By projecting the expected utilization rate of the health plan members at the full cost per procedure, the approximate cost PMPM can be established. Once full costs PMPM have been estimated, the required capitation payments can then be set or negotiated.

Comparison of the Two Methods

The FFS costing method often has an advantage over the cost or budgetary method in that it incorporates factors that are very familiar to the medical group — that is, FFS charges. However, FFS charges are not necessarily a fair representation of the cost of services rendered since they tend to understate the cost of physician/nursing services and overstate the cost of ancillary services, such as lab tests and X-rays. The cost or budgetary method may seem more abstract to the medical group's management and physicians but it does approach the development of capitation rates from an expense standpoint instead of from the revenue or value-of-service view. An understanding of these factors is critically important to group management since MCOs use a cost model rather than an FFS charge model that approximates cost to determine the capitation rates offered to medical groups in agreement proposals. Additionally, one must analyze the impact to cost per clinically integrated episode of medical care delivery when utilization is reduced through the use of good medical management principles.

In summary, capitation rates are principally based in four domains: (1) the MCO's target member population, (2) the MCO's benefit design, (3) the included and excluded medical services covered under contract provisions, and (4) the anticipated service utilization and cost assumptions of the medical group. Since establishing capitation rates is one of the most complex areas in managed care systems, readers are urged to consult other sources to gain a fuller explanation and understanding of this important process. As a starting point, the authors suggest exploring the resources presented in the following section.

INFORMATION SOURCES

The managed care marketplace is changing rapidly and continuously. By the time this book is in print, this chapter will be dated, in part by developments in the mechanisms, technologies, legislation, or other parameters that impact the ways managed care is viewed, measured, controlled, and delivered. Thus, the topic of managed care should be a priority in any medical group financial manager's continuing education. As mentioned before, managed care appears to be gaining momentum in the ambulatory healthcare setting. Leading your group to financial success will include knowing and understanding trends in managed care. The information sources listed below can provide financial managers with a starting point from which to gain access to information germane to the managed care setting. The lists are by no means all-inclusive nor are they intended to represent the best resources available. However, regular visits to at least three or four Web sites, subscription to several newsletters, and reading the latest texts will help the financial manager to stay on top of this dynamic area of practice management.

Web Sites (in Alphabetical Order)

American Association of Health Plans	www.aahp.org
American College of Healthcare Executives	www.ache.org
American College of Physician Executives	www. acpe.org
Centers for Medicare & Medicaid Services	www.cms.gov
Healthcare Financial Management Association	www.hfma.org

Managed Care Connection   www.managedcareconnection.com

Managed Care Digest   www.managedcaredigest.com

Managed Care Information Center   www.themcic.com

Managed Care On-Line   www.mcol.com

Medical Group Management Association   www.mgma.com

Newsletters

Aspen Publishers, Inc. *The Managed Care Payment Advisor* (ISSN: 1093-5061). Frederick, MD.

Atlantic Information Services, Inc., *News and Strategies for Managed Medicare & Medicaid* (ISSN: 1089-6589). Washington, D.C.

Brownstone Publishers, Inc., *Managed Care Contract Negotiator* (ISSN: 1092-8944). Skaneateles, NY.

National Health Information, LLC. *Capitation Rates & Data* (ISSN: 1090-1574). Marietta, GA.

Thompson Publishing Group, Inc. *Healthcare Capitation & Risk* (ISSN: 1091-5826). Washington, D.C.

Additional books and articles are cited in the references section at the end of this chapter.

LOOKING INTO THE FUTURE

Three changes will characterize the face of healthcare delivery in managed care settings in the future: (1) technology, both clinical advances and the explosion of Internet and other communication tools; (2) the continued growth of the ambulatory care marketplace; and (3) the increased importance of patient education.

Technology is likely to continue as one of the key catalysts for change in the managed care marketplace. We may see virtual PCP visits as yet another avenue to control cost. This might include significant electronic health status monitoring at the patient's home and e-mail–based consultations and patient education tools. The Internet holds tremendous opportunities for future developments. Not only could it be a powerful vehicle for a national health information network, it will also facilitate the information exchange between providers, purchasers, and insurers.

The cost-control focus of managed care, combined with the significant advances in technology, drive a growing shift from inpatient to outpatient stays that can now be performed in an ambulatory setting. In addition, some illnesses that used to require referrals to a hospital can now be treated with medication only. Thus, a continued market share expansion in the ambulatory care environment can be expected.

There will be a new focus on patient education. This will go far beyond the traditional patient education on how to administer medicines and how to modify lifestyles to increase or maintain the desired health status. Increasingly, both providers and administrators of medical group practices will have to learn how to teach their patients about managing their own wellness, to assist payers in educating enrollees in how to use the healthcare system most effectively, and to provide educational resources to the capitated populations who have not become patients to the group. In addition, internal professional development is likely to assume more importance as the interrelations of clinical and financial activities grow stronger. It will be a challenge to keep up with the changes and to filter out the most pertinent information that needs to be shared with internal staff to ensure effective patient and practice management.

To the Point

■ The payment system in a traditional FFS system presents providers with a disincentive to contain much of the costs associated with healthcare delivery. The movement toward managed care was seen as an alternative to the inflationary and greatly fragmented FFS system.

■ The managed care delivery system motivates the provider to establish mechanisms to contain costs, control utilization, and deliver services in the most appropriate settings. Adopted methodologies to achieve these goals center on controlling the utilization of medical services, shifting financial risk to the provider, and reducing the use of resources in rendering treatments to patients.

■ The most prevalent managed care organizational forms are health maintenance organizations (HMO), preferred provider organizations (PPO), point-of-service plans (PSP), and exclusive provider organizations (EPO).

■ Since the rise of managed care, a number of new, integrated provider organizations developed. Their main purpose is to bring previously fragmented providers together to deliver healthcare services. Usually, the integrated provider organizations are designed as separate legal entities and include the following organizational forms: integrated delivery systems (IDS), physician-hospital organizations (PHOs), independent practice associations (IPAs), management services organizations (MSOs), physician practice management companies (PPMCs), and ambulatory surgery centers (ASCs).

▪ Entering into managed care contracting has profound impacts on the standards by which providers conduct their practices. The list of principal areas where this impact is most significant includes the following:

  – Access to managed care networks

  – Practice size and structure

  – Price competition

  – Product differentiation

  – Information systems

▪ Within managed care models, there are generally three levels of financial risk that can be assumed by a medical group:

  1. Risk-sharing, where medical groups get paid discounted FFS equivalent rates for services provided to subscribers of a health plan. Related to this model are contractual agreements based on a specified percentage of the RBRVS RVU reimbursement allowable plus the potential for a bonus based on measures of successful performance (relatively low level of risk).

  2. Establishment of a withhold fund or risk pool where a portion of the group's reimbursement amount is diverted into an account controlled by the MCO (intermediate level of risk).

  3. Predetermined PMPM capitation rates where the medical group is paid a per-capita rate per covered patient regardless of the utilization of medical services (high level of risk).

    – Medical group managers are well advised to seek out expert advice before binding their groups to accept high levels of risk.

▪ Before entering managed care contract negotiations, medical groups should develop specific managed care strategies that address all elements of managed care contracting. While every managed care contract differs from one another, many elements are common to these contractual arrangements.

■ Success in a managed care marketplace depends on the level of control a group can exercise over the group's resource utilization and delivery patterns. Common cost-control measures in managed care include the implementation of clinical practice guidelines, outcomes review, well-directed continuing medical education for providers and support staff, and regular contact with purchasers.

■ Negotiating a successful managed care contract requires that medical groups have invested an adequate amount of time and resources in preparation for the process of actually composing the deal. Specifically, understanding the local and national managed care environment, identifying the group's ideal contracting positions and next best alternatives on sensitive issues, determining the full costs associated with each unit of service the medical group renders, and assembling a skillful team of negotiators to look out for the medical group's best interests.

■ To establish capitation rates, there are at least two methods used to determine the costs of services rendered by the medical group and by referrals outside the medical group. These methods are commonly referred to as:

　1. FFS or actuarial method; and

　2. Cost of budgetary method.

■ The topic of managed care should be a priority in any medical group financial manager's continuing education. Regular visits to at least three or four Web sites, subscriptions to several newsletters, and reading the latest texts will help the financial manager to stay on top of this dynamic area of practice management.

■ Managed care of the future will be impacted by further clinical advances, explosion of the Internet and other communication tools, continued growth, and a new focus on patient education. We can expect a plethora of new information sources and information needs in the managed care environment. Keeping up and sharing the most pertinent information will, in part, default to the financial manager.

REFERENCES

1. Todd, M. A. 1996. *The Managed Care Contracting Handbook*, p. 1. Chicago, IL: Irwin Professional Publishing.

2. Schultz, H. A., and Young, K. M. 1997. *Health Care USA,* p. 190. Sudbury, MA: Jones & Bartlett Publishers.

3. Johnson, B. A., and Niederman, G. A. 1996. *Managed Care Legal Issues.* Englewood, CO: Medical Group Management Association.

4. Ibid.

5. Shortell, S. M., Gillies, R. R., et al. 1993. "Creating Organized Delivery Systems: The Barriers and Facilitators." *Hospital and Health Services Administration, 4,* 447–66.

6 Goldmith, J. C. 1994. "The Elusive Logic of Integration." *Health Forum Journal,* 37(5): 26–31.

7. Shortell, S. M., Gilles, R. R., et al. 1996. *Remaking Health Care in America: Building Organized Delivery Systems.* San Francisco, CA: Jossey-Bass, Inc.

8. Johnson, B. A., and Niederman, G. A. 1996. *Managed Care Legal Issues.* Englewood, CO: Medical Group Management Association.

9. Ibid.

10. Ibid.

11. Aaron, H., and Breindel, C. L., 1988. "The Evolution Toward 'Managed' Health Care." *Medical Group Management Journal.* September/October: 63–64.

12. Institute of Medicine. 1992. "United States Committee on Clinical Practice Guidelines." In *Guidelines for Clinical Practice: From Development to Use,* edited by M. F. Field and K. N. Lohr, p. 1. Washington, D.C.: National Academy Press.

CHAPTER 11

Planning and Budgeting

Edited by Robert F. White, MBA

After completing this chapter, you will be able to:

- Understand the importance of planning for the future of a medical group's operations and distinguish between strategic and operational planning.

- Relate the importance and approach of environmental scanning and its role in overall planning.

- Design a practice goal- and objective-setting process within a medical group, and develop and integrate goal and objective statements for use in a medical practice.

- Describe the functions and benefits of budgets in healthcare settings and the components of a comprehensive operating budget.

- Begin the preparatory steps to implement a comprehensive budgetary planning and control system for a small to medium-sized medical group practice.

- Analyze the interplay between physician compensation and the development of an operating budget and the complications of performance-based incentives on the budgeting process.

- Explain the function of a flexible budgeting system and how it differs from traditional static budgets.

- Analyze the simple cost-volume-profit structures of medical groups to calculate the break-even points of the practice and to use the relationships of these variables in assessing the impact on group profits when changes occur in them.

This chapter will provide an overview of the financial planning process that medical groups need to employ or develop in today's dynamic environment. We will discuss the strategic planning and operational planning processes and the approaches that are effective in establishing goals and objectives for future periods of operation. The main focus of the chapter will be to examine the financial budgeting activity that groups should follow to assist them in achieving their short- and long-range goals and objectives. The impact on the budgeting process by physician compensation schemes, especially those involving a combination of salary and incentives, will be examined. Finally, we will illustrate one of the techniques for evaluating the impact of possible future actions on the costs, volume, and profits of group operations when various changes are introduced to the normal operating scheme.

PLANNING STRATEGICALLY AND OPERATIONALLY

Planning is the process by which management looks ahead and develops specific courses of action to attain the entity's goals. Planning involves all activities related to the functioning of the business, such as deciding what types of services to offer, setting fees (prices) for those services, arranging for the proper type and amount of staff to carry out the group's phases of operations, and so on. Sometimes planning is divided into two types: strategic and operational planning.

Strategic planning is the development of a long-range course of action to achieve goals; it usually encompasses periods ranging from five to ten years. Strategic planning involves a continuous process of evaluating long-term changes in the medical group's environment and attempting to assess its effects on the group. The process may identify a concern that can be addressed within the resources of the medical group, or one that requires cooperation with other members of the healthcare delivery system, or one that requires a response in the political arena. In one sense, the objective of strategic financial planning is to avoid unpleasant surprises. From another perspective, it is an attempt to enhance the likelihood of achieving the long-term goals and objectives of the organization. There are definite relationships between the strategic financial planning process, the development of organizational goals and objectives, and the planning and evaluation of activities in the short run. Resource allocation follows, more or less, after goals and objectives have been established, although the planning process often causes a reexamination and revision of goals and objectives once strategic elements are analyzed.

Operational planning is the development of short-term plans to achieve goals identified in the strategic plan. Operational plans, thus, complement the strategic plan and are typically set for time periods ranging from one week or a month to several years. Examples of operational planning are setting the current month's production level of patient service and determining the staffing needs for part-time employees during the next month.

The following discussion of planning will largely focus on the forward-looking aspects of strategic planning. We are not concerned about differentiating between strategic and operational plans per se. Rather, our discussion will deal with both types in a context of planning, in general, without making a distinction as to which type is being addressed. After all, the purpose of all planning is to reduce uncertainty. At times, this can be achieved with a short-term perspective, while at other times, the long-term view must be considered paramount in importance.

IMPORTANCE OF PLANNING

As the composition of group practices continues to change and as competition heightens, planning and formalized approaches to the process become more important to successful operations. Providing a wider breadth of healthcare services will become a larger component of all practices, and this will place new stresses and challenges on the management of groups. Even though it is difficult to predict from a macro sense the specific directions that healthcare policies and procedures will take in the near term (let alone the long view), possible future scenarios must be envisioned in order to plan effectively. Being armed with contingency plans in reaction to future developments will ensure the selection of the best alternative courses of action.

Regardless of whether the planning process is formal or informal, medical practices will benefit from periodically applying the following steps:

- Perform an environmental scan by examining the changes and trends in the healthcare environment:
  - External or outside the medical group
  - Within the medical group

- Develop the goals and objectives of the group:
  - If there is a need for change in the general direction, redefine the goals set previously.
  - Consider the need to reestablish specific targets (objectives) and the dates for accomplishing them.

- Establish short-term operating budgets consistent with goals and objectives.

- Compare actual results to budgets and consider the need for corrective action.

ENVIRONMENTAL SCANNING

Environmental scanning is largely an awareness process used by organizations to systematically examine the surrounding conditions and to identify, quantify, and adopt environmental factors into the planning process. The scan is performed to uncover the most influential factors that can materially affect the organization's strategies — even those that may be beyond the organization's direct control. This knowledge can serve planners well by enabling them to respond to these influences through specific strategies when that is possible, or if responses cannot be developed, to cushion the effects of the forces on the firm's activities if they occur.

The areas to scan are all events, institutions, social policies, and governmental regulations and programs that have an impact on the delivery of healthcare service. The healthcare industry should be reviewed to discover trends or emerging forces that can affect the operation of a medical group. As these factors are identified, an assessment should follow on the degree of importance each has and what effect these items could have on the group's operations.

For example, strategic planning normally has been oriented toward the market for medical services rather than the delivery of services or the design of clinical facilities. The primary questions seem to have been "What medical services are needed?" and "Who will purchase them?" instead of a more traditional strategic question: "What medical services should the group deliver given the environment that exists?" This change in emphasis is needed in today's competitive world of healthcare delivery systems. The shift now is more toward a marketing orientation that anticipates the medical care needs of the population being served. The value of strategic planning is in increasing the ability to diagnose and respond to the changing needs of the marketplace.

To survive and compete successfully, medical groups should be aware of a broad range of possible responses to the many changes that are occurring in the external environment. Groups must be aware of the internal limitations that may affect their long-term ability to respond to the forces of change. Strategic financial planning must assess these external factors along with the internal elements of the group itself.

Planning is closely aligned with control. In fact, many feel that the two processes are intertwined, and planning is merely the first step in a two-fold continuum where control closes the loop on a total unified process. Exhibit 11.1 illustrates the interconnection of planning and control in an organization.

DEVELOPING GOALS AND OBJECTIVES

In the management literature, goals and objectives are sometimes used interchangeably. We prefer to define the term "goals" to mean broad, timeless statements indicating what the organization desires to achieve and "objectives" to mean more specific statements of certain ends that are achieved within a specific time frame.

EXHIBIT 11.1 ■ Illustration of the Planning and Control Process

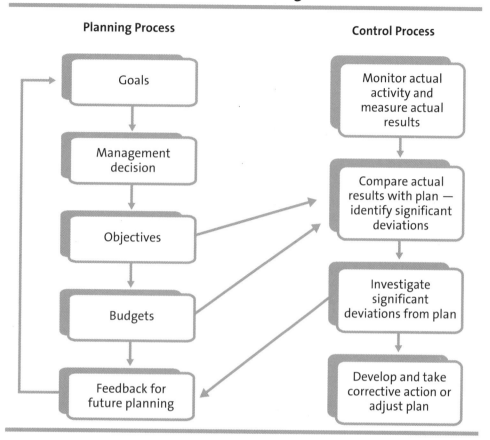

As indicated, goals are long-term and represent endless purposes. Objectives are short-term and flow from goals. Good objectives are measurable and should be stated in terms more specific than goals. Goals should emanate from a common set of shared beliefs that exist among members of the governing body of the medical group. When pronounced, they serve as the main message to the rest of the group about organizational requirements. Organizations should review their goals from time to time, but they should not change frequently. The interrelationship of goals and objectives is often referred to as goals and objectives congruency. In the following section, examples of both terms will be given for a medical practice.

How to Set Goals and Objectives

The first step in setting goals for a medical practice is to answer some basic questions, such as the following:

- What patient groups are going to be served?
- What kinds of services are to be provided?

- What will the group's role and position of leadership be in the medical community?
- What impact will changes in technology have on patient care?
- How large a professional staff does the group want in five years? In 10 years?
- What impact will changes in the local healthcare market have on the group's share of the market?
- Is the general population growing or contracting, and are the population demographics changing?
- Is the physician population growing or contracting, and is the mix of the physician population changing?
- Will the government and other players play a greater or lesser role in the provision of healthcare than they have in the past?

The answers to these questions help in determining a broad statement of direction. There might be a single statement developed — called a mission statement — that signifies what the medical group is all about. For example, the statement might read, "To provide the highest quality of pediatric healthcare in all specialties to patients in the Leesburg, Virginia, area." There will also be several goal statements that will form the set of goals that the physicians and administrators agree are the common targets to which they will commit. Further, the group will examine the relevant variables that relate to the common direction chosen for the practice. This process will aid in setting intermediate-range and short-range objectives.

Objectives are these short- and intermediate-range targets, usually covering a one- to three-year period. These objective statements should be somewhat specific and represent targets for a number of important variables such as units of service to be provided, gross charges, adjustments and allowances, physician compensation, hours of operation, desired cash, and short-term resource balances and capital acquisitions.

The planning process continues through successive steps until the projected targets are consistent with the goals. Such analysis may suggest new services, additional hours of operation, more physicians, or new locations that may be necessary to reach the group's goals. When goals and objectives are consistent, the objectives should represent the best attainable estimates of activity.

Gathering Input for Goal Setting

Goal setting is a process of deciding where the group wants to go. As an iterative process, it is necessary to cycle through a series of repeated exercises of introspection about the group's activities to reach a common direction. To accomplish this during busy daily schedules takes some careful planning and organizing.

A common approach is to devise questionnaires for key staff with pointed questions about issues and subjects sought as the basis for goal setting. The questionnaire should focus on the basic issues the group is attempting to define and should be in an easily answerable format. The thinking must be futuristic, and the framing of the questions must force respondents into that mindset. The design of the questionnaire is most important in gathering the proper kind of information useful to setting goals.

The last element of input on the questionnaire should involve having the respondents identify action priorities. A listing of key areas will allow each physician, board member, and member of management to indicate his or her most urgent concerns. The composite of the individual responses should point to group priorities.

After each member of the professional staff has responded to the questionnaire, goals and objectives must be set. This ideally should be done with all necessary parties present so that differences can be worked out through discussion and collective agreement about which goals can be reached. There may be two sets of goals — primary and secondary. Primary goals should provide overall direction and are overriding in importance. Some of the areas that the questionnaire should provide clear focus for goal setting are:

- Professional services — What services will be offered?
- Human resources — What kinds of personnel should be hired, and what methods should be used to train, develop, and retain them?
- Physical resources — What facilities and equipment will be needed?
- Financial resources — Which funding sources should be used to finance the plans? What are the financial information reporting needs?
- Innovation — What new methods of practice should be employed?
- Productivity — What levels of productivity should be established?
- Social responsibility — What role should the organization play in the local community?
- Salary requirements — How does the wage and salary program align with practice goals and objectives?
- Management information systems — What are management's information needs?
- Compliance — What areas of compliance and accountability need to be further developed?

The goals framed by a group should be based on both the input of the key staff and the results of the environmental scan. Goals that might evolve from this exercise are presented in Exhibit 11.2.

Translating Goals into Objectives

The goal- and objective-setting process is used to expand planning at different levels within the group. At least one time-oriented, specific objective should be set for each of the goal statements. For the timing of the objectives, it is necessary to set priorities for their accomplishment. If resources are limited,

EXHIBIT 11.2 ■ **Example of Medical Group's Goals**

Coastal Medical Center — Goals

Provide superior quality medical care to all patients of the medical group.

Grow within the next five years to a professional staff numbering 25 physicians.

Add a prepaid component, which within five years will grow to contribute a significant portion of the group's revenue.

Expand from a single facility to one having satellite operations.

Provide a formalized capability for intra- and inter-departmental education of doctors and medical staff with educational programs for support personnel.

Maintain financial compensation to physicians and support personnel above the community average.

Positively influence the future of medical care in the community.

the priorities will provide the tangible guidance necessary to develop annual operating plans and budgets.

An example of the objective-setting process for a medical group is illustrated in Exhibit 11.3. Note that the supporting goals in Exhibit 11.3 are designed to further define the primary goal to "provide superior quality medical care."

Objectives are formulated as the last step in the planning process — after individual completion of the questionnaires, joint formulation of the group goals, and establishment of group priorities. Each major area of responsibility in the group should develop its own goals, objectives, and budget proposals that will lead to fulfillment of higher-level objectives and progress toward the primary goal(s).

Attainable objectives cannot be set in a vacuum. Since different objectives are competing for the same resources, they must be tested through the development of budgets of future financial results. If these forecasts show that resources are not sufficient, a priority must be established for each objective. Thus, some objectives will have to be delayed or revised. This iterative process will continue until operating plans are developed that reconcile the priority of objectives with available resources.

Once approved and finalized, objectives must be communicated throughout the group. The budget becomes the medium of communicating objectives by showing what the financial impact will be when all objectives have been achieved.

One step in the budgetary control process is measurement of progress and corrective action when deviations from the plan are significant. Action should be taken to bring operations back to conformity with the plan. However, if

EXHIBIT 11.3 ■ Setting Objectives — Mountain Valley OB/GYN

Primary goal: Provide superior quality medical care

I. Professional services
Supporting goal: To offer comprehensive medical care.
1st objective: To add three general practitioners within six months.
2nd objective: To add all major specialties within five years.

II. Human resources
Supporting goal: To attract and retain only top quality professional and support staff.
1st objective: To train two medical assistants for special procedures within one year.
2nd objective: To train a nurse practitioner to provide a limited range of services in urgent care within two years.

III. Physical resources
Supporting goal: To provide the space and equipment needed to perform high-quality work.
Objective: To provide all standard instruments in each examining room within three months.

IV. Financial resources
Supporting goal: To develop available and flexible sources of funds for all necessary capital needs.
1st objective: To negotiate a line of credit with a local bank for working capital within three months.
2nd objective: To set up a two-year capital budget within one month.

V. Management information systems
Supporting goal: To develop information systems that meet all information needs of management.
1st objective: To develop a financial information system that meets management needs within two years.
2nd objective: To computerize patient appointment scheduling within six months.

VI. Innovation
Supporting goal: To continually explore new areas of service, talent, and methods of medical care.
1st objective: To study and report on the feasibility of subcontracting specialty services with medical insurance carriers in the vicinity within one year.
2nd objective: To establish a marketing plan for the group within one year.

VII. Productivity
Supporting goal: To reward individual doctors for higher than average professional productivity.
1st objective: To initiate a system that tracks individual production on a monthly basis within six months.
2nd objective: To increase professional production by 5 percent within one year.

VIII. Social responsibility
Supporting goal: To take an active role in professional community affairs and to encourage all staff and employees to do so.
1st objective: To achieve 100 percent participation in the state medical society within one year.
2nd objective: To participate in the medical awareness programs in the public schools once per year within two years.

IX. Salary requirements
Supporting goal: To maintain physician salaries and fringe benefits at a level above the community average.
Objective: To increase physician median by $10,000 within two years.

the objectives are no longer attainable, they must be revised to maintain the credibility of the planning process. This revision is essential to establish new priorities among objectives competing for resources. The new priorities, in turn, guide the preparation of revised budgets.

Let's now look at the process of budgeting and how it interrelates with the planning process.

BUDGETING FOR OPERATIONS

Goals and objectives provide the framework for developing operating plans for the coming year. Objectives serve as the bridging mechanism to integrate long-range goals with short-term operating plans. The short-term operating plans are the operating budgets that express these plans in terms of dollars. Many organizations refer to these operating budgets as profit plans since they show the planned activities that the segments of a business expect to undertake in order to obtain their profit goals. However, it is important to remember that not every responsibility center is set up to generate a profit in and of itself.

The major advantage of budgeting lies in its requiring managers to plan in an organized and concentrated way. Since budgets are short-range targets expressed in financial terms, the process demands that the medical group set aside a specific time each year to plan and that these plans be built on already established goals and objectives. In the previous section, the process of goal setting was shown as a valuable exercise for management. But unless goals are translated into objectives and budgets, much of the practice's planning effectiveness is lost. Most medical groups do some sort of planning, even on an informal basis. More groups are formalizing this process by integrating and communicating their carefully crafted financial plans into a single comprehensive document called the comprehensive budget.

To move from an informal plan to a comprehensive budget requires understanding the budgetary process and experience establishing budgeted plans to learn how to adapt them to the nuances of the group's operations. In this section, we will treat budgeting in a broad sense to gain an overall perspective of the process. The next section will delve into the detailed construction of a comprehensive budget, and a later section will address the use of a flexible budget.

Functions and Benefits of Budgets

In addition to the benefits cited above, budgets also serve the following purposes:

- Aid in making and coordinating short-range plans and in communicating these plans to all managers. This becomes more important as the number of responsibility centers or departments grows.
- Serve as a means to motivate managers to achieve the goals of their responsibility centers by providing target indicators.

- Provide an authorization for staff personnel to use and acquire resources during the coming period and to expand existing or implement new activities. Granting such authority demonstrates management commitment to the plan.

- Enable managers to anticipate favorable conditions so that actions can be taken to capitalize on them or, if unfavorable, to minimize their impact.

- Establish benchmarks to control ongoing activities and set criteria for evaluating performance of managers at various levels in the group.

Components of the Comprehensive Budget

A comprehensive budget, sometimes called a master budget, consists of a series of informal projections and a number of formal statements. The components are illustrated in Exhibit 11.4. Each of the numbered steps in the exhibit will be explained below. The exhibit shows that the comprehensive budget is comprised of two major parts:

1. Cash and other short-term resource management systems — the ongoing planning and control systems for managing short-term resources.

2. The formal comprehensive budget, which consists of a profit plan, a cash budget, a capital expenditures budget, and a projected balance sheet or position statement. With the exception of the capital expenditures budget, the comprehensive budget represents projections of the general purpose financial statements covered in chapters 3 and 5.

Steps in the Preparation of the Comprehensive Budget

Exhibit 11.4 illustrates the steps and interrelationships in the preparation of a comprehensive budget. The information assumes a group with both an FFS and a prepaid component in its practice. Each number on the exhibit, described below, indicates a step in the budgeting process.

1. **External information** — The medical group must develop a picture of the environment in which it is operating, including projections of the local economy, anticipated price increases, expected demand for medical services, competition, and any other external influences that are expected to affect the group. The HMOs with which the group is contracting should provide projected enrollment and utilization data.

2. **Physicians' plans** — The physicians/owners must examine both their personal goals and the goals of the group. Through this process, the physicians indicate their expectations and desires concerning personal income levels; changes in hours of service; changes in the style of the group; changes in productivity; planned additions or reductions in the number of providers; and planned changes in the number of nurses, medical assistants, and nonclinical staff. Many of these expectations should be expressed as objectives, which are dated and quantified targets of planned accomplishments.

EXHIBIT 11.4 ■ Illustration of the Comprehensive Budget

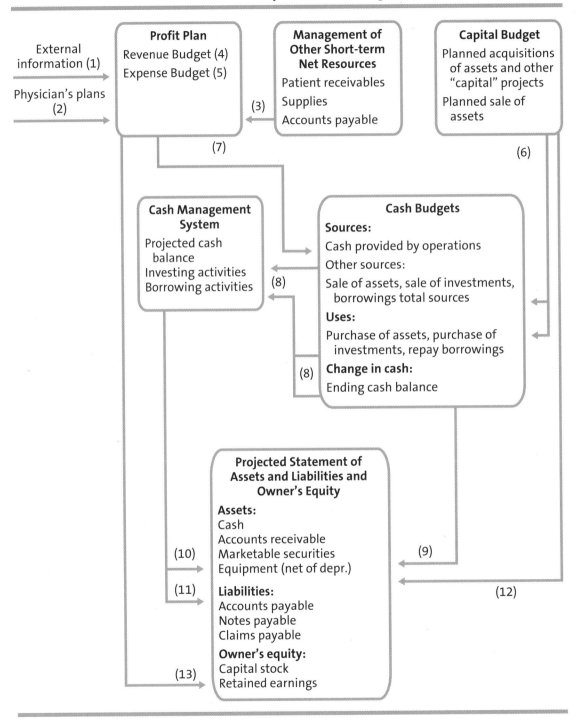

3. **Management of other net short-term resources** — A number of short-term resource control systems are used in any medical group. These systems provide planned levels for patient receivables, supplies, and short-term payables.

4. **Budgeted revenues** — The group's income from prepaid contracts (HMO payments, capitation payments, patient copayments, risk-sharing payments, etc.) and the planned FFS production for each provider may be projected given the changes in the environment, the physician's plans for changes in the style of the group, and the planned level of patient receivables.

5. **Budgeted expenses** — Projected expenses fall into two broad categories, variable and fixed, based on activity changes. Because variable expenses relate to the level of production, variable expense projections are based on the projected production determined in Step 4. Fixed costs are determined by contracts, the level of capacity, and the physicians' plans. Budget preparers need to keep their relevant range in mind when developing their projection (see chapter 6).

6. **Planned acquisition or sale of assets** — Planned acquisition or sale of assets will reflect cash management activities. The cash budget must reflect the expected sources and uses of cash from the purchase and sale of assets. The cash budget should be accompanied by a capital expenditure budget to include all capital expenditures over a specified amount. The amount and timing of these outflows can be critical and place significant demands on short-term resources.

7. **Cash provided by operations** — Budgeted revenues and expenses use the accrual basis and include noncash items (such as depreciation). These must be removed to arrive at cash provided or used by operations. In order to calculate a starting point, expected cash from operations will need to reference operations in the previous year based on your receivables turnaround. For example, there would be no cash flow from a program starting in period 1 of your budget. Cash from operations during your first budget day would be almost entirely attributed to revenue accrued in a previous budget year.

8. **Projected cash balance** — Planned sources and uses of cash are determined in the process of developing the cash budget. The investing and borrowing of cash may be necessary to manage the cash position and finance the capital acquisitions of the group. These activities must be reflected in the cash budget.

Projected statement of assets, liabilities, and owners' equity (Steps 9 through 13) — The interrelation of the steps in the planning process becomes clear when the projected statement of assets, liabilities, and owners' equity is prepared. The beginning statement of assets, liabilities, and owners' equity, along with the changes generated by the previous steps, provides the information to determine the ending individual asset, liability, and owners' equity balances.

9. **Cash balance** — Ending cash balance is a product of the cash budget.

10. **Accounts receivable and marketable securities** — Cash management activities project the amount of estimated collection of accounts receivable and the amount of investment in marketable securities.

11. **Accounts payable, notes payable, and claims payable** — Cash management activities project the amount of accounts payable for supplies, group credit cards, and outstanding bills; the amount of borrowing, repayment, and the resulting balance of notes payable; and the amount of outstanding medical claims payable.

12. **Property, plant, and equipment balances** — The capital expenditures budget determines the changes in the long-lived assets and, with depreciation from the profit plan, the resulting balances of property, plant, and equipment.

13. **Retained earnings** — The profit or loss from the profit plan provides the change in retained earnings.

THE DILEMMA OF THE CASH AND ACCRUAL BASIS

Earlier chapters explained the difference between the cash and accrual methods for keeping records and stressed that the accrual basis produces a better picture of operating results. The issue of cash and accrual measurements often raises problems in the budgeting process. The budget must provide both a planning tool (through the expression of management's plans) and a control tool (by a benchmark with which to compare actual results). On one hand, the budget should reflect what is expected to happen and provide a useful tool for control. On the other hand, the budget must relate to the actual measurements recorded in the accounting system.

Actual activities of the group involve the generation of assets through the provision of medical services to patients and the consumption of assets in providing these services. Because accrual accounting measures revenue in the period that service is performed and measures expenses in the period resources are used, a profit plan prepared on the accrual basis does a better job of reflecting the activities of the group, and therefore provides a better basis for evaluating performance. For a medical group with a significant prepaid component, the use of the accrual basis is the only way to get a proper measurement of the results for a period of time. The natural distortions caused by a lag in collections and payments and the purposeful manipulations of cash payments and collections to reduce the tax burden distort the picture of operations.

As the measurement period is lengthened, to a year for example, these cash-basis distortions are significantly reduced. The value of the annual budget as a control tool, however, is also significantly reduced. Control is exercised before or as an event occurs. Once an action has taken place, nothing can be done to change it. For control purposes, the feedback of information for short periods of time is critical. Nonfinancial data, of course, are needed and used on a daily basis.

Because of monthly distortions caused by cash-basis accounting, most medical groups on the cash basis use a quarterly planning period for their operating budgets, and a balance between the level of distortion on the cash basis and the usefulness of the data is reached. As a medical group becomes more mature in financial planning and control, the accrual basis will often be used for financial planning, control, and other internal purposes, but cash-basis measurements will still be used in the preparation of income tax returns.

THE COMPREHENSIVE BUDGET

This detailed exposition of the comprehensive budget uses accrual accounting principles. Three portions of the comprehensive budget are presented: the profit plan, the cash budget, and the projected statement of financial position or balance sheet. An extended example of a budget for a medical group — Mountain Valley OB/GYN — is given to show how the budget is developed and follows a bottom-up approach.

Sequence for Developing the Comprehensive Budget

After the goals and objectives have been developed and communicated throughout the group, each responsibility center plans its individual activities and prepares a profit plan. Then these individual profit plans are integrated into the overall profit plan for the group. To ensure realistic profit plans for responsibility centers, each manager of the centers should take an active role in planning his or her budget and in follow-up control efforts. These managers' lack of involvement will result in a less-than-maximum level of commitment to the budgeted plans and in the carrying out of the activities that bring about the expected results.

When responsibility centers are intimately involved, a typical sequence in the development of a comprehensive budget includes:

Step 1: Group owners/stockholders of the practice corporation

- State goals and objectives
- Identify budgeting responsibilities
- Project overall activity levels
- Determine resources available

Step 2: Administration

- Further define objectives
- Prepare working documents for responsibility center heads

Step 3: Responsibility centers

- Project activity levels
- Determine staffing

- ■ Project direct costs of responsibility centers
- ■ Compile preliminary profit plan for responsibility centers

Step 4: Administration

- ■ Combine preliminary profit plans into an overall plan
- ■ Prepare cash budget
- ■ Prepare projected statement of financial position

Step 5: Group owners/stockholders of the practice corporation

- ■ Review, amend, and approve the comprehensive budget

The first step in the sequence above involves both the long-range planning and statement of short-term objectives or targets discussed earlier in this chapter. Setting goals, objectives, and the general direction of the practice is top-down planning. Developing the budget is bottom-up planning.

BUDGETING REVENUES

The key element in any operating budget is projecting operating revenues. This is because expense projections, distributions to physicians, cash flow projections, and to some extent capital expenditure projections all depend on the projection of operating revenues. Medical groups use various approaches in estimating future revenues. Three approaches are explained in this section. They are:

1. **Estimate of demand** — Involves a determination of potential demand for the services of the group. It is a useful tool for planning marketing strategy, locating satellite offices, and initiating long-range planning. Because several estimates and assumptions are involved, this method may have a high degree of error. It may, however, provide useful information for long-range planning and can be particularly important for the medical group providing prepaid care to patients who are members of an HMO.

2. **Past activity** — Assumes that the best measure of what will occur in the future is what has happened in the recent past. Only known changes in the group, such as additions or retirements of physicians and scheduled fee changes, are projected.

3. **Estimate the number of procedures or patient visits** — This estimate is based on what is planned by each physician in the group during the budget period. By applying the expected fee schedule to the projection of procedures or visits — adjusted by a collection rate — budgeted production for each physician can be determined. Using this approach, increased efficiency due to other factors (implementation of an EHR, front-end collection plan, etc.) must also be considered to augment revenue.

Unfortunately, the last two methods assume that demand for the group's services will remain constant and that the limiting resource is physician time. As competition increases, the group will be forced to consider its impact and that of other external factors on the group practice.

Projection Based on Estimate of Demand

Periodically, the medical group should assess future demand for its medical services in its geographic area. As a long-range planning tool, this approach assists the group in setting goals and objectives for size and rate of growth. This assessment is comparable to determining its share of the market by an industrial or commercial firm. It is a key planning study when determining the medical needs of the population to be served by the prepaid practice.

The process of estimating demand for the group's services involves four types of data:

1. Economic growth projection of the served area
2. Demographic characteristics of the area
3. Patient usage rates for each department
4. Desired share of the market — that is, the share of potential patient visits that the medical group expects to have in comparison to the competition

This approach is subject to a wide range of error because of the assumptions required. For example, the group must assume both an average patient usage rate and the group's estimated share of the total market — the total number of potential patient visits. Also to be considered in estimating the group's share of the market is the competition from other medical groups. Let's see how this approach might be developed.

Assume that Mountain Valley OB/GYN (MVOB) accumulated the data presented in Exhibit 11.5 concerning the population and medical needs of its service area. The group is located in the east district of a city with a population of about 931,890, which is largely residential. Potential demand for the entire district for the specialties offered in MVOB is estimated to be 26,500 patient visits (Exhibit 11.6). Also, estimated related ancillary tests are 5,400.

What percentage of potential patient visits should the practice plan to attract? One possibility is to assume that the number of patient visits to the group will relate to the percentage of total physicians in the district that are members of the group. For example, with one-fifth of the OB/GYN physicians in the district, MVOB should expect to have 26,500 patient visits. Actually, there were only 22,000 visits to the practice's doctors during the last period. MVOB's share of patient visits for the specialty is presented in Exhibit 11.7. With almost 20 percent of the physicians in the district, the center is serving approximately 28 percent of the estimated demand. This approach is subject to a wide range of error because of the assumptions made: first, average patient usage rate (presented in Exhibit 11.6) and, second, the group's estimated share of total

EXHIBIT 11.5 ■ Data for Determination of Demand

Demographic data

Average education	12.3 years
Average family income	$25,000
Average home value	$75,000

Age and sex distribution summary

Age	Male	Female	Total
Under 15	6,237	6,023	12,260
15–44	9,306	10,038	19,344
45–64	5,443	5,967	11,410
65 and over	1,807	2,719	4,526
Total	22,793	24,747	47,540

Estimated rates for patient visits for fee-for-service patients

Overall	4.3 per year
Under 15	3.2 per year
15–44	3.6 per year
45–64	5.2 per year
65 and over	7.9 per year
Obstetrics/gynecology patients (in addition to regular visits)	.8 per year
Laboratory tests	.5 per year
Radiology procedures	.2 per year

EXHIBIT 11.6 ■ Computation of Potential Patient Visits

Specialty	Population	Average use rate	Potential patient visits
Obstetrics & gynecology	472,858*	0.48	226,972

Ancillary Departments	Potential patient visits	Average usage rates	Ancillary department visits
Laboratory	226,972	0.6	136,183
Ultrasound	226,972	0.25	56,743

Excludes male population under 15.

EXHIBIT 11.7 ■ Estimated Demand — Mountain Valley OB/GYN

Specialty	Potential patient visits	Total in area	Number in group	% of total	Group's share of patient visits	Group's actual patient visits	Group's actual % of potential
		Physicians					
Obstetrics/ Gynecology	226,972	46	9	20%	44,408	53,338	120%

potential patient visits. It does, however, provide a rough estimate of market share and how well the group is competing.

Projection Based on Past Activity

Many groups believe that the best indicator of physician's activity level for next year is their current patient load. This assumes that the conditions for the next year will not change sufficiently and that the productivity of present physicians will not change. It is the method generally used by FFS practices. It assumes that demand for the group's services remains constant and that physician time will be the limiting resource.

The projection starts with each physician's production for the past year or year-to-date (annualized) if the budget is prepared before the end of the year. For example, if the budget for 2005 is being prepared in November 2004 and production of one physician for the first 10 months of 2004 amounted to $164,178, production for 2004 is annualized as follows:

$$\$164,178 \times \frac{12 \text{ months}}{10 \text{ months}} = \$197,014 \text{ annualized}$$

Annualizing in this manner assumes even production throughout the year. Any seasonal pattern must be considered in annualizing the data. For example, in the illustration above, production for the first 10 months is assumed to account for approximately 83 percent (10/12) of annual production. If November and December are the lowest months of production, usually accounting for only 14 percent of annual revenues, production would be annualized at $189,741 ($163,178 divided by 86 percent).

After the current year's data are annualized, expected changes are applied to the current year's data. Changes for a particular physician would include: expected changes in hours of work (e.g., a physician nearing retirement may wish to reduce his or her workload, or a physician may want to expand or contract hours worked for personal reasons), changes in the mix of procedures (thereby changing the average fee charged), or changes in the fee schedule. By applying these changes in the current year's production, the production for the next year can be projected. An example of projecting production by adjusting past activity is presented in Exhibit 11.8.

EXHIBIT 11.8 ■ **Projection of Production Based on Past Activity**

	Actual Quarter 1 (2005)	Changes	Project Quarter 1 (2006)
Physician A	$27,889	Increased production due to additional hours — $837	$31,548
		Increase in fee schedule during 2005 (approx. 10%) — $2,822	
Physician B	$24,122	No changes proposed in activity	$26,534
		Increase in fee schedule during 2005 (approx. 10%) — $2,412	
Total Production	$52,011		$58,082

Exhibit 11.8 involves only one quarter. The process for a year, however, should not be significantly different. Beginning in the new year, Physician A will increase her hours by approximately 3 percent (any significant projected increase in FFS business should be supported by requests for appointments by patients). The major change is to adjust for an increase in fees during the last quarter of 2004. The predictions do not consider the impact of prepaid patients. Past experience indicates what the physicians have done, not what they can do or must do.

Projection Based on Number of Procedures or Patient Visits

A final method of projecting revenues involves estimating either the number of procedures or the number of patient visits each physician expects to handle each month during the budget year. Because of the large number of possible procedures a medical group must deal with, groups generally use the number of patient visits. Another approach is to estimate the number of days each physician will work each month. The disadvantage of projecting only days worked, and therefore, production per day, is that seasonality in patient load is not considered. If good data are available by week or month for the last two years or more, it is possible to consider seasonality in a meaningful fashion. Because the use of either the number-of-procedures or the projection-of-patient-visits method involves estimates by physicians, there will be a stronger attempt by the physicians to meet the target. Therefore, the projections should be more accurate if proper feedback takes place during the year.

To use this approach, the financial manager of the group must provide each physician with a worksheet showing:

■ Number of days the group will be open during each month of the budget year;

■ Number of patients the physician saw each month of the past year;

- Blank spaces for the number of days the physician expects to work each month; and
- Blank spaces for estimated patient visits per month.

The worksheet for a physician is presented in Exhibit 11.9. Use of this worksheet allows the physician to indicate when he or she plans to be away from the practice (for vacations, meetings, etc.) and to show planned changes in practice patterns. Large medical groups may also want to project providers' average sick leaves to ensure seamless continuation of providing services to their patients.

EXHIBIT 11.9 ▪ Worksheet for Projection of Patient Visits — OB/GYN

	Jan.	Feb.	Mar.	Quarter 1 Total	Annualized
Total available working days	21	20	23	64	258
Worksheet as prepared for:					
Physician A					
Previous year revenues					$271,000
Patients seen	648	597	645	1,890	7,619
Average revenue per patient visit					35.57
Estimated working days					
Estimated patient visits					
Average revenue per patient visit					39.13
Estimated revenues					
Completed Worksheet					
Physician A					
Previous year revenues					$271,000
Patients seen	648	597	645	1,890	7,619
Average revenue per patient visit					35.57
Estimated working days	21	20	22	63	256
Estimated patient visits	630	600	660	1,890	7,680
Average revenue per patient visit	$39.13	$39.13	$39.13	$39.13	39.13
Estimated revenues	$24,649	$23,475	$25,823	$73,947	$300,484
Summary for Practice (7 providers)					
Previous year revenues					$1,626,000
Patients seen	3,888	3,582	3,870	11,340	45,360
Average revenue per patient visit					35.57
Estimated working days	21	20	22	63	256
Estimated patient visits	4,536	4,179	4,515	13,230	52,920
Average revenue per patient visit	39.13	39.13	39.13	39.13	39.13
Estimated revenues	177,473	163,506	176,652	517,631	2,070,524

Revenue per visit inclusive of $0 revenue OB visits and delivery fees

It also allows the financial manager and medical director to identify potential staffing problems. Because this schedule reflects only working days and patient visits, it will not necessarily meet the demand for the group's services. How will the prepaid patients be served? It should be easy to add 8, 13, and 20 expected prepaid patient visits during the first three months; however, any projected significant increase in visits needs to be accommodated with additional resources and/or an illustrated increase in operational efficiency.

BUDGETING EXPENSES

Cost behavior patterns were covered in chapter 6. The importance of knowing about these patterns for a particular medical group cannot be overemphasized. As previously discussed, the four patterns of cost behavior are (1) variable, (2) fixed, (3) mixed or semivariable, and (4) step-fixed. Variable costs change in proportion to changes in activity, while fixed costs do not change as activity changes. Some costs exhibit both characteristics (mixed), while other costs increase in stair-step fashion (step-fixed). A useful concept in estimating specific expenses in the budgeting process is to identify the flexible budgeting formula for each expense and to apply it in making expense projections.

The Flexible Budget Formula

The flexible budget formal is a mathematical statement of the relationship between activity and costs. It is as follows:

Fixed Costs + (Variable Cost per Patient × Number of Patient Visits) = Total Costs

By expressing costs as fixed or variable, the flexible budget formula allows costs to be projected for any activity level. For simplicity, a straight-line relationship between activity level and cost level is assumed. Also, it is assumed that all costs can be identified as fixed or variable costs; mixed or semivariable costs must be separated into the fixed and variable components. This model is best applied to a small practice segment with relatively defined services.

To illustrate the application of the formula, the following example is given:

FC $139,633 + (VCPP $1.47 × NOPV 5,000 = $7,350) = TC $146,983

With the budget formula for each element of cost as shown above, the total costs for any level of activity can be projected by substituting the number of visits in place of NOPV in each formula equation. For example, if 5,000 tests are performed, the four individual costs would be $8,633 for building rent, $120,000 for salaries, $7,350 for supplies, and $11,000 for equipment rental. Total costs are $146,983 when 5,000 visits are performed, resulting in a cost per visit of $29.40 ($146,983 divided by 5,000 visits).

The unit cost of $29.40 is correct only at the 5,000 level. Suppose that the number of visits dropped to 1,000 per month. If the cost behavior patterns remained unchanged, what is the unit cost at the 1,000 visit level? Total costs equal $139,633 plus $1.47 per visit, or $1,470, resulting in a $141.10 cost per visit, an unacceptable volume level.

With these flexible budget formulas, costs can be projected when developing an operating budget and profit plan. Also, at the end of a period, actual costs incurred can be compared to the proper budgeted measure using the actual activity level experienced by the use of the flexible budget formulas.

Exhibit 11.10 lists the costs of Mountain Valley OB/GYN, classifies them by behavior pattern, and indicates the flexible budget formula based on last

EXHIBIT 11.10 ▪ Classification of Costs — OB/GYN

Costs	Cost behavior pattern	Flexible budget 20×4 (average month)	Expected changes in 20×5	Fixed	Variable	Total 20×5 Costs	Total 20×4 Costs
Physician salaries	Programmed fixed	$62,500 per month	Increase on Jan. 1, new physician, to $72,917	$72,917		$72,917.00	$62,500.00
Physician benefits	Programmed fixed	a) 20% of salaries	a) increase to 22% of salaries	$16,042		$16,041.74	$12,500.00
		b) 2% of salaries for meetings and professional development	b) increase to 5% of salaries	$3,646		$3,645.85	$1,250.00
Staff salaries	Programmed fixed	$24,000 per month	increase at anniversary dates (2.5%)	$24,600		$24,600.00	$24,000.00
Staff benefits	Programmed fixed	15% of salaries	18% of salaries	$4,428		$4,428.00	$3,600.00
Supplies	Variable	$1.40 per patient visit	5% increase to $1.47 per patient visit		$7,350	$7,350.00	$7,000.00
Equipment rental	Committed fixed	$4,000 per month	No change	$4,000		$4,000.00	$4,000.00
Professional liability insurance	Committed fixed	$2,000 per month, per physician	Add for new physician, no rate change	$14,000		$14,000.00	$12,000.00
Staff salaries average increase of 5% on anniversary date, project even spread of dates, 50% discount.				$139,633	$7,350	$146,982.59	$126,850.00

Equipment rental based on existing contracts for ultrasound and laser equipment.

| | | | | | | $29.40 | $25.37 |

year's (2004) costs. For purposes of projecting fixed costs, they are identified as committed or programmed in the exhibit. Committed fixed costs arise from long-range decisions and usually remain unchanged for long periods of time. Examples of committed fixed costs include depreciation of buildings and equipment, lease expense, insurance, and property taxes. Programmed fixed costs are set by short-range decisions and changed by management action. Programmed fixed costs are usually stair-step in pattern and include most of the staff salaries, employee benefits (particularly professional development), repairs, and marketing costs.

Seasonal expenses (such as utilities) and fixed expenses that vary from month to month (such as telephone) should be projected by applying the expected increases to monthly amounts for the previous year. In addition to the expenses, adjustments and allowances must be considered. In the example, they are approximately 6 percent of production. The previous year's flexible budget formula for total costs was: TC = \$119,850 per month + \$1.40 per patient visit. Considering the expected price and rate increases, the current flexible budget formula for total costs becomes TC = \$139,633 + \$1.47 per patient visit. Further discussion about the flexible budgeting will be presented later in this chapter.

BUDGETING PHYSICIAN COMPENSATION

Administratively speaking, a straight salary system is clearly the easiest to budget. It is easy to project and requires little data analysis during the year. The downside is that by choosing straight salaries, the practice foregoes a significant opportunity: Physician compensation can be a powerful tool to influence physician behavior. Every system should be in line with the practice's overall strategic goals and promote existing or desired professional values, but ultimately, the system's ability to support the recruitment and retention of physicians is the criteria by which it will be evaluated. Creating a committee comprised of clinicians and the practice's physician and administrative leaders to discuss and design a compensation model is advisable. This will ensure good communication and will increase the probability of physician satisfaction with the resulting compensation structure. The committee needs to start its project by understanding what the historic accounting data really mean. For budgeting purposes, which will determine the affordability of the compensation packages, the following questions need to be asked:

- First, what are the market forces predicted for the coming budget year?
- Second, are there corporate changes that will influence the future accounting detail?

Equally important in the structure of the compensation plan are underlying corporate structures, policies, or legislation that may impact feasible compensation structures, and how the compensation formula will promote the goals and objectives of the practice's strategic plan.

Administrators and physician leaders must take the utmost care in designing their particular compensation system. It is recommended to model any proposed compensation system to ensure it enforces the desired behavior and to assess any negative consequences. Drastic changes should be implemented with great caution and only with considerable forethought on the benefits and liabilities of the proposed compensation plan. The best systems are the ones that are in place for long periods of time. Practices that change compensation systems annually seldom recognize benefits from any incentives to change physician behavior embedded in the compensation plan.

Many medical groups opt for a combined system that includes the following:

- **Base salary** pays the physicians for the core requirements of their job.
- **Incentive compensation** compensates for special achievements or for increased levels of productivity. Items considered for incentive compensation should be aligned with the practice's strategic goals and objectives.
- **Bonus compensation** enumerates a reward for achieving the group's overall business goals.

HOW PHYSICIANS ARE COMPENSATED

The general allocation of net income and especially the bonus compensation to physician compensation must be differentiated by the group's organizational structure.

- **In a sole proprietorship, partnership, or a professional corporation,** the income portion available for physician compensation is usually revenue after operating costs minus staff salary expenses for midlevel providers. While midlevel providers contribute to the revenues, they are seldom considered partners or shareholders in a healthcare organization. The allocation of the remaining balance may take the form of profit sharing or stock options. Remember that retained earnings will come out of the same balance. No matter what route the practice takes, tax implications of all options should be addressed before disbursing income to the owner.
- **Not-for-profit organizations** (tax-exempt) cannot simply divide their net income amongst the physicians because the earnings of the organization may not in any way inure to the benefit of a private person. In addition, federal law requires that compensation be "reasonable." The competitiveness of the salary can be established through physician compensation comparison surveys. Related to the issue of reasonable compensation is the recommendation to cap the maximum annual amount of incentive pay. This precaution will help safeguard the organization's IRS tax-exempt status.

As Koeppen et al. describe, tax-exempt healthcare organizations can allow physicians to participate in the group's performance through the following tools: (a) revenue growth measures that index bonus compensation based on achieving budgeted growth projections; (b) market share performance measures that index bonuses based on increasing market share penetrated as expressed by covered lives; (c) utilization control indexes to compensate for achieving the practice's resource utilization objectives; and (d) quality management scores that index total quality and outcome targets.[1] These scores are becoming increasingly important for practices as insurers and other organizations have begun to analyze them for use in contract negotiations and reimbursement models.

While financial managers will mostly think about cash compensation, it is feasible to include other compensation facets to develop a competitive, successful compensation package. Some physicians may be just as motivated by increased continuing medical education benefits, retirement dollars, or nonmonetary values such as preferred parking or a choice of free holidays. No matter which compensation model a medical group practice adopts, it is strongly recommended to ask the group's board and/or legal and tax advisory counsel to review the model to ensure full compliance with any regulatory requirements.

Estimating the Level of Compensation

If the medical group implements a productivity-based compensation scheme, the budget planner must develop a flexible budget that includes several production levels and the corresponding physician compensation amounts. In the managed care environment, where compensation might be tied to the number of patients assigned to a particular primary care physician, lower levels of resource use might be rewarded by a compensation model because the reimbursement is based on a patient-per-month count versus the amount of services rendered. It is important to not overcompensate for reduced production because a practice should avoid extreme negative correlation between production and compensation. The outgrowths of such a system may include downcoding by physicians to avoid compensation "penalties."

Fitting Compensation into the Overall Budget

Designing an effective model is only the beginning of the budgeting process. The financial manager must then determine the total amount of money projected to be available for physician compensation. The challenge is further complicated by a potential need to combine the incentives of an FFS and a capitated environment. The following step-by-step method assumes the group only deals with a limited amount of capitation and decides to compensate similarly for services provided for capitated patients and for FFS patients. While this is in part driven by the organization type the practice operates under (see above), the following steps apply in principle:

Step 1: Agree on a fee schedule or an RVU scale to determine the value of each service and the different amounts of work needed to complete each service.

Step 2: Determine the monthly amount of money projected to come into the practice through each capitated contract. Use the HMO projected covered lives minus the set-aside-for-IBNR HMO claims.

Step 3: Tally the monthly revenues determined in Step 2 for all capitated contracts.

Step 4: Project the income adjusted by bad debt, contractual allowances, and risk pool withholdings from FFS for the remaining resources.

Step 5: Deduct the total amount needed to cover all operating expenses.

The remaining balance indicates the total amount available for physician compensation and incentives. The compensation formula will then determine the amount after operating expenses to be allocated to the individual physicians. The fee schedule or score will help determine production-based incentives.

Good compensation plans are simple and easy to explain. If the physician does not understand the compensation schedule, it is unlikely to motivate desired behaviors. In addition to the diffusion of cause and effect, undue administrative burden makes it unrealistic to incorporate more than a few tracking benchmarks. Useful benchmarks include clinical outcomes, staffing levels, patient satisfaction scores, compliance rate of providers, participation in administrative tasks, patient-base growth, and resource utilization. It is also advisable to consider different compensation plans for primary care physicians and specialists. However, none of these decisions is all or nothing.

Bonus payments are typically not part of the budget because the resources used for bonus compensation should be based on excess income after the budgeted physician salaries. As for all budget line items, the physician compensation section needs to be adjusted at least mid-year. Although — based on the significance of this expense — it is recommended to either perform routine quarterly adjustments or to revisit the physician compensation budget item whenever the practice introduces other significant changes to its operations.

PREPARING THE BUDGET PLAN

The profit plan integrates budgeted revenues and budgeted expenses to show the net income or contribution income for the total practice or for segments of the practice. Planning, control, and decision making are most effective when the profit plan and subsequent performance reporting are related to responsibility centers. Most medical groups are organized along responsibility center lines, with each medical specialty a separate responsibility center.

Responsibility Center Profit Plan

Using the revenue projections and cost behavior patterns developed in Exhibit 11.10, a profit plan is presented in Exhibit 11.11. The profit plan shown in Exhibit 11.11 and in later exhibits will include figures for each of the three months in Quarter 1 and for the total year (Quarters 2, 3, and 4 are omitted to simplify the exhibits). Only expenses directly traceable to the responsibility center are included in the responsibility center's profit plan.

EXHIBIT 11.11 ■ **Profit Plan — OB/GYN**

	Jan.	Feb.	Mar.	Quarter 1 Total	Annualized
Gross Charges	$236,631	$218,008	$235,536	$690,175	$2,760,699
Adjustments and allowances (25%)	$(59,158)	$(54,502)	$(58,884)	$(172,544)	$(690,175)
Net Revenue	$177,473	$163,506	$176,652	$517,631	$2,070,524
Operating Expenses					
Physician salaries	$72,917	$72,917	$72,917	$218,751	$875,004
Physician benefits	$16,042	$16,042	$16,042	$48,125	$192,501
Staff salaries	$24,600	$24,600	$24,600	$73,800	$295,200
Staff benefits	$4,428	$4,428	$4,428	$13,284	$53,136
Supplies	$6,668	$6,143	$6,637	$19,448	$77,792
Equipment rental	$4,000	$4,000	$4,000	$12,000	$48,000
Professional liability insurance	$14,000	$14,000	$14,000	$42,000	$168,000
Total Expenses	$142,655	$142,130	$142,624	$427,408	$1,709,633
Gross Margin	$34,819	$21,376	$34,028	$90,223	$360,891

Prepaid Practice Profit Plan

It is critical for the group entering a prepaid practice to establish accountability for its prepaid contract. Each medical and ancillary responsibility center providing service to prepaid patients should be given FFS equivalent credit for patient visits or procedures performed in the responsibility center. This rewards each responsibility center with a satisfactory revenue measure. It does not, however, provide an evaluation of the prepaid practice. A separate responsibility center should be created for this purpose.

Revenues in the prepaid practice responsibility center are the capitation payments from the HMO. Expenses include the cost of service provided to prepaid patients, expressed in the FFS equivalents, and the cost of outside referrals if the practice is at risk for them. If there are incremental costs traceable to the prepaid practice (e.g., a nurse or clerk assigned to utilization review and control), these costs should be included in the profit plan of the prepaid practice and in subsequent reporting.

The real cost for inside services is the cost PMPM. The difference between the FFS equivalent for service provided to prepaid patients and the real cost of serving the patients is included in the reports of the medical and ancillary responsibility centers. The cost PMPM should be included as a note to the profit plan of the prepaid practice.

Compilation of Responsibility Center Profit Plans into a Profit Plan for the Group

The purpose of the profit plan for the group is to forecast whether total revenues will be sufficient to cover total expenses and provide an adequate level of income. Production (FFS gross charges), adjustments and allowances, and net revenue are presented as single amounts for the entire group. Expenses, however, are presented by responsibility centers. An alternative presentation would be to list the contribution (revenues minus direct costs) of each responsibility center, then deduct common costs from the total contribution for the group. Presentation of total production (including capitation) has been chosen because most medical groups want to see total revenues for the group in the budget and in the income statement.

The profit plan may be prepared several times, using different projections of production and expenses, if the physician-owners are not satisfied with the overall income level. To meet the target income level, it may be necessary for individual responsibility centers to consider cost reductions, charging higher fees or increasing productivity levels.

PREPARING THE CASH BUDGET

The second part of the comprehensive budget is the cash budget. This budget shows the anticipated sources and uses of cash for the coming year. Chapter 7 presented the development and use of the cash budget extensively. In terms of timing, the cash budget is developed after the profit plan is prepared and the capital expenditures are finalized. Ideally, both the profit plan and the cash budget should be structured as "rollover budgets," adding a new month at the end of each month (and a new quarter at the end of each quarter) and always showing the next three months and the next three quarters. In this way, the profit plan and cash budget are always current.

Groups that engage in increasing levels of prepaid contracting need to be aware of certain cash flow nuances arising from these contracts. For example, the lag in cash outflows resulting from IBNR claims for outside referrals is sufficiently significant that the impact of the lag on the cash budget should be understood. Measurement of cash flows for outside referrals is the "other side" of measuring IBNR claims. The typical FFS medical group does not have a liability for services provided outside the group. The medical group that has agreed to provide services to members of an HMO on a capitation basis typically has a liability for physician services performed outside the group. The need for estimating outstanding claims and the presentation of several examples of how this liability can be measured are covered in chapter 8.

Exhibit 11.12 shows the budgeted revenue as it will arrive as cash in the practice. Taking seasonality of revenue out of the equation for simplicity, we can track the anticipated flow of cash in the door from past and present operations. The percentage of revenue realized in each period can be developed through use of historical data, historical collection rates, and any current trends in managed

EXHIBIT 11.12 ■ Revenue Realization — Cash vs. Accrued Budget

Month	Gross Charges	January	February	March	April	May	Collections June
July	$—	$—	$—	$—	$—	$—	$—
August	—	1,500	—	—	—	—	—
September	—	4,500	1,500	—	—	—	—
October	—	9,000	4,500	1,500	—	—	—
November	—	45,000	9,000	4,500	1,500	—	—
December	—	60,000	45,000	9,000	4,500	1,500	—
January	236,631	35,495	70,989	53,242	10,648	5,324	1,775
February	218,008	—	32,701	65,402	49,052	9,810	4,905
March	235,536	—	—	35,330	70,661	52,996	10,599
April	236,631	—	—	—	35,495	70,989	53,242
May	218,008	—	—	—	—	32,701	65,402
June	235,536	—	—	—	—	—	35,330
July	236,631	—	—	—	—	—	—
August	218,008	—	—	—	—	—	—
September	235,536	—	—	—	—	—	—
October	236,631	—	—	—	—	—	—
November	218,008	—	—	—	—	—	—
December	235,536	—	—	—	—	—	—
Totals	$2,760,700	$155,495	$163,691	$168,975	$171,856	$173,321	$171,254

Expected Cash Collections Percentages

Month 1	Month 2	Month 3	Month 4	Month 5	Month 6	Totals
20%	40%	30%	6%	3%	1%	100%

Assumption: Charges were flat at 200,000 per month in previous year.

care contracts or operations (upfront collections, etc.). This "executive window" report can provide management with an instantaneous comparative assessment of accrued versus actual revenue for the business unit/practice.

PREPARING THE PROJECTED STATEMENT OF ASSETS AND LIABILITIES (BALANCE SHEET)

The third and final step in developing the comprehensive budget is the preparation of a projected statement of assets and liabilities, or a balance sheet. Exhibit 11.5 illustrated the flow of data through the profit plan and cash budget to the projected statement of assets and liabilities. When the cash

July	August	September	October	November	December	Totals	Revenue Outstanding	Accrued Revenue
$—	$—	$—	$—	$—	$—	$—	$—	$—
—	—	—	—	—	—	1,500	—	—
—	—	—	—	—	—	6,000	—	—
—	—	—	—	—	—	15,000	—	—
—	—	—	—	—	—	60,000	—	—
—	—	—	—	—	—	120,000	—	—
—	—	—	—	—	—	177,473	—	177,473
1,635	—	—	—	—	—	163,506	—	163,506
5,300	1,767	—	—	—	—	176,652	—	176,652
10,648	5,324	1,775	—	—	—	177,473	—	177,473
49,052	9,810	4,905	1,635	—	—	163,506	—	163,506
70,661	52,996	10,599	5,300	1,767	—	176,652	—	176,652
35,495	70,989	53,242	10,648	5,324	1,775	177,473	—	177,473
—	32,701	65,402	49,052	9,810	4,905	161,871	1,635	163,506
—	—	35,330	70,661	52,996	10,599	169,586	7,066	176,652
—	—	—	35,495	70,989	53,242	159,726	17,747	177,473
—	—	—	—	32,701	65,402	98,104	65,402	163,506
—	—	—	—	—	35,330	35,330	141,322	176,652
$172,790	$173,587	$171,254	$172,790	$173,587	$171,254	$2,039,853	$233,172	$2,070,525

budget is developed, many of the ending balances of assets and liabilities for the statement of assets and liabilities are produced. For example, projection of the cash payments lag for incurred but unreported claims also produces the balance of the liability for incurred but unreported claims.

The major purpose of the projected statement of assets and liabilities is to tie the planning documents together and show the estimated financial position at the end of the planning period. Are the physician-owners and the creditors satisfied with the balances and the relationships presented in the projected statement of assets and liabilities? If the group has active cash management, a strong credit and collection function, and a good supply control system, the balances on the projected statement of assets and liabilities should produce very few surprises.

Using the Budget

When budgets are adopted and placed into operational use, it is important to be aware of what is likely to occur. A budget is a target derived from an informed estimate of what future events will likely be. Even though group management attempts to achieve the planned levels of activity, revenue, and expenses, seldom are they identical to these plans. There are usually five reasons why deviations in actual and budgeted results occur:

1. More or fewer patients are seen than planned.
2. The pattern of cash collections is changed.
3. Price changes occurred in fees and/or in expenses.
4. The group is either more or less efficient with regard to the budget in the use of resources.
5. Changes occurred in the level of short-term resources such as the supplies inventory.

One of the major problems in the control process is to differentiate the effects on the budget for variances that arise from these five and other reasons. If a significant change in activity is accompanied by excessive use of resources, there may be a tendency to attribute the inefficiencies to the change in activity. This inference is illustrated by the example in Exhibit 11.13. This example presents budgeted and actual results for the first quarter of 2005 for one satellite office of Mountain Valley OB/GYN, which is staffed by one physician.

During the quarter, economic conditions in the community caused a reduction in the actual number of patient visits from the budgeted level. If the mix of services did not change, how well did the Crater Lake office perform? There

EXHIBIT 11.13 ■ Operating Statement — Crater Lake Office

	Quarter 1, 2005		
	Budget	**Actual**	**Variance**
Gross charges	$ 120,000	$ 100,000	$ (20,000)
Operating expenses:			
Physician salary	$40,000	$40,000	$—
Staff salaries	15,000	14,500	500
Laboratory services	15,000	12,000	3,000
Medical supplies	8,050	9,000	(950)
Rent and utilities	5,000	6,000	(1,000)
Other expenses	14,000	14,000	—
Total expenses	$97,050	$95,500	$1,550
Contribution to common costs and income	$22,950	$4,500	$(18,450)

was a 16.7 percent reduction in gross charges ($100,000 actual gross charges are 16.7 percent less than the budgeted gross charges of $120,000) but only a 1.6 percent reduction in expenses of $97,050. Was the office efficient in controlling expenses?

To answer the questions, one must first know how much actual expenses should have decreased because of decreased activity. The original profit plan (budget) was prepared for $120,000 gross charge level of activity. To evaluate performance, a new operating budget should be prepared for the $100,000 actual level of activity. By removing the change in activity from the budget, one can then focus on the variances due to price changes and operating inefficiencies. A budget revised for change in activity is called a flexible budget or a performance budget. Except for the change in activity, the same assumptions are used to prepare both the profit plan and the performance budget. Exhibit 11.14 presents the actual results for the quarter (gross charges of $100,000) compared to a performance budget established at the $100,000 activity level. Only laboratory services and medical supplies are assumed to be variable expenses; all other expenses are assumed to be fixed. In the revised performance budget, laboratory expenses and medical supply expenses are reduced in the same proportion as the level of gross charges (83.3 percent of the original budget). All other expenses are considered fixed and remain the same in the revised budget as they were originally.

The performance budget shows that the Crater Lake office should have contributed $6,790 (rather than $22,950) to the income of the group. Total deviations from plan now amount to $2,290. These may be partly explained by excessive costs in medical supplies, rent, and utilities. On the favorable side, the time of nurses and medical assistants and laboratory services were reduced

EXHIBIT 11.14 ■ Actual Operations Compared with Performance — Crater Lake Office

	Quarter 1, 2005		
	Budget	**Actual**	**Variance**
Gross charges	$100,000	$100,000	$—
Operating expenses:			
Physician salary	$40,000	$40,000	$—
Staff salaries	15,000	14,500	500
Laboratory services	12,500	12,000	500
Medical supplies	6,710	9,000	(2,290)
Rent and utilities	5,000	6,000	(1,000)
Other expenses	14,000	14,000	—
Total expenses	$93,210	$95,500	$(2,290)
Contribution to common costs and income	$6,790	$4,500	$(2,290)

(demonstrating that some fixed expenses are not "fixed" if management wishes to change them).

THE FLEXIBLE BUDGET

The comprehensive budget described above can be prepared either in a static form, where volume is assumed to be unchanging, or in a flexible form for different levels of volume activity. With the exception of service volume, all assumptions will be identical in either a static or flexible budget. In reality, the flexible budget is prepared as a series of static budgets, each reflecting a different level of activity that sets forth the appropriate details of revenues and expenses at each activity level.

It is difficult for any healthcare organization to accurately estimate activity volume. Projecting activity volume for a medical group practice is no exception. The volume of activity depends on a number of external and internal forces, many of which are not entirely within management's control. Fluctuations from planned activity volume will cause variances from budgeted revenues and expenses. When it is difficult to estimate future activity volume and when costs vary in response to volume changes, use of the flexible budget provides an excellent approach to both planning and performance reporting.

The Nature of Flexible Budgeting

The development of flexible budgets in a fairly simple situation was demonstrated in the last part of the section on comprehensive budgeting coverage. In a more extended way, the flexible budget accommodates changes in number and type of patient encounters and in volume of procedures. For planning purposes, a flexible budget enables management to analyze costs based on a series of individual volume forecasts coupled with estimates of fixed and variable costs for each type of medical group activity. For performance reporting, a flexible budget allows responsibility center managers to evaluate periodically how budgeted resource consumption (costs) compares with actual production (like the previous example for the Crater Lake office). It also provides a structured tool to answer two of the most common budget variance excuses — "our volume estimates were off" and "our patients were sicker than we budgeted for and required more services." Both of these are common managerial problems with static budgeting.

The value of flexible budgeting is perhaps best observed through the advantages and disadvantages of static and flexible budgeting approaches. These are shown in Exhibit 11.15.

REQUIREMENTS FOR FLEXIBLE BUDGETING

To prepare a flexible budget, determining an appropriate unit of service is one of the most complex requirements. An output measure (unit of service) must be identified for each responsibility center and for each activity within

EXHIBIT 11.15 ■ Advantages and Disadvantages of Static and Flexible Budgets

Static Budgets

Advantages	Disadvantages
Simple and easy to understand. May be manually prepared.	Cannot easily be adjusted to reflect actual activity levels.
Time required to prepare and monitor is somewhat less than with a flexible budget.	If actual activity level varies widely from budgeted activity level, it becomes very difficult to analyze discrepancies caused by changes in volume, prices, and efficiency.
Can be a meaningful tool for measuring performance if actual level of activity is reasonably near budgeted level.	Explanations for variances are often blamed on volume changes rather than on more controllable factors.

Flexible Budgets

Advantages	Disadvantages
Can be adjusted to reflect actual activity levels.	Requires more time and resources to develop and update.
Easier to obtain meaningful variance analysis.	Requires additional training and usually requires a computer to process the effect of changes in activity level.
	Generally a higher level of sophistication is required by the group's administrative, financial, and operating personnel to properly utilize the budget.

a responsibility center that adopts flexible budgeting. Unit of service may be defined at various levels of detail, depending on the needs and resources of the medical group. At a greater level of detail, units of service can be defined at the procedure level within the responsibility center. The degree of detail selected will affect the complexity of the data collection process and, consequently, the investment necessary to implement and maintain the database. The greater the level of detail, however, the greater the opportunity for exercising management control.

With regard to preparing a flexible budget of expenses, the simplest measure of resource utilization and related costs is a procedure. There are three approaches to developing the cost of procedures. They are:

1. Unit of service approach
2. Relative value unit (RVU) approach
3. Standard cost approach

Unit of Service Approach to Procedure Costing

Under this approach, each procedure performed equals one unit of service. Our objective is to compute the average cost of resources used per procedure for each responsibility center. The calculation is simple — total center costs divided by total center procedures.

The location where the costs are collected and where the procedures are performed must be identical. For example, to calculate the cost per procedure for a medical group's clinic facility, the total costs of the facility are divided by the number of procedures performed in the facility. Normally, this will exclude all procedures performed on inpatients.

The result of this calculation is a single cost amount — a macro-measure representing the average cost of resources consumed to produce a single unit of service. It is considered a macro-measure because the per-unit cost is calculated without regard to the relative intensity (mix) of services. A change in procedure mix between periods can have a significant impact on the costs incurred. A macro-measure will not permit procedure-mix variance analysis.

Other unit-of-service definitions more appropriately define the activity within an individual responsibility center. For example, the number of prescriptions filled is the normal measure of pharmacy activity. A list of responsibility centers and their typical unit-of-service measures are shown in Exhibit 11.16.

EXHIBIT 11.16 ■ Typical Unit of Service Measures

Responsibility center	Unit of service
Physician's practice	Procedure or patient encounter
Emergency services	Procedure or patient encounter
Surgery	Operating room hour or encounter
Psychiatric services	Patient encounter
Pharmacy	Prescription
Laboratory	Laboratory test
Physical Therapy	Workload measurement unit or number of patients
Occupational Therapy	Workload measurement unit or number of patients
Respiratory Therapy	Procedure
Speech Pathology	Session
Audiology	Procedure
EKG/EEG	Procedure
Radiology/Imaging	Radiology/imaging procedure
Patient Reception	Number of patients or number of appointments
Medical Records	Number of patients or number of appointments
Building Operations and Maintenance	Square feet
Data Processing	Number of transactions
Administration	$1,000 of operating revenues

In a simplified organization, an application of the unit-of-service costing for obstetrics/gynecology could be calculated as follows:

■ Determine total ambulatory care procedures performed in the responsibility center:
   – Total obstetrics/gynecology procedures = 1,000

■ Determine total direct costs of the responsibility center:
   – Total obstetrics/gynecology direct costs = $20,000

■ Divide total responsibility center direct costs by total procedures:
   – $20,000/1,000 procedures = $20.00 per procedure.

This approach does not recognize, however, the different degrees of effort related to each type of procedure or encounter. Because different procedures require significantly different effort, expertise, and related resources, an RVU approach to measuring costs may be more appropriate.

Relative Value Unit (RVU) Approach to Procedure Costing

This approach eliminates the impact of procedure-mix fluctuations and provides a more refined method of projecting and managing costs. It uses a relative value scale with weighting factors for each procedure or group of procedures performed within a responsibility center. Actual weighting may be based on many factors such as time to complete the procedure, training and education costs, difficulty of procedure, cost of resources used, malpractice insurance cost, or any combination of such factors.

To calculate procedure costs under this method, procedure volumes are multiplied by their respective RVUs and totaled. The total costs of the responsibility center are divided by the total of all RVU weights to determine a cost per RVU. The cost per RVU is then multiplied by each procedure's RVU weight to determine a cost per procedure. See Exhibit 11.17 for an example.

The RVU approach requires more effort but offers several advantages over the unit-of-service approach. First, the cost and resource information is more detailed — each procedure is assigned a specific cost, not an average cost. Secondly, the RVU approach isolates changes in costs due to changes in procedure mix as well as changes in volume. Isolating the impact of procedure mix allows management to focus on cost performance regardless of volume and procedure mix changes. The effort involved in the RVU approach can be reduced by costing only the procedures that are performed frequently or by using a computer software package that performs the calculations.

Standard Cost Approach to Procedure Costing

The third method of costing procedures uses expected levels of time and resources that are consumed in performing a procedure. The expected levels of effort can be based on the historical experience of the group or, in some cases, they can be adapted from "industry standards" such as Resource Based Relative Value Scales (RBRVS). This is discussed in detail in chapter 7.

EXHIBIT 11.17 ■ RVU Calculation

Step 1. Determine total RVUs associated with procedures performed in the responsibility center.

Procedures performed in obstetrics/gynecology CPT-4 code	Number of occurrences	Individual RVU weight	Total RVUs
59030	1	10.0	10
59020	1	5.0	5
58100	75	8.0	600
59430	100	10.0	1,000
90040	900	4.5	4,050
90060	965	10.0	9,650
Totals	3,162		26,483

Step 2. Divide total responsibility center cost by total RVUs.

Direct costs	Responsibility center total RVUs	Cost/RVU
75500	26483	2.85

Step 3. Multiply the cost/RVU by the RVU weight for each procedure.

Procedure	Cost/RVU	RVU Weight	Cost/procedure
59030	2.85	10.0	28.50
59020	2.85	5.0	14.25
58100	2.85	8.0	22.80
59430	2.85	10.0	28.50
90040	2.85	4.5	12.83
90060	2.85	10.0	28.50

This approach, in essence, develops a standard cost per procedure and provides a measure of the expected resource requirements associated with each procedure. The standard amounts of labor, supplies, and equipment are determined by studying the requirements for delivering patient care in the medical group's particular setting. Once determined, the required resources are extended by the current unit costs (labor rates, supply prices, and capital expenses) and the amounts totaled to arrive at the standard cost for a specific procedure. For certain applications (e.g., establishing fee schedules), a measure and an allocation of overhead costs per unit of output also are required.

The level of detail may be constrained by available source data (such as supply detail records). For example, a medical group with limited computerized analysis capability may budget labor costs as averages, regardless of skill level. In a more detailed system, the labor requirements may be identified individually by the skill level of each person involved in performing the procedure. Likewise, supply costs may be identified as a single average cost of the supplies used or be listed by the individual cost of the items consumed.

The level of detail in each group's cost management system should be determined by the planned management applications and by the resources available to implement and maintain the system. For example, systems that are designed primarily for income distribution and fee setting will typically require less detail. However, systems used for production monitoring and control will require a finer level of detail, such as identifying the skill levels of the labor component.

Regardless of the level of detail used in the system, costs must be first separated into their fixed and variable components (chapter 6). As noted previously, this is very important to the flexible budgeting concept because variable costs are affected most by changes in volume. The flexible budgeting approach becomes more appropriate as the ratio of variable costs to fixed costs increases and as the volume of patient care fluctuates. Consult chapter 7 if additional information is desired about the development of standard costs for purposes other than budgeting and for other illustrations on the use of RVUs in cost determination.

FLEXIBLE BUDGET VARIANCES

Once flexible budgeting has been accepted and established, it has the potential to become a valuable performance-reporting tool. At the end of each reporting period (usually monthly), the actual expenses can be compared to the flexible budget's prediction of expenses for the actual patient activity level achieved. To accomplish this, the original monthly budgeted volumes are replaced with the actual patient activity volumes. The budgeted variable unit costs are multiplied by the actual activity volumes to obtain the "flexed" budget amount for variable costs. This amount is then added to the budgeted fixed costs to arrive at the total flexed budget cost, which then can be compared with actual costs for analysis purposes.

Any differences between the flexed budgeted costs and the actual costs relate to how well resources were matched to the level of output during the reporting period. The differences, called flexible budget variances, typically pertain to how well the individual responsibility center managers have run their departments. As the year progresses, the flexible budget may be modified to incorporate actual changes in employee wage rates, material costs, and overhead costs. This flexible approach to budget management provides a meaningful tool to monitor financial performance and take corrective action at the earliest warranted stage. However, it requires a significant level of available cost data and careful consideration of projections on both variable and fixed cost components.

COST-VOLUME-PROFIT ANALYSIS

Cost-volume-profit (CVP) analysis offers a macro-level approach to examining the effects on profits that result from changes in volume of revenue or production, fees, costs, and profits. It is a commonly used tool that provides management with useful information about running a business or medical practice. CVP analysis aids in establishing budgets by assessing the impact on costs, volume of service, and profits when changes are contemplated in any of these three variables. Also, CVP analysis can be used in setting fees, selecting the mix of services to be offered, and choosing among alternative delivery strategies. This analysis is a complex matter since these relationships are often affected by forces entirely or partially beyond the control of management. Nevertheless, CVP analysis in some relatively simple situations can be of great value in providing insights into possible results from adopting individual or combined changes in the cost structure, fee arrangements, and volume load of the practice.

Contribution Margin Concept

One relationship between cost, volume, and profit, which is especially useful in business planning because it gives insight into the profit potential, is the contribution margin concept. The contribution margin is the excess of revenue over variable costs and expenses. The deduction of fixed costs and expenses from the contribution margin equals the operating income or loss. To illustrate, examine the following income statement for the Kathryn Hailey Medical Group prepared in a contribution margin format:

Kathryn Hailey Medical Group	
Gross charges	$1,000,000
Variable costs	600,000
Contribution margin	$400,000
Fixed costs	300,000
Operating income	$100,000

The $400,000 contribution margin is available to cover the fixed costs of $300,000. Once the fixed costs are covered, any remaining contribution margin adds directly to the operating income of the group.

Contribution Margin Ratio

The contribution margin can be expressed as a percentage. The contribution margin ratio, sometimes called the profit-volume ratio, indicates the percentage of each revenue dollar available to cover fixed costs and to provide operating income. For the Kathryn Hailey Medical Group, the contribution margin ratio is 40 percent, as shown by the following computation:

$$\text{Contribution margin ratio} = \frac{\text{Sales} - \text{Variable costs}}{\text{Sales}}$$

For example:

$$40\% = \frac{\$1,000,000 - \$600,000}{\$1,000,000}$$

The contribution margin ratio permits a quick determination of the effect that an increase or decrease in revenue volume will have on operating income. To illustrate, assume the management of Kathryn Hailey is studying the effect of adding $80,000 in revenue volume. Assuming the ratios of variable and fixed costs remain the same, multiplying the contribution margin ratio (40 percent) by the change in revenue volume ($80,000) indicates an increase in operating income of $32,000 if the additional volume is obtained. Again, the utility of this calculation depends on the assumption that the fixed cost components would remain the same despite the increase in volume.

Unit Contribution Margin

Similar to the contribution margin ratio, the unit contribution margin is also a useful relationship for analyzing the profit potential of proposed expansions of services. The unit contribution margin is the dollars available from each unit of revenue to cover fixed costs and provide operating profits. For example, if Kathryn Hailey's average fee per patient is $20 and its unit average variable cost is $12, the unit contribution margin is $8 ($20 − $12).

Both the contribution margin ratio and the unit contribution margin can be employed in analyzing a critical level of operations in any business — the break-even point. Let's examine this next.

BREAK-EVEN POINT ANALYSIS

The break-even point for any business is that level of operations at which revenues and all expired costs are exactly equal. At this level, a business will neither realize an operating profit nor incur an operating loss. Break-even analysis can be applied to past periods, but it is most useful when applied to future periods as a guide to business planning, particularly in situations that involve the expansion or curtailment of operations. In such cases, the analysis is concerned with future prospects and future operations and hence relies on estimates. The reliability of the analysis is greatly influenced by the accuracy of the estimates.

The break-even point can be computed by means of mathematical equations that indicate the relationships between revenue, costs, and volume or graphically by various charts. Each of these approaches is explained below.

Break-Even Analysis through Equations

The break-even point may be determined by an equation that divides fixed costs by the unit contribution margin. To illustrate, assume a laboratory charges an average of $6.00 per test and incurs an average variable cost per test of $2.74. Further, assume the laboratory's fixed costs per month total $9,040. The use of the break-even equation would produce a break-even point of about 2,800 tests per month, calculated as follows:

$$\text{Break-even point for number of tests} = \frac{\text{Fixed costs}}{\text{Contribution margin per test}}$$

For example:

$$\frac{\$9,040}{\$6.00 - \$2.74} = 2,773 \text{ tests}$$

To show how this kind of analysis can be useful, assume that the laboratory has been requested to contribute $1,000 per month for administrative services performed by the main clinic of the practice, in addition to covering all costs in the laboratory. How many tests would be required for the laboratory to break even under this new set of assumptions? As indicated below, the answer is an increase in tests to about 3,080 per month:

$$\frac{\text{Required number of tests to generate required contribution}}{} = \frac{\text{Fixed costs} + \text{Allocated costs}}{\text{Contribution margin per test}}$$

For example:

$$\frac{\$9,040 + \$1,000}{3.26} = 3,080 \text{ tests}$$

Break-Even Analysis through Graphs

Perhaps for some, the easiest way to visualize and understand cost-volume-profit analysis is graphically — through a break-even chart or a profit-volume chart. A break-even chart shows much more than the point at which an organization or a practice will break even. It provides a picture of profit or loss at all levels of activity within the relevant range of activity.

Returning to the laboratory example above, we saw that the break-even point was 2,773 tests per month. In Exhibit 11.18, the break-even point is that point at which the revenue line crosses the total costs line. The areas marked with "R" on the chart indicate the relevant range, that is, the range over which it is known that the cost-volume-profit relationships are valid. Any projection below or above the relevant range may not be reliable because there is no experience on which to base the projection. From the graph, it is possible to determine the profit of 4,000 tests (a profit of $4,000) and at 2,000 tests (a loss of $2,520), or any other level of activity within the relevant range.

Another form of the break-even chart is the profit-volume chart. By plotting only the contribution margin, the profit or loss is easily determinable at any level of activity with a single line. At zero activity, the loss is equal to fixed costs. The profit-volume chart for the laboratory is also shown in Exhibit 11.18. The break-even point, the profit at 4,000 tests, and the loss at 2,000 tests are the same as shown on the earlier break-even chart.

The benefits of graphing the break-even point on charts can be borne out by the following examples. If the group is dissatisfied with the predicted results for the laboratory, there are at least three possible courses of action: (1) increase the fee per test, (2) increase the volume of tests, or (3) decrease the costs. Exhibit 11.19 shows the impact of cost and fee changes. The long, dashed line in the upper chart shows the impact of decreasing fixed costs by $2,000. The break-even point decreases to about 2,160 tests. The short, dashed line in the lower chart shows the impact of decreasing variable costs or increasing fees by $0.50 per test. Both a decrease of $0.50 per test in variable cost and an increase of $0.50

EXHIBIT 11.18 ■ **Illustration of Break-Even and Profit-Volume Charts**

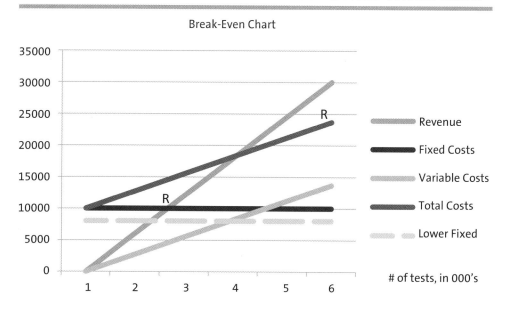

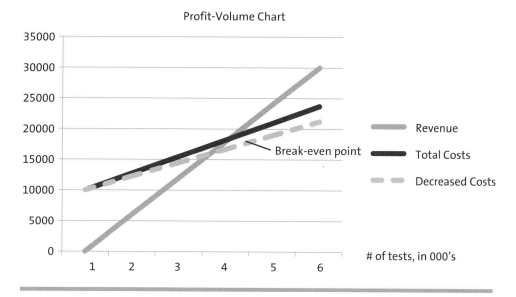

per test in fees will increase the contribution margin by $0.50 per test. The slope of the line is increased, dropping the break-even point to about 2,400 tests.

Financial managers often opt for using profit-volume charts for presentations to their management but use equations for detailed and precise calculations of break-even points. In addition to providing more precision, they also afford the ability to deal with several changes at one time.

EXHIBIT 11.19 ▪ Illustration of the Impact of Cost and Fee Changes

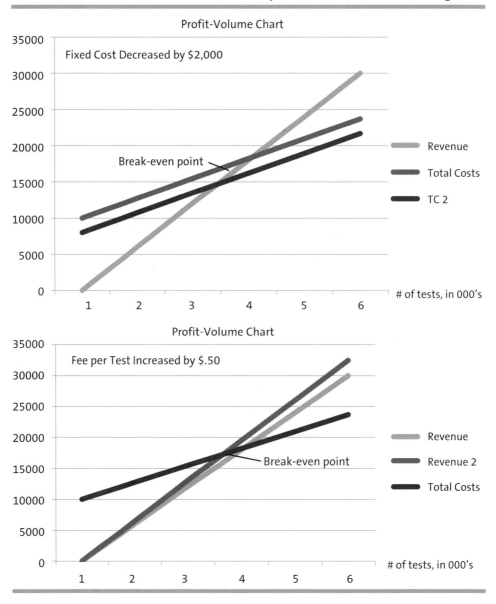

COST-VOLUME-PROFIT ANALYSIS FOR A PREPAID PRACTICE

If the number of prepaid patients is used as the measure of activity, the break-even chart for the prepaid practice will look much like the typical break-even chart. The break-even chart shows the number of patients at which the plan will break even and the profit or loss at any level of activity. However, a not-so-subtle change occurs as the plan matures. If a constant number of prepaid patients is assumed, as may be found in a mature plan, there is a dramatic change in relationships. The total costs include the fixed costs of the practice, the variable cost per patient visit, and the variable costs for referrals and hospitalization. Because revenue is fixed and cost is increasing as the prepaid patients make more visits, the practice shows a profit below the break-even point and a loss as additional activity is incurred above the break-even point. To change this result, capitation payment increases must be negotiated or operating costs must be reduced.

The prepaid practice is rewarded for efficient use of resources. Anything the practice can do to minimize the use of the practice's resources (yet provide quality care) will tend to increase the practice's income. In contrast, the FFS group practice is rewarded for increasing patient visits, and therefore, revenue.

Cost-volume-profit analysis for a combined FFS/prepaid group is further complicated because revenue and cost data are in different terms. The capitation payments are on a PMPM basis; the FFS revenue and cost data are developed on a per-procedure or per-patient visit basis. For example, assume the following data for Costal Medical Center's satellite office.

Capitation payment for services performed at the satellite office passed on to the satellite office	$7.34 PMPM
Capitation payment for other services provided by the group and for referrals outside the medical center	$9.47 PMPM

Cost of operating satellite office
   Direct costs:

Fixed costs per month	$15,000.00
Variable cost per visit	$3.00
Allocated costs from medical center for administration and support (14% of capitation)	$1.19
Expected utilization	.3 visits per PMPM

If the variable costs are translated into PMPM data, the cost-volume-profit analysis may use enrolled members as the measure of activity. In this example, the variable cost per visit of $3.00 translates to a $0.75 PMPM (0.3 visits × $3.00 = $.9 divided by 12). The contribution margin per-member per-month is then calculated as $6.075 ($7.34 − $.075 − $1.19). The break-even point becomes 2,469 members as evidenced below.

$$\text{Break-even point} = \frac{\text{Fixed costs per month}}{\text{Contribution margin PMPM}}$$

For example:

$$\frac{\$15,000}{\$6,075} = 2,469 \text{ members}$$

As different types of procedures are added to this type of analysis above, the complexity of the calculation increases.

To the Point

■ Planning is the process by which management looks ahead and develops a specific course of action to attain the entity's goals. Strategic planning is the development of a long-range course of action to achieve goals and usually encompasses periods ranging from five to 10 years. Operational planning is the development of short-term plans to achieve goals identified in the strategic plan, and they range in time from one week or month to several years.

■ Medical groups benefit from planning regardless of whether the process is formal or informal by following these steps:

   – Perform an environmental scan

   – Develop goals and objectives for the group

   – Establish short-term operating budgets consistent with the goals and objectives

   – Compare actual results to budgets and consider the need for corrective action

■ Goals are broad, timeless statements indicating what the organization desires to achieve. Objectives are more specific statements that support and flow from goals that become ends to pursue in order to achieve the goals. Good objectives, as well as goals, should be measurable.

■ Operating budgets, sometimes called profit plans, are the short-term operating plans of the medical group expressed in terms of dollars. Among the advantages of this budgeting process are the following: requires managers to plan in an organized and focused way; aids in integrating short-range plans with long-range directions; serves as a communication device of management plans to all segments of the group; motivates managers to achieve their agreed-to targets embodied in the budget; and establishes benchmarks to control ongoing activities and set criteria for evaluating the performance of managers.

■ A comprehensive budget, sometimes called a master budget, consists of a series of informal projections and a number of formal statements. There are two major parts: First, the planning and control systems for managing cash and other short-term resources. Second, the formal, comprehensive budget, which consists of a profit plan, a cash budget, a capital expenditures budget, and a projected balance sheet or position statement.

▪ There are several steps usually followed in preparing a comprehensive budget that include (1) developing a picture of the surrounding environment; (2) gathering the expectations of the physicians and other providers; (3) projecting revenues and expenses; (4) budgeting for cash; (5) preparing a capital expenditure budget; and (6) summarizing the results in a set of financial statements.

▪ To project operating revenues, medical groups use three approaches in estimating future revenues — (1) estimating the total demand for the group's services on a broad basis, (2) making base projections based on past activity data, and (3) using estimates of procedures or patient visits.

▪ Using a flexible budgeting formula to estimate expenses provides a way to better match actual results with appropriate budget amounts based on the actual level of activity achieved by the group.

▪ The profit plan integrates budgeted revenues and budgeted expenses to show the net income or contribution income for the total practice or for segments of the practice.

▪ A flexible budget is a series of static budgets (which assume no change in volume) reflecting different levels of activity by setting forth the appropriate details of revenues and expenses at each activity level. This type of budget allows for more accurate comparisons of actual results with appropriate budgeted amounts and leads to better evaluations of performance.

▪ In budgeting expenses for clinical responsibility centers, three approaches to develop the cost of procedures are used: (1) the unit-of-service method, (2) relative value units (RVUs), and (3) standard cost.

▪ Cost-volume-profit (CVP) analysis is an evaluation of the effects on profits that result from changes in volume of revenue or production, fees, costs, and profits. The analysis provides insights into how changes in these three variables can affect each other and be useful in managing the practice.

- Two relationships in CVP analysis are the contribution margin concept — the excess of revenue over variable costs and expenses — and contribution margin ratio — the percentage of each revenue dollar available to cover fixed costs and provide operating income.

- The break-even point is the level of operations at which revenues and all expired costs are exactly equal and where there is neither an operating profit nor an operating loss.

REFERENCE

1.   Koeppen, L., Mess, M. E., Trott, K. J., & Yazvac, L. S. 1997. "Aligning Incentives for Success." *Physician Executive* 23(1): 14–18.

CHAPTER 12

Identifying, Analyzing, and Improving Sensitive Areas of Operations

Edited by Sarah J. Holt, PhD, FACMPE

After completing this chapter, you will be able to:

- Describe how financial analysis is used for appraising medical group operations.

- Specify the measurement criteria and reports for the various types of responsibility centers.

- Develop approaches to evaluating the performance of total group operations, profit center contributions, and cost center results.

- Create a descriptive picture of the policies, orientations, and activities that highly successful medical groups follow, and identify the key financial and nonfinancial indicators to track the performance.

- Summarize the nature of provider profiling.

- Identify the software package, DataDive, and how its contents can assist in evaluating medical group operations.

- Analyze the operations of a medical practice in order to improve productivity, implement cost reductions, and increase the income potential of the practice.

- Identify the sources of assistance that financial managers may use to help solve organizational problems.

A major part of the financial management process involves analyzing the performance of group management during the last operating period. Analyzing actual performance is best accomplished by comparing it to planned activities selected by the group at the beginning of the period. An operating budget enables this comparison, which links the processes of planning and control, and is referred to as performance reporting. It furnishes the following benefits to the group:

- Identifies responsibility
- Calls attention to problem areas
- Offers a means of assessing the results of implemented decisions

Performance reports are not an end in themselves. Once the degree of variance from plans is determined — either positive or negative — management can adjust performance or the expectations of the group's management.

There are two basic focal points for analyzing the areas of group operations: (1) financial measures and (2) nonfinancial indicators. The financial analysis should include assessing performance along three dimensions:

1. Evaluating responsibility centers
2. Meeting goals and objectives and the operating budget
3. Comparing group operations with external norms and other groups

The nonfinancial areas include the clinical aspects of the practice and are just as important as financial areas. Both points will be covered in this chapter.

Provider profiling will also be discussed using the DataDive online application. Finally, practice approaches will be highlighted to bring about improved operations and increased performance results, including the use of consultants.

FINANCIAL PERFORMANCE ANALYSIS

Responsibility Center Performance Evaluation

In chapter 6, the concept of responsibility accounting was introduced. Each type of responsibility center is evaluated based on the level of responsibility assigned to each manager in the group. For example, if a responsibility center treats patients, then it will probably be labeled a profit center. A center that does not treat patients would probably be called a cost or expense center. Furthermore, if a satellite office is largely free standing and has a discrete quantity of assets that it uses in patient care, it could be called an investment center. For each type of center, the performance measurement criteria would be different, as follows:

▪ Profit center evaluator might be a profit measure, such as a contribution margin.

▪ Cost or expense center measure might be meeting the operating budget.

▪ Investment center criterion might be a return-on-investment indicator.

Some general questions that group management would like to have answered about the performance of responsibility centers are:

▪ How did each center perform for the period?

▪ If it is a profit center, to what degree did it meet or exceed its profit plan?

▪ If it is an expense center, to what degree did it meet its budgeted expenses?

▪ What factors caused the actual results that varied from the plan?

▪ If there is a prepaid component to the practice, what indicators can be used to assess performance in this area?

▪ What other criteria can be used to evaluate the overall performance in the managed care phases of the practice?

Accounting information that helps to answer these questions must be organized so that revenues and expenses are traced to profit and investment centers and expenses are traced to cost or expense centers. In this way, revenues and/or costs become the indicators of performance for each responsibility center manager. Under responsibility accounting, the responsibility center is the unit within an organization that can and should exert control over the performance and consumption of its own resources. Two examples of this would be a pediatrics department of a group that is designated as a profit center and a laboratory connected with the group that is treated as a cost center.

For the medical group with a small prepaid component — less than 25 percent of the total practice — it is probably sufficient if revenues and costs of the prepaid component are treated as a separate responsibility center. Other responsibility centers in the group would report FFS equivalent amounts as revenue surrogates for providing care to the prepaid patients. The effect of this is twofold:

■ Responsibility for treating prepaid patients in a cost-effective manner is diffused throughout the group, and no one individual or responsibility center is clearly accountable for their care. The primary care physician comes closest to having full responsibility for a particular patient's care when serving in a gatekeeper role. However, no one person has a similar responsibility for the entire prepaid practice.

■ Performance is expressed in terms that are meaningful in the FFS environment, and financial results are monitored in these terms. On the other hand, the prepaid environment requires different performance and outcome criteria, which are expressed in terms that are not necessarily consistent with FFS practice.

Thus, with less than 25 percent of its revenues from prepaid care, the above effects are not significant in distorting the picture of operating results for the group.

However, when prepaid revenues exceed 25 percent of a group's total revenues, it becomes necessary to change the group's reporting format as well as the rewards system for physicians. One option is to switch from crediting individual responsibility centers with FFS equivalents to crediting the centers with a pro rata share of the capitation revenue for physician services. Similarly, instead of being charged to a single responsibility center for prepaid care, the cost of outside referrals would be charged to the responsibility center of the referring physician. On the surface, this may not seem to be a significant shift; however, it represents a shift from the FFS orientation of increasing production to an orientation toward managing costs within a fixed income amount. This may lead to the individual physician becoming a responsibility center for cost control. The unit of performance measure would then become the cost PMPM.

GOALS AND OBJECTIVES AND BUDGET PERFORMANCE EVALUATION

Measuring goals and objectives must be an important part of any performance evaluation system. If the group sets a profit goal or some other financial target, there should be a periodic assessment, at least annually, to see if the financial goal has been met. If nonfinancial goals and objectives are also established, measures for comparing actual results to these plans must also be established to evaluate the performance of the total group as well as segments.

The operating budget is the primary tool to evaluate financial performance organizationally and departmentally. Comparison of actual results with budgeted amounts may show deviations from the plan for any or all of the following reasons:

■ A change in activity from the planned level of activity

■ More or less efficiency in the use of practice resources

■ Changes in the price of resources purchased

■ Incorrect assessment of the cost composition of providing services

Since departures from budget cannot be attributed solely to any one of the above reasons, causes of budget variances are often difficult, if not impossible, to determine.

Evaluating Profit Center Performance

The manager of a profit center, also called a contribution center, is accountable for both revenues and costs. In this regard, financial performance is measured by the achievement of a budgeted profit — or contribution toward common costs. Performance reports should include only those costs and revenues over which the profit center manager has control. All items beyond the control of the center manager should be excluded. However, for other purposes, such as fee setting, it may be necessary to include a fair share of indirect costs to arrive at a full cost of the center's services.

Evaluating the Total Group Performance

As mentioned in chapter 11, one problem with evaluating performance with a comparison of the prior year's results or a static budget is the effects of changes in activity and deviations due to changes in efficiency and prices. We can isolate the changes of activity by adopting the concept of performance budgeting, that is, a budget prepared to reflect what revenues and costs should have been at the actual level of activity during the period.

Inherent in the preparation of a performance budget is the concept of variable and fixed costs. In the example presented in chapter 11, a flexible budget was developed for a medical group by applying variable and fixed behavior patterns. That flexible budget must be adjusted for programmed fixed costs that are seasonable and for a different time period (quarterly rather than monthly).

Analyzing Cost Center Performance

Cost centers do not generate revenue; they support the revenue-producing responsibility centers or the group as a whole. Examples of these cost centers include the medical support group, the data processing department, occupancy, and use, as well as administration. Frequently, they are referred to as support centers.

A performance budget can be used when fixed and variable components of expenses in cost centers can be identified. In cost centers where fixed/variable cost relationships cannot be determined, the budget becomes a maximum authorization to spend. Here, performance reports are used to ensure that the center does not go over budget without prior approval. The report is not designed to assess the effectiveness or efficiency of the department's operations. When this type of budget is used to assess efficiency, the staff may be motivated to spend less and report favorable variances. Such variances may arise because the budget was padded, or the quality of patient care was reduced. In this case, budget control is exercised by requiring prior approval of budget overruns, perhaps in excess of some percentage allowance. Periodic reports then serve to keep the administrator informed of the current status.

EXTERNAL COMPARISONS PERFORMANCE EVALUATION

The third dimension of operations analysis involves a comparison of current group financial data with compatible information about other similar groups. There are few sources that collect and report on the financial operations of medical practices in a fashion enabling periodic comparison of performance. MGMA offers a report called *Performance and Practices of Successful Medical Groups*. This tool describes business methods used by medical groups selected as being "better performers" compared to similar organizations. Using this tool provides medical groups with some insight about business practices that yield the greatest efficiencies so that groups are encouraged to emulate effective, proven ways of operating a medical practice. Comparison data drawn from the MGMA Cost Survey reports based on prior-year are also presented that reflects key financial measures that help track the achievement of superior results (http://www.mgma.com/pm/default.aspx?id=9302).

The *Performance and Practices of Successful Medical Groups Report* includes the following features:

- Performance measures of better-performing medical groups in four functional areas:
  - Profitability and cost management
  - Production, capacity, and staffing
  - Accounts receivable and collections
  - Patient satisfaction
- Narrative sections relating the experiences of subject matter experts to identify relevant management practices that lead to success
- Comparison measures of "better performance"
- Success stories of better-performing medical groups with accounts of the management practices used to achieve the superior results

An interesting aspect of this report is that it provides an overall portrait of a successful group practice based on certain policies and actions. Such a picture would include the following practices and orientations:

- In general, these groups employ formal strategic planning, rigorous financial management, and customer-focused innovations to meet the challenges their market presents.
- Their cultures are marked by open communication, effective compensation mechanisms, trust between physicians and administrators, and high levels of physician job satisfaction.
- Administrators and physicians respect the roles and skills of one another and recognize the value of each individual's contributions.
- Positive group values are inculcated in new physicians, including the necessity for hard work and cooperation among all group members.

- Compensation is based on productivity, although some income distribution formulas include financial incentives to encourage efficiency in managed care or the time to see more patients.

- There are extensive investments in quality management and information systems, particularly those with a high proportion of managed care revenues.

- These groups usually employ more staff than the norm, mostly in direct patient care or physician support positions, such as nurses, nursing assistants, and medical assistants.

- These groups install excellent billing and collection procedures, use annual budgets to track performance, and employ cost accounting techniques to increase physician awareness of practice costs.

- Practice administrators and most of the physicians have a good grasp of finances, competitive positions, and performance goals — without having to dig them out of files or a computer system.

- These groups display a commitment to serving customers — patients, insurers, employers, and group physicians.

- They adopt the latest technical innovations, such as patient portals, to enhance patient retention.

KEY INDICATORS OF SUCCESS

As mentioned, the report covers success indicators in four areas: profitability and cost management; productivity, capacity, and staffing; accounts receivable and collections; and patient satisfaction. Important financial indicators are listed in each of these areas with the values for the better performers contrasted with a total value of the group sampled. We will briefly summarize each of these sectors.

Profitability and Cost Management

In this area, factors attributing to exceptional performance are cited. They are:

Cost accounting — These groups implement detailed cost accounting systems to gain a better understanding of the costs of treatments and procedures by type of service, practice site, department, or division and physician. These systems also provide data for detailed reports, allowing managers to enhance planning and control of relevant activities.

Transaction costing — This approach assigns costs to each function or transaction associated with care delivery. Based on relative value units, more accurate costing information is created to aid in decision making.

Zero-based budgeting — Zero-based budgeting requires managers to justify each budgeted item and accurately project expenses that will be generated during the year. Better performers frequently use this method instead of preparing incremental budgets that simply apply a uniform factor to existing budget components for the prior year.

Physician incentives — High-achieving groups frequently include physician incentives to provide compensation formulas that encourage physician efficiency and control costs. Typically, they also use physician profiling and cost accounting methods to identify higher-cost providers.

Effective managed care contracting — Effective groups use sophisticated management practices for negotiating and monitoring managed care agreements and have an awareness and command of their cost structures to enable negotiating favorable contract rates.

Coding effectiveness — These practices emphasize coding procedure training, develop explicit coding processes, and succeed in carrying them out well. Also, they recognize the need to standardize the interpretation of care delivery across multiple clinic sites.

Improved service delivery — Better-performing groups adopt strategies that optimize each provider's style and standards of delivery and are constantly experimenting with different strategies. In addition, computerized scheduling systems help identify over- or under-utilization of resources and allow the creation of management reports that document accurate patterns of patient care delivery.

These high-performing medical groups also present an interesting financial operating picture that includes the following characteristics:

- Higher revenue per physician
- More procedures per physician
- Lower cost per procedure
- Lower debt ratios
- Higher asset turnovers (more revenue per total assets)

Many statistical indicators are provided in this section with numerous breakdowns by medical group type, such as family practice, primary care single specialty, multispecialty, and so on. These include:

- Operating cost per procedure (inside the practice)
- Total operating cost as percentage of total net medical revenue
- Total operating cost per FTE physician
- Total physician cost as percentage of total net medical revenue
- Total physician cost per FTE physician
- Revenue after operating cost as percentage of net medical revenue
- Revenue after operating cost per FTE physician
- Total net medical revenue per FTE physician
- Nonsurgical operating cost per procedure

Productivity, Capacity, and Staffing

Achieving superior production and capacity performance in a medical group begins with physician productivity — based on patient visits, encounters, and procedures, all of which generate revenue. Further, production is a function of capacity. Highly productive groups optimize capacity by making the most efficient use of their resources and attending to the following:

Infrastructure — High-performing groups utilize their existing infrastructure capacity effectively by having larger amounts of gross charges per square foot and smaller numbers of square feet per physician. Investment in a greater number of examination rooms and locations increases a group's capacity and potential for production.

Policies and procedures — They must be clear, concise, centralized, and automated. Patient records, documentation, and coding procedures receive focused attention. Physicians are skilled in coding and engage in continuous quality improvement processes. These skills are used to maximize operational efficiencies.

Staffing — Creative uses of staffing lead to increased productivity. These groups delegate certain responsibilities to the lowest level feasible and use midlevel providers to supplement physicians. Clerks and assistants complement the nursing staff by doing certain patient-related activities.

Hiring and training — In recruiting physicians, careful attention is paid to work-ethic compatibility and productivity expectations. Training, both for physicians and staff, is essential for demonstrating efficiency opportunities.

Physician compensation methods — Effective compensation arrangements lead to high performance. These groups have determined which measures of productivity to track. They also have well-defined and reasonable performance standards and have resolved the cost allocations dilemma.

Information systems — Successful groups use information systems and technology to improve productivity and increase capacity. Functions used include: computerized patient scheduling, electronic patient records, online encounter information, and immediate access to test results. Also, online information about physician performance enables them to evaluate their efforts and make appropriate adjustments when necessary.

Although there are only four indicators in this area, the report provides them in a wide array of breakdowns — again, largely by type of medical group. These indicators are:

- ▪ Total support staff per FTE physician
- ▪ Total gross charges per FTE physician
- ▪ Square feet per FTE physician
- ▪ Procedures per FTE physician

Accounts Receivable and Collections

Although accounts receivable usually constitutes the single largest balance sheet asset, its records are frequently undermanaged. The better-performing medical groups view accounts receivable and collections from a system-wide perspective.

They view receivables management as a total practice process starting with scheduling a patient's visit to the final collection for services. These groups tend to be proactive and invest in the "front-end" of their operations, such as setting up new patient accounts, preauthorizing services, and capturing and entering charges. Their systems are designed to incorporate the complexities of third-party payers and the managed care environment. And they invest in and allocate appropriate and adequate staff to perform important functions.

The following are some of the particular practices that high-achieving groups use:

Adjustments and write-off policies — These are both written and consistent. Also, they have separate policies covering contractual and noncontractual write-offs and adjustments. These groups also understand the transaction costs involved in billing and collections that help formulate an effective small balance write-off policy to avoid incurring costs that exceed anticipated collections.

Preauthorizations — Investing in this front-end effort results in cleaner and higher-quality accounts receivable, fewer denials of care and nonpayment by insurers, and faster collections. Specialty groups must be proactive in this area.

Charge capture — Successful groups quickly enter charges and minimize uncaptured charges. Unbilled charges represent a substantial opportunity cost that largely goes undetected. Better-performing groups enter charges within 24 hours of outpatient services and 48 hours for inpatient services.

Electronic data submission — The best groups submit claims daily using electronic claims submission for all third-party payers that accept the transmission.

Integrated systems — High-achieving groups enhance manual processes with the use of integrated clinical and billing systems.

Reports and analysis — Better-performing groups understand the importance of timely and consistently reported information in managing receivables; thus, they develop and use tailored management reports to control and measure performance, such as aging reports, unbilled revenue reports, write-off and adjustment reports, and key charge procedure reports.

Four key indicators are used in monitoring the accounts receivable and collections of high-performing medical groups. Similarly arranged by type of group, they are:

- Percentage of total accounts receivable from 0 to 60 days old
- Adjusted FFS collection percentage
- Number of months gross fee-for-service charges in accounts receivable
- Total accounts receivable per FTE physician

Patient Satisfaction

Retaining patient satisfaction at high levels is perhaps the most important element in maintaining and building a group's capacity. In better-performing practices, all functions interfacing with patients are fully staffed, and patient relationships are closely monitored by management.

NONFINANCIAL MEASURES OF PERFORMANCE

Most performance evaluations focus on financial information taken from the basic accounting data in the financial management system. But an overall analysis of a medical group's operations should also include nonfinancial information since money only reflects one aspect of resource utilization. The quantitative element not expressed in financial terms has equal importance. Thus, nonfinancial measures should be integrated with a sophisticated financial management system for an overall balanced picture of group operations.

There are different types of nonfinancial performance measures. The easiest to obtain include these aggregates:

- Number of patient visits
- Number of procedures performed
- Number of physicians
- Number of physician days
- Number of employees
- Number of employee days
- Number of hours worked
- Number of laboratory procedures
- Number of hospital days
- Quantity of supplies used or purchased

Standing alone, any one of these aggregates is not very useful. However, over time and in combination with other information, they can show important trends that can be compared with past history or with data from other groups.

Thus, a more useful type of nonfinancial performance measure combines separate indicators to show various relationships. The most common relationship involves the level of activity and use of resources per FTE physician. Another involves resources used per patient visit or procedure. Some of these common indicators are listed below:

- Number of scheduled physician office hours
- Number of various procedures performed
- Number of missed appointments
- Number of hospital days per physician by specialty
- Turnover of employees
- Number of calls completed to patients reminding them of regular checkups
- Number of patients referred to outside specialists
- Data related to promoting the practice (e.g., results of using advertisements)

- Monthly average number of prepaid plan members
- New enrollees: Total during quarter
- Disenrollees: Total during quarter
- Prepaid capitation payment per 1,000 members per month
- Prepaid charges (FFS equivalent) per 1,000 members per month
- Outside physician referral expense per 1,000 members per month
- Outside laboratory referral expense per 1,000 members per month
- Outside X-ray referral expense per 1,000 members per month
- Inpatient admissions per 1,000 members per month
- Average length of stay per inpatient admission
- Physician outpatient encounter per 1,000 members per month

PROVIDER PROFILING

Beyond the use of financial information to analyze and improve practice operations, it may be useful to embrace broader measures of performance evaluation. Utilizing broader measures of performance evaluation provides important indicators of performance, such as physician/provider profiling. Profiles or capsulized summaries of the nature of treatments are developed for clinical and economic performance that serve as benchmarks or desirable modalities with which to evaluate and improve the delivery of services. Sources of variation in practice patterns are identified, quantified, and communicated to providers to discourage unnecessary variation and rationalize the delivery process. Profiling has the potential of becoming an important educational tool. Profiling also holds promise as a cost control mechanism for delivery and insurance systems.

The Nature of Profiling

Profiling is defined as a process using epidemiological methods to collect, analyze, and use provider practice data.[1] It focuses on and analyzes patterns of care rather than specific clinical decisions. The practice pattern of a single physician or a group of physicians is frequently expressed as a rate that incorporates measures of resource utilization (costs or services) or of outcome (functional status, morbidity, or morality) that is measured over a defined period for a defined population.[2]

Developing valid profiling information requires that the developers of a new system address the following questions:

- What data will help the physicians and will lead to better service of the patients?
- What are the other legitimate information needs that go beyond the physician's requirements?
- What information does the practice already receive from other external sources (reports from HMOs and insurance carriers)?

▪ What other information needs are currently unmet? What data and which resources are needed to turn raw data into useful information?

It is key to aim the development process at enhancing the effectiveness of care and not to focus on cost reduction to the point of decreasing the quality of care. Physician profile developers should include both clinicians and administrators as part of the development team to profile a clinic's activities. This is not only important to ensuring a good understanding of how physicians deliver care, but also to facilitating the buy-in of all parties for this all-encompassing project. Gaining the support of all participants early on will enhance the clinic's later attempts to turn its profiling analysis into change for improved physician behavior.

Further, making valid judgments about "practice styles" is fraught with arguable premises. These include the following:

1. Data collection, such as administrative and billing data, may not be collected in a rigorous fashion and may contain sampling errors.

2. Knowledge of what constitutes "average" or "desirable" behavior is not available nationally, with only the profiles of local physicians being accessible for comparison.

3. There is variation in the type of patients who are treated, depending on the severity of illness. Additionally, profile development is complicated in that once practice-based norms are available, they do not necessarily reflect clinically appropriate medical care. Only norms based on sound practice guidelines that are grounded in scientific evidence can reflect appropriate care.

Despite these caveats, developing and transmitting provider-level performance measures can be an important component of the effort to improve the efficiency and effectiveness of healthcare delivery. We must recognize, though, that developing valid provider profiles is a difficult and time-consuming process.

Data Compilation

The objective of provider profiling is to present the same type of indicators for the profiled provider and for a peer group of participating providers with comparable demographics (i.e., specialty, years in practice, gender, etc.). After comparison, a search is made for outlying patterns of practice (significant differences between the performance of the profiled provider and the peer group). If an outlier exists, the provider should then be presented with more detailed data to identify possible reasons for why there was a difference from the norm. If the result of the drilled down report leads to the assessment that a change in a physician's behavior would improve the quality of care — or would maintain the desired quality of care while decreasing the cost of care — change in the mode of delivery should then be the responsibility of the provider.

Data are the driving force of profile development. However, before data are selected, clear identification and prioritization of the objectives of profiling are imperative. A provider group, a health plan, or other healthcare entity may embark on developing provider profiles for a number of reasons. Setting objectives at the outset establishes criteria for data selection, determines the analytic dimensions of the data, and enables the group to assess the scope and expense of the profiling effort. Developers need to be wary of common one-size-fits-all assumptions. Objectives will determine the profile subjects, the mode of analysis, and the type of data to be collected. For example, provider profiles support evidence-based medical management, and quality improvement objectives emphasize clinical data presented in terms of process and outcome measures for member and patient populations. Profiles oriented toward resource efficiency, cost reduction, or improved profitability typically focus on the financial dimensions of provider decisions about resources expended in patient care. Profiles that meet requirements for accreditation, like HEDIS, or reinforce employer-group satisfaction and member retention imply still different criteria for data selection, measurement tools, and reporting style.

For any physician-profiling objective relating to quality and/or cost purposes, the following data elements constitute the database:[3]

- Unique patient identifier
- Diagnostic information — usually provided by using ICD-9-CM/ICD-10-CM
- Procedural information — derived from Volume III of ICD-9-CM/ICD-10-CM, CPT, and/or HCPCS codes
- Level of service information — usually obtained from evaluating CPT codes
- Charges for services ordered by the physician or the healthcare entity
- Results of information derived from additional studies, such as patient satisfaction surveys and measurement of patient health status

Data sources currently used to develop provider profiles include the following:

1. Patient enrollment and eligibility systems
2. Billings claims and encounter data
3. Clinical and service code data
4. Financial data
5. Patient-derived information

The type of profiling report the practice wishes to generate will govern the data requirements and resources.

Composition of Provider Profiles

The scope of data required to support provider profiling and the way data are organized and treated analytically vary substantially depending on the type of provider, the provider's relationship to members and patients, and the analytical tools deemed appropriate for measuring achievement of the desired objectives. Another variable is the nature of the entity undertaking the profile development. Thus, the type of provider and the nature of the using organization both play a major role in the selection and formulation of data to form the profiles.

Further, particular profiles may be constructed as profiling individual practitioners within a specialty or as interacting participants within a practice group or clinic. If the units for comparative analysis are groups, a designation must be made whether it is a single- or multispecialty group. This clarity is important because primary care physicians (PCPs), in such areas as family practice, internal medicine, and pediatrics, are often considered members of multispecialty groups, sometimes joined under the same administrative umbrella by specialists in obstetrics and gynecology. Single-specialty groups are more common for referral care, such as a cardiology practice. Each of these configurations poses a challenge for data availability, selection, and analytic treatment.

Another distinction for profiling purposes is the role of physicians. For instance, there are some who are accountable for an assigned panel of members and are financially at risk for all or a substantial portion of the member's care for all types of services (PCPs). Then there are those physicians who are accountable only for the patients to whom they deliver care.

It is useful to contrast the makeup of the profiles for the primary care physician and the specialist.

Physician Profiles

The term *physician profiles*[4] usually denotes profiles for primary care providers. These profiles require data on all assigned members, including those who have not had a service during the profiling period and data from claim and encounter systems from all providers for all types of care. It should also include a summary of members' demographic characteristics. The data should be assembled to report on the percentage of members who had no claim and on the average length of eligibility and rate of turnover among the assigned panel. Utilization data can be misleading for a physician whose members are all recent enrollees compared to one whose panel has well-established relationships because the calculation of rates of service are based on services PMPM.

A comprehensive PCP profile also presents summary utilization and financial information on the members' rates of use of hospital inpatient and outpatient resources, primary care and referred medical and surgical services, prescription drugs, and other resources. This information may be complemented by selected utilization and cost highlights, such as key improvements in reducing emergency room visits and increasing rates of preventive care services.

The profiles also include each PCP's direct contribution to the members' overall resource consumption and incorporate data only from the PCP's own claim or encounter records. Some examples are: What specific services did this PCP deliver to the patients, and what percentage of the overall member panel's needs did the PCP meet? To assemble these data, the organization will need to decide how to aggregate individual CPT codes or CPT codes in combination with ICD-9 diagnosis codes and put them into medically meaningful units that communicate a clear picture of patients' care experience. This type of profile allows the evaluation of performance against expectations at a number of different points, such as whether a PCP appears to supply 50 percent or 90 percent of the panels' ambulatory care or whether every asthmatic child is always referred to specialists. Profiles of specialists are very difficult to develop, which is in part because of a lack of access to specialist data.[5]

Outlook for Profiling

Provider-profiling data are basically for providers. Observers conclude that the best results from its use are obtained when profiling data are initially used internally. Data should be blinded to focus on improving care rather than finding the shortcomings of individual physicians. After the data have been carefully scrutinized, analyzed, and appropriately summarized, a blinded version can be disseminated externally to all providers who participate in a health plan or other business entity and ultimately made available to outsiders.

Researchers assert that the results of provider profiling as it affects measures of resource utilization are dependent on the following characteristics of profiling systems:[6]

- By type of physician profiled (specialties, although most have been family or general practice)
- In setting (hospital or group practice)
- Intervention (peer comparison, informational)
- Frequency (daily, weekly, to every three months)
- Study design (uncontrolled, controlled)
- Measures of resource utilization (number of laboratory tests, total charges, costs, number of prescriptions)

To fully assess the impact of profiling, rigorously designed and carefully performed studies with an eye toward evidence-based practices are required. In the move to establish this indicator as a useful tool, the primary goal of provider profiling must be kept in mind. That is, profiling should involve the development of information useful to clinicians and clinical managers in evaluating practice patterns. Primary emphasis should be placed on demonstrating the effectiveness of care and not on the efficiency of production. The restoration or improvement of patients' functional health status should constitute the real outcome of the care.

Areas that will be continually addressed in the development and use of evidence-based management and used for profiling include new and better techniques of measurement and reporting of resource usage, clinical outcomes, quality of life, overall patient care outcomes, and patient satisfaction. Decisions must be based on a foundation of solid research. As the demand for accountability in healthcare increases, so will the use of provider profiling.

ANALYZING PHYSICIAN SERVICES AND PRODUCTIVITY

DataDive

MGMA developed a tool to analyze physician services and the productivity of medical groups. It is a personal computer–based software package called DataDive, which analyzes physician productivity based on the number and complexity of procedures performed.

DataDive measures physician productivity on a work-performed basis and generates information by weighting procedures with a relative value scale similar to what we have discussed. Because a relative value scale can assess the comparative difficulty of various medical procedures, such a measure of physician productivity is consistent among groups, physicians, and providers over time. DataDive utilizes the CMS Resource-based Relative Value System (RBRVS) for productivity measurement and cost analysis because the RVUs are segmented into the three components: provider work, practice expense, and malpractice. Other relative value scales do not offer a similar RVU breakdown by components.

Information produced by DataDive can be analyzed at three different levels — group, specialty, and provider. This allows users to get customized data depending on the type of information desired. Examples of data that can be obtained through DataDive include:

- Comparisons of case intensity — calculated by dividing the total number of relative values by the total number of patients, as well as procedures/patient
- Comparisons of procedure complexity — calculated by dividing the total number of relative values by the total number of procedures
- Comparisons of provider productivity — measured by the total number of relative values for each full-time equivalent (FTE), encounters/FTE, patients/FTE, and procedures/FTE

When comparing provider productivity, the terminology used must be clearly defined. An FTE is defined in DataDive as the number of clinical hours the practice considers to be the minimum for its normal clinical workweek. Clinical work refers to the time that the provider devotes to patient care and supporting activities, such as medical records updates, consultation with other providers, preparation for clinical and/or surgical procedures, patient telephone contacts, and so on. For example, a physician who performs 80 percent clinical work and 20 percent administrative work would be classified as a 0.8 FTE.

When considering the encounters/FTE and patients/FTE, one needs to remember that patient encounters differ. Encounters are determined by the number of times a patient is seen by a provider at a facility regardless of how often those visits occur. Patients are defined as the total number of unique individuals who receive services from the medical practice each month or reporting period. Thus, a unique patient is one who is counted only once per month regardless of the number of encounters or the number of times that the patient sees a specific physician or midlevel provider.

The term *procedure* is often used in relation to procedures/FTE and procedures/patient. Procedures are services provided during a month or cycle that are identified by CPT codes. A procedure is one that is documented as a current CPT stipulated annually by the federal government in the *Federal Register*.

Practice management can use DataDive provider-productivity information in negotiating with third-party payers, evaluating new reimbursement mechanisms, monitoring utilization, and establishing methods of compensating physicians based on individual and overall organizational performance. A popular method for compensating physicians is based on the work component of the relative value unit. DataDive allows for easy work-only analysis for each physician through its work-analysis component.

IMPROVING OPERATIONS

This section highlights approaches that groups take to make their practices more efficient and profitable. Our summary will be oriented toward practical ideas and will provide a framework for financial managers to use in striving to make their practices more competitive in today's ever-changing markets.

Improving operations involves three types of change efforts. They can be classified as:

1. Improving productivity
2. Implementing cost reductions
3. Increasing income potentials

Although all these categories seem to point primarily to financial efforts, quality is still an important factor and will occupy equal footing on the hierarchy of medical group objectives.

Within each category discussed, quality improvement is implied. In approaching these efforts of improvement, the financial manager must conduct analyses, evaluate alternatives, and decide on courses of action with the joint participation of the physicians in the medical group. In addition, the governing body must be involved and approve any major changes affecting operations, organizational structure, and future directions of the group.

Improving Productivity

Productivity is concerned with the way in which resources are used to produce services or product. In discussing productivity, it is most often done in the context of a relationship between inputs and outputs. When measuring productivity, the reference is to a ratio between inputs, or resources used, and the outputs, or the services produced. There are five basic types of resources involved in delivering healthcare services. These are:

1. Labor
2. Supplies
3. Equipment
4. Facilities
5. Capital

Since rendering service is a labor-intensive industry, focus is on the productivity of labor.

To monitor productivity, two types of information should be the focus of attention:

1. The trend in the ratio of inputs to outputs
2. The comparison of the actual ratio of inputs to outputs to the expected ratio or the standard

The monitoring of productivity ratios should occur regularly by calculating and comparing them to standards on a biweekly or monthly basis. Examples of these ratios include nursing time per clinic visit, therapist time per physical therapy treatment, and medical supplies per ambulatory surgery procedure.

What is the process of measuring and managing productivity? How should a medical group go about undertaking an analysis of its operations so that it can obtain an understanding of how productive they are? Once information about its state of productivity has been compiled, how can the group start to make changes and establish standards for managing future productivity? The group needs to perform an operational review.

Operational Reviews

These reviews entail a comprehensive analysis of a specific department, area, or free-standing entity. Through this review, areas are identified where productivity improvements can be directed. The analysis covers five areas, which are:[7]

1. Organizational analysis
2. Functional analysis
3. Facility analysis
4. Staffing analysis
5. Material analysis

Organizational analysis — This analysis includes the evaluation of the organizational structure within a department or area. The evaluation relates to the responsibilities and roles of all professionals in the area and whether they are appropriate to the area's workload. For example, a medical group may be growing rapidly and adding physicians every few months. Each physician is provided with an appointments secretary to handle the clerical needs of his or her practice. During an organizational analysis, it became evident that the practice had too many appointments secretaries for the workload of the group. As part of the analysis, a new organizational arrangement was developed that consolidated several appointments positions, and the group established a central appointments center.

Functional analysis — The purpose of this analysis is to determine the types of activities being conducted in the department or area being studied. Each activity should be broken down into its various tasks and work steps. The frequency with which each work step is performed and who performs it should be delineated. The review of each work step should involve the following questions:

- When is it performed?
- How often is it performed?
- Where is it performed?
- Who is performing it?
- Is it necessary to perform this at all?

After analyzing each of these elements for each step, changes and improvements through this functional analysis should be initiated. When these modifications prove to be effective, then they should be established as the productivity standards in the area. For example, several months ago, a medical group upgraded its computer system to handle billings, collections, and registrations. A number of tasks that had been performed manually were eliminated. During the functional analysis, the reviewers discovered that the manual procedures necessary under the old system were still being performed, although they were not required now. Because of the functional analysis, the redundant tasks were identified and eliminated.

Facility analysis — The focus of this analysis is to evaluate the appropriateness of the size and layout of the physical space in a department or area. This phase is particularly important for fairly large medical groups that require a large number of treatment rooms for outpatients, ambulatory surgery, and outpatient radiology. When performing this analysis, the capacity of the existing facilities needs to be calculated and compared to the present and planned workload. Care should be taken to conduct this study over a sufficient span of time to ascertain the usage requirements during different parts of the week, month, or season.

An operational review was conducted in a medical group's laboratory facility that carried out a large volume of outpatient tests. The space used by the laboratory had been assigned over 15 years ago and had gradually grown as more and varied types of tests were added to the workload of the laboratory. Most of the rooms had fixed counters, and as new equipment was purchased, it was placed in the same space that had been occupied by the old equipment. The laboratory's manager was now requesting a significant expansion of the laboratory's space. When the facility analysis was undertaken, it revealed that remodeling the existing space (such as removal of walls and fixed counters) could improve the laboratory's workflow and reduce its staff. Additionally, with changes to the existing facility, the expansion would not be necessary.

Staffing analysis — Most individuals are familiar with this component. In performing this analysis, estimates of the time required to carry out the department activities are made. Also, the historical, current, and future staffing levels should be reviewed in relation to the workload. The scheduling of staff should be evaluated and compared to the volume of work.

The administrator of a medical group started to receive complaints that the staff at a satellite outpatient radiology center was being overworked. Yet, after reviewing historical staffing and workload levels, the number of employees seemed to be more than what was needed to handle the current patient load. After reviewing the operations at the center, it was discovered that the patient scheduling caused the productivity problems. The majority of patients were scheduled at two peak periods, in the early morning and late afternoon. During these times, the staff was required to perform continuously at top speed; but at midday, they had very little to do. The staffing analysis demonstrated the need for improving patient scheduling and staff scheduling, as well. There was a reduction in the number of staff members to better match the workload.

Material analysis — This fifth component of operational analysis deals with supplies and equipment. Three areas comprise this segment: (1) the distribution systems for supplies, (2) the determination of supply inventory levels, and (3) the adequacy and maintenance of equipment. For most medical groups, material analysis is not significant. But where supplies and equipment are major resources used in delivering services, such as large clinics or practices, it can be a valuable area for review.

A large clinic conducted a material analysis of its operations. A number of problems were uncovered, including the practice of purchasing supplies from a number of different vendors in order to satisfy physician preferences, purchasing supplies in quantities larger than necessary to ensure that quantities on hand were adequate, and not using the manufacturer of the equipment to service the items but employing an outside source that charged more than the manufacturer. Once these costly practices were identified, corrections were made to modify these activities.

When conducting operational reviews, the financial manager should seek assistance from someone outside the department who has experience in productivity measurement and management. This ensures objectivity and independence in the review process. Outside consultants may be used in these instances.

TYPICAL AREAS WHERE PRODUCTIVITY GAINS CAN BE ACHIEVED

Improving productivity involves lowering the ratio of inputs to outputs in the studied department or area. The ratio will decline if either the required inputs are decreased or the outputs produced are increased. The nature of the particular problem will dictate the approach to be followed to achieve productivity improvements. A series of techniques, covered below, have proved effective in enhancing productivity levels. They are not meant to be all-inclusive but merely illustrative of what is possible in certain situations.

Improve Scheduling

Scheduling modifications for patients, staff, and physicians are probably the most important way to improve the medical group's overall productivity. The overriding goal of an efficient scheduling system is to ensure that patients, staff, and physicians are all available at the appropriate times.

In patient scheduling, it is important for the workload to be distributed as evenly as possible throughout the entire day. Peaks and valleys in the load should be avoided. Usually, this even distribution is difficult because many patients prefer to have their visit prior to or after their work hours. Thus, patient visits are very light at midday. A technique often used is to emphasize to patients that waiting times are almost nonexistent between 10:00 a.m. and 2:00 p.m. A key in patient scheduling is the decorum of the appointment scheduler on the telephone. Telephone lines available for patients to reach the office must be sufficient. Some flexibility must be allowed to "work in" emergency patients into the schedule or have the scheduler respond with a suggestion for the patient to see an alternative physician if care is needed immediately.

For staff scheduling, the appropriate staff members should be available to match patient schedules. Sufficient numbers of staff need to be available during the peak workload period. Excess staff during lighter patient-load periods may be cross-trained and assigned to complete duties that are essential to organizational efficiency. Also, part-time employees may be assigned to work only during the peak period.

The final schedule consideration is physicians. Like patients and staff, physicians must be present to match the schedules of the other two. Since physicians are a key ingredient in the triumvirate of players, communication of their availability is critical to the entire scheduling process. In fact, communication among all three types regarding their availability and inability to meet committed times is essential for the system to function effectively.

Staff Support Levels

Labor cost is the most significant expense of the medical group. Considering both the salary and benefits costs, staffing usually represents about one-half of the group's total expenses. Yet, maintaining staffing at the proper levels to ensure maximum efficiency and meet every contingency represents a difficult challenge for the administrator and financial manager.

To accommodate growing outpatient and ambulatory service volumes, some managers are setting their staffing levels to meet expected workloads rather than existing workloads. This strategy has been employed because of the rate of increase in patient volume and the reluctance to turn patients away or have them wait a long time for appointments. As long as volume is consistently increasing, this is a low-risk strategy. However, in the changing environment, although volumes are increasing, the number of competing providers is rising, too, perhaps even faster than patient volume. Volume increases for some practices may be at a slower rate than previously, or the volume may have stabilized. In this case, staffing for a higher expected workload can be very risky. There are also negative implications for productivity. It becomes a problem because employees feel comfortable with the expected work effort when they are overstaffed. When volume increases or when staff is reduced to meet lower current workload levels, employees begin to feel overworked because their expectations about productivity and the required work effort appear to have changed.

As in many businesses today, medical practices need to develop approaches for handling workload increases without adding full-time staff until the higher workload level has been maintained for at least six months and appears it will continue into the future. One option is to hire part-time staffers who are willing to accept flexible hours. Some groups have negotiated part-time contracts for temporary staff members. Another alternative is develop a flex-time scheduling system that has people starting and ending at different times during the day and week.

If adequate staffing levels cannot be worked out, physicians and managers may need to evaluate the option of turning away patients rather than increasing the staff to provide the demanded services. Managers must evaluate the benefit of having patient services available on demand at all times. This action involves a financial and a nonfinancial decision as to whether the incremental volume justifies the addition of staff and whether the services can be rendered in a cost-effective manner.

Human Resource Management

High morale, efficiency, and organizational loyalty are characteristics that most managers strive to achieve in their staff members. While salary and benefits are important, the working environment and how workers are treated always rank high in preferences among employees in polls about their working relationships with employers. The improvement of productivity can be obtained by paying attention to these factors in the management of staff and physicians.

The administrator, financial manager, and governing body should strive to create a climate where each staff member is personally motivated to be as efficient and effective as possible. The main factors that make up such a climate are well-articulated set of goals and objectives for the group, clearly defined roles and responsibilities, and equitable treatment of all employees. Eliciting the input of staff is vital for establishing a productivity-oriented climate in two ways:

1. Having staff identify possible changes in work flow or work steps that increase efficiency: Usually, those persons who perform the work are in the best position to specify changes to improve productivity. Staff members need encouragement to offer these suggestions, and management needs to be open and listen to them objectively and responsively.

2. Establishing productivity standards in each area with the assistance and input of the staff: These standards should be realistic and achievable with a reasonable amount of effort. Having the participation of staff will ensure acceptance of and commitment to the standards.

Improving the Functional Design of Facilities

Many medical groups provide services in physically inadequate space. This may be the case because of the rapid growth in medical service demands. Frequently, the work flow arrangements are poorly designed, and treatment areas are inefficient. For certain ancillary services, such as radiology and physical therapy, there may be an insufficient number of dressing rooms for outpatients or none at all. Also, in outpatient surgery, separate areas for patient changing, preparation for surgery, and acute- and step-down recovery may not be provided. These facility constraints limit the number of patients who can be served and will likely decrease the staff's productivity.

In facility layout, the need for reasonable integration of diagnostic and therapeutic support services exists. The availability of on-premises ancillary services and departments can be convenient to both physicians and patients. With proper investigation and analysis of costs and controls, ancillary departments might prove to be cost efficient if located within the facility of the medical group. This also has the effect of sharing any cost and productivity gains with the patient since outpatient groups' fees may be lower than fees charged by external service organizations. Undertaking such an option requires capital investment. The amount of the investment must be compared with a realistic estimate of the potential increase in revenue or the possible decrease in the costs of ancillary services considering the time value of money before the project is pursued.

Physician Incentives

Physician compensation plans are multifaceted and tailored to the physicians of each medical group. Most seem to be structured to accomplish two ends: reward effort and maintain the integrity of the group. Experience has shown that an initial change from an equal distribution arrangement to even a limited-incentive scheme will result in a measurable increase in productivity. Sometimes, this increase happens even before the change is actually implemented, as members anticipate past productivity to be an initial baseline. Interestingly, it has also been observed that after the initial thrust, subsequent changes that allocate greater individual incentive do little or nothing to increase productivity.

Surveys of MGMA members have shown that an incentive factor is present in most compensation plans. Apparently, the prospects of greater monetary rewards serve as a motivator to greater productivity. Exercise caution since these systems can become disruptive to team-effort efficiency, cohesiveness, and patient service if the incentives are perceived as inequitable.

Systems and Procedures

No medical practice can operate efficiently without well-designed systems and procedures. It is essential that subsystems be designed to ensure that the right chart arrives before or with the patient, that charges for patient services are correctly made, that patient account information is complete and accurate, that laboratory orders and report slips are correct, and so on. In some cases, the penchant for properly designed systems and subsystems and their procedures is so great that the systems become the object of over-attention, and patients become secondary to a bureaucratic structure. The objective of high productivity is to ensure an optimum balance between the system functions and work flow.

IMPLEMENTING COST REDUCTIONS

A primary responsibility of the financial manager is to constantly seek ways to improve the profit and cash available for distribution to the physician owners. There are many avenues that can be taken to increase revenues, reduce contractual and bad debt allowances, and lower the cost of operations. To have an ongoing effort that focuses on continuous profit improvement requires a process that has been referred to as cost management.

Cost Management

Cost management is a continuous process or system of planning, monitoring, and controlling the cost of operations to meet the strategic directions of the medical group. It provides a logical and organized approach to balancing profitability, quality, and mission-related objectives. The function of a cost management system is to use the concepts of responsibility accounting, cost accounting, budgeting, and financial reporting in an integrated fashion to achieve profitable operations, primarily through cost reductions.

The process of managing costs necessitates that a proper chart of accounts be established for the medical group. In previous chapters, we pointed out that the MGMA standard chart of accounts has been designed to collect the proper cost data in the accumulations necessary to meet management's needs. This standard chart enables the comparison of the medical group's cost data with other groups. The cost management system includes setting a profit target for each year that has been developed by a consensus of physician-owners and management and that is acceptable to the group. There must be a budgeting system that translates the next year's plans and programs into a monetary expression of these intentions. Budgets should be prepared for each site level of the group, for each medical specialty and individual physician, and by the function of the medical group. Performance reporting must be set up to compare monthly actual expenses with planned expenses. Variations for each cost category should be analyzed, and departures, both favorable and unfavorable, should be explained. Performance reporting and variance analysis form the foundation of information upon which financial managers will react to initiate cost reduction efforts.

Objectives of Cost Management

There are many objectives for implementing a cost management program. The primary one is profit improvement. Others will follow from the medical group's other goals and objectives. Some will result from the position of the medical group in the marketplace — that is, its market share — and from the strategic direction of the group. For example, if physician incomes are declining or are flat, profit improvement will be a key outcome of cost management. If a group's market share is declining, a strategy of the group may be to become more cost efficient in the delivery of care to purchasers of healthcare, such as employers. If a medical group is contemplating entry into managed care systems, the assumption of risk requires not only utilization control, but also cost control for services provided to patients. If the group's medical business plan calls for expansions by acquiring or merging with other group practices, cost management may be one means of making available additional dollars for the pursuit of strategic objectives. With increasing competition for patients, medical group managers must understand cost behaviors and must implement methods to control them. These environments and group-specific factors will dictate what an effective cost management program must provide to the group.

In the next section, we will summarize some actions that medical groups have taken in the application of cost management techniques.

Personnel Costs

To reiterate, one of the largest cost factors in a medical practice's operations is support personnel. The annual cost of support personnel is a significant percentage of collected revenue. The control of these costs involves the assessment of staffing levels from the standpoint of demonstrated need. Centralizing certain functions, such as appointments, transcription recording, and receptionists, are examples where cost savings can be effective. Under the centralization philosophy, only nurses remain as departmental employees, with receptionists, appointment staff, and medical records personnel being assigned to one or two departments that, space permitting, may be contiguous to or in the same general area for several departments. With a centralized appointment desk, all appointments are made by one or two persons, which replace a considerable number of individual staff members who have been serving one or a few physicians.

Another approach to reducing personnel costs is to analyze whether the duties of various staff members are matched to the skills needed to perform certain functions. In some instances, overqualified or more expensive personnel are hired to do jobs that can be done by others. For example, hiring a medical technician instead of a registered nurse can save some salary dollars. Also, new people should be employed because of their skills and experience, not their professional titles. On the other side of this analysis, sometimes it is more cost effective to pay for a more experienced person than to select less expensive help who have to be trained. For example, an individual with knowledge of collections and claims processing who can maintain and improve cash flow is more valuable than a trainee who lets reimbursement lag while learning the job.

Another area that is receiving greater attention is the cost of employee benefits. Changes in various benefit programs that are being explored include creative health plans, 401K retirement programs, and cafeteria benefit plans.

Some other steps that reduce staff costs include the following:

- Limit the number of RNs on hand at any time, using them only for tasks requiring their training and skills.
- Cross-train the staff to fill in for temporary vacancies, vacations, and illnesses, thus avoiding temporary help and "floater" employees.
- Avoid overtime work by keeping office hours on time and staggering staff work schedules.
- Move payroll to an outside payroll service, thus reducing manager and accounting time demands.
- Inventory and reduce clerical and clinical supplies.

These items may be a significant element of cost, especially for large medical groups. Supply costs can become excessive through waste, pilfering, and uncontrolled purchasing. There should be one person in charge of ordering and monitoring supplies. Incoming orders should be checked, and invoices should be filed and matched against vendor bills. Inventory should be kept at adequate levels and reordering systematized. Ordering items at the last minute, particularly in small quantities, is expensive. Discounts are offered, usually, on volume purchases, but adequate storage space must be available.

Some practice procedures to control supply costs include:

- Evaluate the accounts payable system to see if it needs to be strengthened. Fraudulent practices can easily occur when employees collude with vendors.
- Comparison shop since there can be vast differences in vendors' charges for the same supplies and services. If a reliable supplier is found, establish good relationships for continued competent service.
- Inventories of clinical supplies should have expiration dates where applicable. Monitor any wastage due to expiration and adjust orders to eliminate such waste.
- Keep supplies locked up except during office hours.
- Negotiate for a year's requirements of supply items at competitively bid prices, making sure to reopen the process each year.

Facilities and Equipment

The costs related to facilities and equipment represent the second largest overhead cost area. These occupancy costs, which total more than 10 percent of a group's gross income, include rent, leases, depreciation, and maintenance. But financial managers rarely perceive this area as a candidate for cost reduction. One way might be the following: a large cross section of the public and employers say that daytime service hours are inconvenient. A great opportunity exists to improve both market share and overhead costs by initiating expanded hours. This seems practical since medical group facilities are probably used at less than 70 percent capacity.

Regarding equipment maintenance, comparison shopping for maintenance agreements is recommended, as charges vary greatly. All agreements should be scrutinized to ascertain whether they are necessary. Service contracts may be more expensive than an occasional repair bill or replacement cost. For equipment acquisitions, the financial manager should avoid being wed to one equipment brand or one distributor and retain the ability to negotiate price and terms. Also, leasing should be investigated as an alternative to purchasing equipment.

When more office space is needed, the group should hire competent designers and architects with medical practice expertise to design the area for maximum efficiency. If the group has excess office space, it should explore subletting options, especially for days, nights, and weekends when the practice is not using it. Also, negotiations with landlords should be firm to achieve better terms, including repainting, carpet replacement, and limited rent escalation clauses.

Other Areas

Other actions to consider in order to reduce costs are:

Telephone

- Monitor telephone bills, especially long distance calls, to see if they are justified.
- Review costs to see if switching to another telephone system is warranted.
- Have only the number of lines needed by the group, or restrict some lines to incoming calls so that others are dedicated solely to outbound calls.

Laboratory fees

- Be critical of the use of hospital laboratories. If their charges are higher, explore other outside providers.
- See if a referral laboratory will place a technician in the office of the group at its cost to secure the group's business.
- Recognize that volume discounts may be available from outside laboratories.

Legal and accounting

- Move most accounting functions in house, using a computer to reduce referral work to the outside accountant.
- Strongly negotiate for reduced fees with the outside accountant and lawyer, and obtain advance agreements on fees and time deadlines for the specific work they perform.
- Shop around for competent, lower-priced retirement plan administrative services.

Physician-level benefits

- Have one person coordinate all ordering of professional books and journal subscriptions to avoid duplication among group members.

- Choose professional meetings critically and avoid those not promising meaningful content and counsel.

INCREASING INCOME POTENTIALS

This alternative emphasizes the enlargement of the revenue stream to improve operations. The old, traditional assumption was that there was always an adequate number of patients available to be served. The healthcare seller's market has been transformed into a competitive arena that is much like the markets for most goods and services today. Medical groups are being urged to approach their practices as businesses and to perform all the managerial techniques followed by managers of commercial enterprises. The principles of marketing need to be adopted and followed so the group can be competitive and occupy a strong position in the local marketplace.

Some of the more subtle approaches that groups have undertaken embrace the preparation and distribution of patient brochures aimed at presenting the advantages and attractiveness of the medical group's service capacities to potential patients and managed care group audiences. Some groups have even used radio and television advertisements to attract greater patient volume. The most successful efforts have been based on comprehensive market analysis and planned marketing strategies.

Some possible directions that marketing strategies have taken include:

- Establishing satellite offices and using shared space
- Creating ambulatory surgical centers
- Increasing production and physician exposure
- Outsourcing unprofitable activities

Establishing Satellite Offices and Using Shared Space

Since patient convenience and time availability are becoming customer issues that need to be addressed, medical groups have established satellite offices to increase business. With a few changes in their work patterns, physicians can cover an additional facility and greatly extend their exposure to areas where a small group might not be as flexible. Changing referral patterns and the increase of hospital-based offices have resulted in referring patients to physicians who serve the hospital or have offices connected with the hospital (which a satellite might become).

Satellites must be established in profitable locations with minimum overhead burden. Population growth in the area of the satellite should be checked. A marketing survey should be made to identify the growth potential for patients using demographic analyses. For example, the group might decide to cater to a certain age group. What is the composition of the age group in the area planned for the satellite office? How many primary care physicians, who can refer patients to the specialty group practice, are there in the locale? Is a hospital readily available? These are only some of the questions that should be researched and answered before a decision is made about the satellite.

Shared space may be another avenue to explore in areas that may not be able to support a full-time satellite facility but where a need for a specialty still exists. Often, it is possible to work with a primary care physician for shared space. Some groups have made these arrangements in small towns, and physicians travel there one day a week on the local physician's day off, using his or her personnel. In this way, a satellite can be established at a very low cost with a potential for later expansion.

Creating Ambulatory Surgery Centers

Setting up a satellite operation is similar to establishing an ambulatory surgery center. However, a great deal of research and planning are necessary prior to creating this center. Many surgical procedures handled in hospitals could be performed in such a center, providing savings to the patient and insurer. While surgery fees remain the same, the lower charge for space, supplies, and attending personnel would provide added revenue to the medical group.

A feasibility study is recommended to evaluate this option. It should cover the estimated number of procedures that could be performed on an outpatient basis. A pro forma set of financial statements should be developed showing the estimated surgery charges and costs for operating this center. Once the financial feasibility is affirmed, it is necessary to contact the local department of health to obtain a certificate of need as well as their approval on the specifications they prescribe. Medicare regulations need to be consulted to determine their requirements since payment for procedures completed at ambulatory surgery centers may have to be approved separately. Also, the state licensing board must be contacted because it is necessary to comply with their specific requirements. After all approvals are secured and the financial projections indicate a potential profitable venture, the center project should be launched.

Increasing Production and Physician Exposure

Increased production can result from the establishment of an incentive reward system for stimulating physician productivity. As mentioned previously, most medical groups experience an increase in revenues from physicians who have been motivated by the possibility of greater income that is tied to productivity measures. This seems to have positive effects on all physicians participating in a group setting.

Another method for income enhancement is the increase in referrals from other physicians through greater exposure to the local medical community. This can be accomplished by making hospital visits during the times that offer maximum visibility to other physicians. If contacted for a consult, physicians should respond as soon as possible so that the discharge of the patient will not be delayed. The consult should be followed up with a letter to the referring provider as quickly as possible, and the patient should be returned to that physician as soon as treatment is concluded. In addition, good marketing exposure can also be created through public speaking, hospital committee work, and church and community activities.

Outsourcing Unprofitable Activities

A careful analysis of single-standing service procedures may lead to the conclusion that it would be more economical to buy the service from an external source. When preparing the analysis, financial managers should include all relevant cost detail. Thinking about this scenario from the point of view of creating options will lead to the best decision possible. In other words, managers should not decide on whether to outsource but whether to choose option A, B, C, or D. If outsourcing is selected, practices are advised not to outsource mission-critical functions because they need to maintain full control over how the tasks are completed to ensure the desired quality and quantity standards. Once this decision is made to entrust a different organization with the fulfillment of a particular practice need, it will free staff time. This may lead to the reassignment of staff.

MONITORING THE PULSE OF THE PRACTICE

Whether a medical group has a simple financial management system or a sophisticated one, group management members must filter through the maze of financial information and concentrate on a few key variables so that they can obtain an overall picture of the practice. Furthermore, close monitoring of operations necessitates that these few variables be available and studied on a monthly basis. Collectively, they enable the financial manager or administrator to track important activities and to react to signals quickly before a condition becomes potentially damaging to group operation. Milner has compiled a list of 16 items that form these key variables. They are:[8]

- Number of new patients
- Number of new patients referred by the Yellow Pages or other advertising efforts
- Number of new patients referred by particular physicians or healthcare plans
- Number of no-shows
- Number of patients from a particular zip code
- Volume of various ancillary services or tests performed in the office (e.g., X-ray, echocardiograms, stress tests, ultrasounds, visual fields, etc.)
- Volume of surgical procedures performed by type
- Number of patients admitted to the hospital
- Number of statements mailed
- Number of insurance forms filed
- Total number and amount of accounts sent to collection

- Total number patients whose balances have been outstanding for more than 120 days, and amount of balance
- Total charges, adjustments, and payments recorded
- Total expenses of the practice for the month
- Checkbook balance
- Total of all bills that have yet to be paid by the practice

With the use of the computer and special programming, these data can be conveniently organized and reported at intervals set by the financial manager.

SOURCES OF ASSISTANCE

The major source of assistance for financial managers is the professional consultant who has experience in the healthcare industry, especially in working with medical group practices. Other sources may be colleagues who are employed with other medical groups, hospitals, or healthcare entities. Usually, each individual develops a special relationship with one or two other persons and, over time, a deep sense of trust and mutual understanding grows and matures among them. Another source of professional information and relevant data for the financial manager is MGMA's publications. The *MGMA Connexion;* various surveys, such as the Cost Survey and Physician Compensation Survey; and other financial services, such as DataDive, provide a wealth of current information that is vital for keeping abreast of current events and for comparing a medical group's operations with that of peer organizations. For more information, please consult MGMA's Web site at www.mgma.com.

Since consultants are perhaps the major source of expert assistance to financial managers, we will mention several aspects of their role and the type of help they render. By definition, a consultant provides professional advice as a service to the entity that engages him or her in that role. There are many different types of consultants, and each performs a variety of services. Let us examine the major kinds of services these professionals perform for medical groups.

CONSULTING SERVICES TO MEDICAL GROUPS

Bohlmann classifies consulting services provided to medical groups into four types, as follows:[9]

1. Third-party opinion
2. Task orientation
3. Comprehensive study
4. Facilitation

Third-Party Opinion

This service requests the consultant to provide an opinion on a specific issue. The issue may be very narrow in scope or could be a subset of considerations identified in the broad context of a larger problem. The opinion may be needed by the medical practice because it has limited knowledge about the subject or it may need a validating response to an issue it already has developed an impression about. The consultant or firm may be a consulting generalist or have recognized special expertise in an area. In each case, the medical practice has defined the scope of its needs and sought to match these with an appropriate resource.

Task Orientation

This consulting engagement combines advice with a specific, deliverable objective. Here the definition of the consultant is merged with the scale of advice. For instance, an architectural firm may be engaged to render advice about the feasibility of a clinic facility at a specific site. The same firm may be engaged later to produce working drawings and supervise construction. The feasibility phase was entered into as a separate project with a defined goal. The study was undertaken with a full understanding about the deliverables and fee. In this case, a functional resource consultation is applied to task-oriented advice, in contrast to a task-oriented project.

Comprehensive Study

This study deals with a broad-scope engagement where the client medical group requests advice on a variety of issues. Specific areas may be designated, and they may not be related. On other occasions, the goals of the engagement may be somewhat undefined because the client is unable to fully articulate the nature of the problem or direction of the issue. In these cases, the consultant assists the client in exploring the problem and defining its nature and possible solutions. At the end of each engagement, the consultant typically submits a formal report to the client providing details of the problem assessment and recommended corrective actions. Operational assessments and process reengineering projects are examples of common comprehensive studies.

Facilitation

The role of a facilitator is to act as an intermediary in a meeting of various groups. The facilitator helps to structure an agenda, leads the group in discussions, and steers the group toward a successful termination of the meeting(s). The facilitator might be asked to moderate meetings and help two divergent parties or groups resolve their differences. In this case, the facilitator is selected jointly by the dissident parties. Sometimes, the task or project of the facilitator is vague because the medical group is uncertain of the type of assistance needed. The facilitator in this role must lead the client through a series of steps to uncover the nature of the problem and to assist members in addressing and solving the problem(s) brought to light. Typical facilitation engagements include strategic planning, mergers, and new organizational formations. A skilled facilitator will also be a valuable resource to resolve conflicts because of their outsider status.

TYPES OF CONSULTANTS AND THEIR ROLES

There are consultants for almost any type of activity. Levels of expertise span a broad spectrum of understanding and specialization. There are individuals with significant reputations as well as firms that have compiled reputable records for valuable work performed for a variety of clients. For example, MGMA's Health Care Consulting Group is comprised of a team of expert management consultants, virtually all of whom have significant practice management experience. The group provides a range of services, from improving practice operations and providing strategic planning facilitation to designing physician compensation plans and implementing performance turnarounds for integrated delivery systems. For more information about the group, visit their Web page at www.mgma.com/consulting.

When a financial manager needs to employ a consultant, the best source for determining whom to engage would be the informal network of other medical group managers and colleagues who might have firsthand experience with certain individuals or firms. Once names are identified, MGMA may be able to provide specific information about these contacts, or the association may be able to provide a consultant from its staff. The best information about consultants is obtained from previous users of their services. Before selecting any particular consultant, solicit and evaluate several sources of reference from prior users.

In addition to MGMA's Health Care Consulting Group, other consultants are included in the following list:

Accountants — There are large national accounting firms as well as small area accounting firms that have very qualified experts in the healthcare industry. Caution needs to be exercised in assuring that the individual who is assigned to the medical group has sufficient experience in the type of service being requested. If there is a mismatch, the group should contact the firm and request a qualified replacement.

Management consultants — A wide array of individuals are in this category. Professional directories of consultants might be a good starting point to locate one in the special area in which assistance is needed. There are national and local consulting firms, some with broad-based experience in multiple industries. Others specialize in the healthcare field and are likely to provide the most relevant level of assistance. Again, the MGMA Health Care Consulting Group is also a recognized and valuable resource.

Lawyers — When legal problems arise, lawyers are essential. There are large partnerships and small ones located in all major cities. Some lawyers specialize in healthcare matters and some have subspecialties within the field such as reimbursement, Medicare fraud and abuse, managed healthcare negotiations, antitrust, and professional liability issues.

Actuaries — These specialists are needed in developing retirement plans and related benefit programs. Consulting actuaries are connected with insurance agencies and brokerage houses. They are also recommended when medical groups begin their entry into prepaid contracts in the managed care phase of the practice.

Computer consultants — Frequently, salespersons are referred to as consultants in this area. There are knowledgeable individuals who are not employed by a computer firm and consult independently. Also, persons from accounting or consulting firms can provide expert advice on computer selection, programming, software options, and networking arrangements. Again, caution should be exercised in ensuring that the advice giver is free of a specific product interest and that the advice is objective and appropriate to the needs of the group.

Architects/designers — When a medical practice undertakes the design and working-drawing phase of a facility construction project, an architect or designer is frequently engaged to give advice independent of the specific project. Services range from feasibility studies to situations where an architect may serve as an outside adviser to a medical practice or primary architectural firm. There are usually qualified architects and architectural firms available in most cities.

Marketing specialists — The range of services in this area may be as narrow as advice on a specific advertising program or as broad as a multifaceted marketing strategy program. In these cases, the distinction between giving advice and providing service is fuzzy. When entering into broader strategy issues, the competence of the consultant should be carefully evaluated.

Managed healthcare experts — There are a growing number of individuals who offer specialized assistance in all types of delivery systems. Their work ranges from plan development and contracting to detailed operations and reporting.

Contract managers — Some consulting firms offer managers to be employed by healthcare entities on a part-time or advisory basis. The line between contracting services and bonafide consulting may become blurred in these arrangements.

To the Point

■ The analysis of actual performance is best carried out by comparing it to the planned activities that the group decided to follow. Referred to as *performance reporting*, it is accomplished with an operating budget.

■ To analyze areas of medical group operations, one should look at financial measures and nonfinancial indicators. The financial analysis should include three areas:

   — Evaluating responsibility centers

   — Meeting goals and objectives and the operating budget

   — Comparing group operations with external norms and other groups

■ The performance measurement criteria for three different types of responsibility center are:

   — Profit center evaluator, which might be a profit measure, such as a contribution margin

   — Cost or expense center measure, which might be meeting the operating budget

   — Investment center criterion, which might be a return-on-investment indicator

■ To measure the overall performance of the entire medical group, the original operating budget should be adjusted for the actual level of volume reached before actual results are compared with the adjusted budget. This budget is called *performance budgeting*.

■ To measure the performance of cost centers also requires the use of adjusted budgets for the actual volume level of activity achieved before comparing actual expenses to budgeted amounts.

■ MGMA's *Performance and Practices of Successful Medical Groups Report* provides performance measures of better-performing medical groups in four areas:

   1. Profitability and cost management

   2. Productivity, capacity, and staffing

   3. Accounts receivable and collection

   4. Patient satisfaction

■ Overall analysis of a medical group's operations should include nonfinancial information as well as financial indicators. The easiest nonfinancial performance aggregates are: number of patient visits, number of procedures performed, number of physicians and physician days, number of employees and employee days, number of hours worked, number of laboratory procedures, and quantity of supplies used or purchased.

■ More useful nonfinancial performance measures involve level of activity and use of resources per full-time equivalent physician. Another measure relates to resources used per patient visit or procedure.

■ Profiling is defined as a process using epidemiological methods to collect, analyze, and use provider practice data. It focuses on and analyzes patterns of care for a single physician or group of physicians. The practice pattern is expressed as a rate that incorporates measures of resource utilization or of outcome that is measured over a defined period for a defined population.

■ A tool to analyze physician services and productivity of medical groups is DataDive developed by MGMA. The service analyzes physician productivity based on the number and complexity of procedures performed for the entire medical group subscriber, each specialty, and each physician within the group. DataDive utilizes CMS's Resource-based Relative Value Scale (RBRVS) with a breakdown of relative value units (RVUs) into provider work, practice expense, and malpractice components. The statistics include:

  – Improving productivity — requires a medical group to conduct operational reviews of a specific department area and the entire organization

  – Implementing cost reductions — personnel costs, clerical and clinical supplies, and facilities and equipment

  – Increasing income potentials — establish satellite offices and use shared space, create ambulatory surgical centers, increase production and physician exposure

■ Monitoring the pulse of the practice can be achieved by examining financial and nonfinancial key variables on a regular basis, at least monthly.

■ Financial managers can obtain assistance for medical group problems from consultants, other medical groups' managers, colleagues, and mentors. MGMA and its publications, as well as the MGMA Health Care Consulting Group, can be helpful, too.

REFERENCES

1. Tran Z. V., and Burman, D. 1999. "Introduction: The Story of Profiling." In *Physician Profiling: A Source Book for Health Care Administrators*. San Francisco, CA: Jossey-Bass, Inc.

2. Ibid.

3. Goldfield, N. 1999. "Harvesting Data for Physician Profiling — The Administrative and Clinical How's." In *Physician Profiling: A Source Book for Health Care Administrators,* pp. 34–35. San Francisco, CA: Jossey-Bass, Inc.

4. Ruben, M. S., Braun, P., and Caper, P. 1999. "What Data Are Needed for Physician Profiles?" In *Physician Profiling: A Source Book for Health Care Administrators,* p. 9. San Francisco, CA: Jossey-Bass, Inc.

5. Smith, N. S. 1999. "Laying the Foundation for a Profiling System." In *Physician Profiling: A Source Book for Health Care Administrators,* p. 5. San Francisco, CA: Jossey-Bass, Inc.

6. Tran, Z. V. and Burman, D. 1999. "Introduction: The Story of Profiling." In *Physician Profiling: A Source Book for Health Care Administrators*. San Francisco, CA: Jossey-Bass, Inc.

7. Budd, G. B. 1988, February. "Productivity: The Challenge for Ambulatory Services." *Journal of Ambulatory Care Management*, 2–6.

8. Milner, D. E. 1992. "Topics in Office Management: Monitoring the Pulse of the Practice." *Journal of Medical Practice Management*, 29.

9. Bohlmann, R. C. 1991. "Consultants: Selection and Use." In A. Ross, S. L. Williams, and E. L. Schafer (Eds.), *Ambulatory Care Management,* p. 384. Albany, NY: Delmar Publishers.

CHAPTER 13

Tools for Managing Operations

Edited by Michael O'Connell, MHA, FACHE, FACMPE

After completing this chapter, you will be able to:

- Explain the benchmarking process and the benefits and applications relevant to medical practices that use them.

- Participate in an initial effort to benchmark elements of a medical group's practice.

- Describe the basic concept of quality and total quality used in business and healthcare.

- Explain the current quality efforts being pursued by the Centers for Medicare and Medicaid including value-based purchasing (VBP) and HCAHPS.

- Articulate the essence of total quality management (TQM) principles and operational processes and compare them with the traditional approaches used in quality control efforts.

- Assist in the initial establishment of a total quality management effort within a medical practice and evaluate its effectiveness after implementation.

The healthcare field is in the midst of profound and pervasive change. At this writing, many ideas about the possible directions and scope of change are being widely discussed and disseminated throughout the healthcare field, especially in the areas of healthcare reform. While everyone agrees that the goal is to improve the operations of all medical providers, to increase access to medical services, and to reduce the acceleration of healthcare costs throughout the industry, there are many differences in opinion on how to achieve these outcomes.

Today, there are many more measures of success that healthcare leaders are accountable for. Some of these measures are revenue over expenses (profit), timely access to a provider through a same-day appointment, turnaround time for services or results, percentage of medical errors, and cost of alternative services. A successful medical group must provide high-quality care at a competitive price with a strong orientation toward service. In this chapter, we will discuss two major areas that are impacting the operations of a medical practice — benchmarking and quality of care.

These changes affect all members of the medical group, and the medical practice administrator and team will be key individuals serving on many quality improvement teams. In addition, they are often called on to provide the financial detail needed to benchmark the practice. It is critical for the team to be "quality literate" and emerge as leaders to implement change.

BENCHMARKING

A benchmarking movement continues to sweep America. Every day, healthcare groups are sharing data, learning from others how to improve a system or process, and developing new benchmarks and score cards to share information. According to Wikipedia,

> Benchmarking is the process of comparing one's business processes and performance metrics to industry bests and/or best practices from other industries. Dimensions typically measured are quality, time, and cost. In the process of benchmarking, management identifies the best firms in their industry, or in another industry where similar processes exist, and compares the results and processes of those studied (the "targets") to one's own results and processes. In this way, they learn how well

> *the targets perform and, more importantly, the business processes that*
> *explain why these firms are successful.[1]*

It is thought that the term *benchmarking* was first used by shoe cobblers to measure a person's feet; the cobbler would put a foot on a bench and mark it up to make the shoe pattern. Benchmarking measures performance using customized key indicators (e.g., cost per patient visit, staff hours per surgical procedure, test result turnaround time, or billing errors per 1,000 medical claims), resulting in a performance metric that is compared to others. Also commonly known as "best practice benchmarking" or "process benchmarking," this management tool is used to evaluate various aspects of their processes related to best practices or the processes of those within a peer group defined for comparison. This effort allows medical groups to develop plans for how to make improvements or adapt specific best practices with the goal of increasing performance. Benchmarking is usually a continuous process in which medical groups continually seek to improve their practices.

Benchmarking fits closely with the total quality management (TQM) process by assisting in the establishment of goals and objectives that medical practices set to improve their processes. The process of benchmarking begins by first evaluating a medical practice's own operations to pinpoint its weaknesses. Then efforts are made to identify, study, and imitate similar operations that other organizations use. This process has proven successful in many industries outside of healthcare. Some medical groups have catapulted ahead of their competitors almost overnight, and some have even surpassed the performance levels or benchmarks set by their mentors.

Building on the concept of strategic planning, benchmarking takes the next step toward execution by examining not only numbers but also processes. It provides the answer for "how" strategies that have been selected can be successfully implemented. The "how" is the process used by the most profitable and productive producers and deliverers of the product or service being benchmarked.

Benefits and Advantages

Medical practices that have accepted and employed benchmarking practices have discovered that emulating the best can revitalize nearly every facet of their operations. Robert Camp listed five areas of corporate activity where benchmarking has affected operations most profoundly. They are:[2]

1. **Meet customer requirements** — When the best competitors are studied, accurate information on consumer demand and the current responses within the industry are obtained. And, most importantly, strategies for meeting and exceeding customer requirements become known by the benchmarker.

2. **Set relevant, achievable goals** — Once the benchmarker is able to match well-defined customer requirements with proven business practices, the emulator can feel confident that their goals are on target and realistic.

3. **Develop accurate productivity measures** — By evaluating their internal operations against optimum standards, managers and workers of the benchmarker develop a better understanding of company strengths and weaknesses, together with the will to change areas where necessary.

4. **Be competitive** — The practice of benchmarking challenges the status quo and turns an organization's focus inside out by replacing internal viewpoints with external perspectives. This comparison may be a motivating experience. For example, leading companies can generate new products up to two and a half times faster than the industry average and at half the cost. By adopting proven practices of organizational leaders, companies can bypass the usual trial-and-error learning curve and jump ahead to a competitive advantage.

5. **Adopt industry best practices** — When the success stories of the studied corporate leaders are documented, executives and managers of the benchmarker can easily justify support for the adoption of the best practices even when major changes are necessary. When a cross-section of managers and employees are included on the benchmarking study team, the process to be emulated receives broad-based enthusiasm for adoption.

Requirements for and Types of Benchmarking

While the process of benchmarking sounds simple and promises great rewards, there is no quick fix. It is costly, laborious, and entails an ongoing process similar to continuous quality improvement. To be successful, benchmarking needs the following prerequisites:

▩ **Strong management commitment** — Top management's involvement and support are crucial to successful efforts because considerable resources are required, and changing organizational goals is part of the process. Change is difficult and needs senior leadership's commitment and support.

▩ **Complete understanding of the medical practice's operations** — To discern what makes the other medical practice the best, the emulator needs to know its own operations in great detail. To incorporate the ideas of the other medical practice, managers must know their own operations well enough to customize the best practices to fit their system.

▩ **Openness to change and new ideas** — If a medical practice has a parochial attitude and is averse to change and new ideas, this bias will work against imitating others' practices. To build a competitive edge demands open minds and a desire to implement necessary changes.

▩ **Willingness to share information with benchmarking partners** — Once the benchmarking medical group is allowed to study a target medical group and absorb information to use and emulate that group's actions, it should be willing to share its experiences, problems, and solutions with the original targeted medical practice. Of course, as in any sharing of information, trade secrets need to be protected.

▪ **Dedication to continuous benchmarking efforts** — After the initial effort to benchmark has begun, the process should continue, and the medical practice should continue to measure its performance against the best.

Today benchmarking has expanded from manufacturing industries into service, financial industries, and governmental agencies. (For example, the Internal Revenue Service targeted American Express on billing and Motorola for accounting practices.) The process has been adapted to a variety of specific uses and situations. There are three categories on which most benchmarking efforts are centered:[3]

1. Competitive benchmarking

2. Cooperative benchmarking

3. Collaborative benchmarking

Competitive Benchmarking

This type of benchmarking is the most difficult to implement because most medical practices are reluctant to share trade secrets with direct competitors. Some medical groups even try to steer benchmarkers off track with misinformation. Yet many groups do share some information with competitors for mutual benefits, just not the most critical information. For example, medical groups may provide an office tour and visit, but no cost data are exchanged. With the visit and other data obtained from external sources relating to the target medical group, the benchmarker can get quite close to what it needs. External sources may include public records, industry publications, the medical group's workforce, suppliers, and outside consultants. In this type of effort, the goal is to find out what the competitors are doing, how, and how well to compare their practices with the benchmarker's operations.

Cooperative Benchmarking

Even though discovering what one's competition is doing is essential, many successful benchmarking efforts begin by targeting a company outside an organization's own industry and focusing on a particular business practice or function. Some experiences have shown that the more diverse a company's benchmarking partners, the better the result. For example, the Association for Benchmarking Health Care links the needs of healthcare management to processes and techniques to identify leading cross-industry practices. Through the exchange of data gathered in benchmarking surveys, members will be able to benefit from the experience of many entities in the industry. Benchmarking can be learned from other industries in many areas including capital projects, e-mail management, and succession planning.

When benchmarking partners are not competitors, both often respond with a great amount of information. Frequently, new ideas are gained from looking at a successful practice in an industry completely separate from the benchmarker's setting and tailored to the needs of the medical group's situation. Also, a company that compares itself only with its direct competitors is only "playing catch-up." Cooperative benchmarking might lead to new innovations that cause the emulator to leap-frog over its competitors.

Collaborative Benchmarking

Collaborative benchmarking is an alternative to the orthodox approach because it involves a limited exchange of data within an ad-hoc consortium or organizations. The focus is on statistics primarily (how much), rather than the actual work practices (how). Thus, the result may not be as helpful as full-blown studies. However, with new database clearinghouses that now describe best practices online, collaborative benchmarking may well become a fruitful exercise. Because participants remain anonymous, the process can offer valuable insights into a competitor's operations.

MGMA provides collaborative benchmarking services by producing five major survey reports and numerous specialty reports. The major reports are:

Cost Survey Report

The *Cost Survey Report* is available for specific specialties and observes individual, nonacademic medical practices. Other reports use the individual provider or management professional as the unit of observation. The Cost Survey Report provides data on organizational expenses, revenue, and operational and output indicators and is broken out in two versions: single-specialty and multispecialty. The other reports review individual compensation and productivity measures.

Physician Compensation and Production Survey Report

This report is the gold standard for data on physician compensation and production. In fact, with data on more than 44,000 providers representing more than 1,800 organizations, it's the largest sample available. This report includes individual physician performance and compensation data, including collections, work RVUs, nonphysician providers, and more.

Management Compensation Survey Report

This report includes thorough compensation information for many practice leaders, including physician-executive positions, compensation by experience level and education, compensation for managers of integrated delivery system practices, and retirement contributions.

Performance and Practices of Successful Medical Groups Report

The *Performance and Practices of Successful Medical Groups Report* looks at better-performing practices and their characteristics. It includes data from the Cost Survey as well as articles profiling better-performing practices.

Academic Practice Compensation and Production Survey for Faculty & Management Report

The *Academic Practice Compensation and Production Survey for Faculty & Management Report* is limited to academic departments and practice plans. This report also includes some departmental and practice plan characteristics, as well as benchmarks for research, clinical care, and education.

Interactive Reports: Cost Survey and Physician Compensation and Production

The two interactive report products are available for the *Physician Compensation and Production Survey Report* and the *Cost Survey Report*. Both allow users to export data and include more data points and levels of information.

MGMA's *Physician Compensation and Production Survey: 2011 Report Based on 2010 Data*, which includes data from 59,375 providers in 2,846 groups, spotlights the critical relationship between compensation and productivity for providers. This report includes:

- Demographic categories ranging from geographic region and practice setting to years in specialty and method of compensation
- Various performance ratios illustrating the relationship between compensation and production
- Comprehensive and summary data tables that cover many specialties
- Data on collections for professional charges and work RVUs

The report is used to:

- Conduct peer comparisons to evaluate the performance of your individual physicians and nonphysician providers
- Develop physician compensation and production targets for your providers
- Assess your compensation methods for compliance
- Track provider compensation trends by specialties

MGMA offers benchmarking resources to help the medical practice administrator, including complimentary Webinars, tools, an online community, video case studies, and articles. They can be accessed at www.mgma.com/pm/default.aspx?id=9238.

THE BENCHMARKING PROCESS

Each benchmarking effort should be a carefully planned and tailored project that every company designs to meet its desired objectives. However, studies of successful experiences show that most follow a certain pattern that Robert Camp has summarized in 10 steps that cover five phases, from planning through maturity:[4]

Planning

1. **Determine what to benchmark.** This is a difficult part of the process. A medical group needs to examine its production processes carefully and determine where bottlenecks or problems are occurring. Also,

management needs to be aware that to build competitive advantage, it must focus solely on factors that will advance the organizational mission and really make a difference in performance.

Problems in operations cannot be identified unless one possesses a thorough knowledge of one's own operations. Even then, it may be difficult to discern problem areas until a company's modus operandi is compared to the best practices of others in the industry. For this reason, some medical groups benchmark across a wide variety of functions to discover exactly where they fall short. Usually, however, benchmarkers narrow their focus as much as possible, concentrating on areas that most affect customer values, company performance, and, ultimately, competitive status. Nearly any issue, process, or function can be benchmarked.

Some suggest that the start of benchmarking might begin with activities that:

- Account for a large part of your cost or value chain

- Differentiate the medical practice from its competitors

- Frustrate employees

If positive changes are made in these areas, profit is likely to increase, market credibility will be enhanced, and group pride and commitment are likely to result.

2. **Identify the best medical practices in those areas.** This step involves detective-like work. It should begin with a search of public records including databases and publications. Names of companies known for their expertise in a particular area or business practices can be uncovered through a keyword search of online databases. (If multiple practices are being benchmarked, each one may need a study of a different company.) Next, talk with industry experts; the medical practice's employees, customers, and suppliers; and others knowledgeable about the areas or business practices being targeted. Ask whose products, services, or business practices are similar in some way to the benchmarking organization's. A benchmarking consultant may be helpful in this step.

All likely candidates should be researched thoroughly, as this step is crucial to the entire process. You may not be able to obtain much information from the competitors themselves. Even if a medical group is planning a cooperative benchmarking effort outside its industry, it is still wise to find out as much as possible about its competitors. Competitors may be benchmarking, too, and the medical group needs to know what changes they are planning. Once the research has been completed, the list should be narrowed to fit the travel budget, and then the top targets should be approached to request a meeting and possibly a site visit.

The chances of getting a heavily solicited benchmarking partner to work with a requesting medical group are increased if your practice can communicate the following:

- Knowledge of benchmarking — Assure the targeted medical group that your company is serious about employing sound techniques of benchmarking. You will be received more favorably than you would be if your medical group were merely snooping around. Most partners know what real benchmarking is all about.

— Offering something in exchange — Not all medical practices have processes that others want to learn from, but those that do and are willing to share will find more doors opening as a result.

3. **Collect data to measure both your own and your benchmarking partner's performance.** Before collecting any data, the group first must decide what kinds of measurements it needs to best illuminate the practices and how best to collect that sort of data. The value of benchmarking is lost if benchmarkers bring back irrelevant or inaccurate measurements from the targeted medical practice. It is always best to center the search on factors that relate to cost, quality, and timeliness.

Another critical facet in benchmarking is the careful selection of the fact-finding team. There should be a team comprised of a benchmarking "guru" who knows the process thoroughly, a senior manager, a line person who understands the targeted activity, and a change leader with the authority to implement the recommendations. Including line managers and workers as team members ensures broad support for changes. Finally, enough time should be allowed for data collection. Schedules should remain flexible to fit the partners' availability. The search needs to concentrate on the processes behind the numbers.

Analysis

4. **Determine current performance "gap."** When all data are in, the medical group should compare common denominators. (At this point, benchmarkers may find that they have been using inferior measurement methods and must reassess their own processes to obtain usable statistics.) This comparative analysis will reveal any performance gaps between your operations and best-in-class practices.

5. **Project future performance levels.** Using current data on performance, the medical group should project the targeted company's performance level three to five years down the road. That becomes the medical group's benchmark(s).

Integration

6. **Communicate benchmark findings and gain acceptance.** Before the medical group integrates its partner's best practices into its internal operations, it should present and promote the benchmarking results to win support for change at all organizational levels.

7. **Establish functional goals.** Based on all information collected and the insights from analyzing it, the medical group's team should recommend whatever changes it deems necessary to achieve the benchmarks inspired by the targeted medical group. In doing so, strategies should be

formulated on how to present them to senior management, especially if they have to be sold on the process. These recommendations should be incorporated into a statement of operational principles and distributed throughout the medical group.

Action

Action is the real reason for benchmarking. Without action, benchmarking is merely an intellectual exercise. A team's success is judged solely on the improvements it makes.

8. **Develop action plans.** Assisted by line managers and employees responsible for the targeted processes, the medical group should set objectives and devise specific plans for meeting them.

9. **Implement specific actions and monitor progress.** With benchmarks, objectives, and action plans in place, the transformation of processes can begin. Progress must be monitored, and rising performance levels should be reported to all employees.

10. **Recalibrate benchmarks.** Because market forces and business practices are constantly changing, the medical group should plan to reevaluate and recalibrate benchmarks at set intervals. This recycling is part of the continuous improvement effort of TQM. Benchmarking should not be a one-time event but a continuous process.

Maturity

The benchmarking process reaches maturity when benchmarks have been met or exceeded, and the medical group has earned recognition as an industry leader. At this point, the targeted best practices have been fully integrated into operational processes, and benchmarking has become an essential way of life for the medical practice. Especially when engaging in cooperative or collaborative benchmarking, the process should incorporate communication, timeliness, intermediate goals, and reporting requirements that participants formally agree on at the onset of the project.

HEALTHCARE MODELS OF BENCHMARKING

Benchmarking in healthcare represents the formalization of certain comparative efforts such as MGMA's Physician Services Practice Analysis Software program, the American Hospital Association's benchmarking surveys, and the Health Care Financial Management Association's 14 financial indicators published each year. As a formal process, benchmarking goes beyond knowing what others do and what their indicators are to *understanding* what others do and learning from their practices.

Benchmarking embraces a new tendency or willingness for healthcare professionals of all backgrounds to break through some traditional barriers by following several guidelines:

- ▪ Aggressively seek out change.

- ▪ Go outside the healthcare industry to find the best practices that can ultimately help to improve the quality of healthcare delivery.

- ▪ Identify sources of variance.

- ▪ Implement continuous quality improvement processes.

- ▪ Establish a basis for continuously evaluating customer needs and expectations.

According to Madeline Hyden, MGMA-ACMPE Web content writer/editor, she used benchmark data to determine connections between EHRs and more effective care.[5] She learned that 63.54 percent of better performers use problem lists as a part of EHR functionality and that 56.25 percent of better performers have EHRs that integrate with practice billing and claims systems. Integrating an EHR with the practice management system (PMS) is challenging with limited training time and room for error. However, integration improves front and back office efficiency, decreases errors, and can eventually improve the bottom line, thus giving credence to the reasons why high-performing medical groups pursue EHR integration. Integrated systems prevent having to enter patient demographic information twice (once in the PMS and again in the EHR), and automated EHR alerts encourage more complete claims without missing information. This reduces denied claims and improves reimbursement rates. Hyden suggested that before purchasing and implementing an EHR, make sure it interfaces with a current PMS and any other devices or office equipment. She also learned that 55.21 percent of better performers have EHRs that offer functionality for drug formularies. This prescription drug list that covers specific healthcare plan details enables users to electronically check if drugs are in a patient plan's formulary. Similar to problem lists, meaningful use requirements mandate that practices have access to at least one internal or external drug formulary during their EHR reporting period.

This study offers some insight into the validity of benchmarking efforts to improve physician performance. More studies can be implemented to determine effective administrative, clinical, and financial tools to increase the effectiveness of benchmarking.

THE QUALITY FOCUS

An increasing share of attention through U.S. and global businesses is centered on the term *quality*. Healthcare is also receiving extra scrutiny through the insistence of patients, payers, and industry members shopping for quality healthcare at the best price. In fact, many vocal individuals assert that as competition increases among healthcare providers, the difference in the cost of services between providers will shrink, and physicians, hospitals, and clinics will be judged on the quality and value of their services.[6] The term also has been applied to managing a practice, and Kaiser states that to survive in the new age, quality management of a practice is as important as quality medical care.[7]

Quality Defined

Can we really provide a definition of *quality*? According to Business Dictionary. com, quality is a measure of excellence or a state of being free from defects, deficiencies, and significant variations brought about by the strict and consistent adherence to measurable and verifiable standards to achieve uniformity of output that satisfies specific customer or user requirements . . . the totality of features and characteristics of a product or service that bears its ability to satisfy stated or implied needs.[8]

In *Merriam-Webster's Dictionary*, quality is a "peculiar and essential character, an inherent feature, property; a degree of excellence, grade."[9]

For many people, quality cannot be defined in principle because it has no essence and is abstract. The word itself is abstract like the words "knowledge" and "beauty." As a result, "quality" definitions will bear resemblance to each other; however, none of the definitions will be the definitive definition.

Quality in the eyes of industry is all about measurement. So instead of spending time wrestling with a definition, many organizations identify what they want their medical group to look like once quality is better (e.g., fewer missed appointments, improved patient satisfaction, fewer billing errors). The focus is not to wrestle too much with defining quality but to produce quality. And an organization can produce quality even if a definition of quality doesn't exist.

Quality assurance (QA) is a broad concept that focuses on the entire quality system including suppliers and ultimate consumers of the product or service. It includes all activities designed to produce products and services of appropriate quality. According to the American Society of Quality (ASQ), QA includes all those planned or systematic actions necessary to provide adequate confidence that a product or service will satisfy given needs.[10]

Quality control (QC) has a narrower focus than quality assurance. Quality control focuses on the process of producing the product or service with the intent of eliminating problems that might result in defects. According to ASQ, QC includes the operational techniques and the activities that sustain a product or service's quality and that satisfies given needs.[11]

Quality management is the totality of functions involved in the determination and achievement of quality (includes quality assurance and quality control).[12]

Another account lists eight attributes that might be perceived as requirements from the customer's point of view:[13]

1. Aesthetics
2. Conformance
3. Durability
4. Features
5. Perceived Quality

6. Performance
7. Reliability
8. Serviceability

These definitions relate to services as well as to products. They describe quality not as a static end result but a continuous process of improvement. It is not a bull's eye but a moving target. In a sense, quality is what is theoretically possible, minus some small allowances for life's imperfections. Quality is meeting the customer's expectations and thereby gaining total customer satisfaction.

When quality is applied to business operations, several useful concepts become acceptable and are employed to provide evidence of quality attainment:

- **Product portfolio** — Quality in existing products (services) and in new product design means providing a commodity that appeals to customers by satisfying their particular needs to a greater degree than a competitor's product. This product should be introduced in the shortest possible length of time from design to manufacture with zero redesign reiterations.

- **Zero defects** — Zero defects are achieved when a process produces no waste of material, capacity, or time. Zero defects are part of the continuous improvement process that is measured by statistical process control (SPC) and design for manufacturing processes; in medical practices, examples include zero surgical errors and zero infections.

- **On-time delivery** — Quality in this context requires the producer to deliver all products (services) on time to all customers at all times. On-time delivery is a function of many things, but in manufacturing, cycle time is the most important concept to understand. Cycle time is defined as the time that elapses between order entry and shipping the product, including downtime within and between organizational departments; in medical practices, this could apply to turnaround time for lab results or time to get a bill paid.

- **Total quality service** — Total quality service refers to the many customer needs that are provided in a professional, timely, and courteous manner. Services are provided even when there are no contractual obligations to do so. Total quality empowers every employee to add value to his or her medical practice's products or services so that they meet the real needs of the customers.

- **Six sigma** — Six sigma is a relatively new way to measure how "good" a product is. It is based on the identification of defects that are introduced into a product or work element and the systematic reduction of these defects. It operates on the premise that as we eliminate defects from our activities, we will realize tremendous opportunities in reducing cycle time and cost and improving quality, reliability, and overall customer satisfaction.[14]

Evolution of Total Quality

According to ASQ, the quality movement can be traced back to the thirteenth century when individual craftsmen organized into unions. This model continued until the 1800s when factories developed and incorporated quality processes in quality practices with a focus on product inspection. By the 1940s and the advent of World War II, total quality was born with quality gurus Joseph M. Juran and W. Edwards Deming, who focused on creating improvements in system processes by the people who used them rather than improvements in the actual product. The explosion of TQM occurred in the 1970s by the U.S. industry in direct response to Japan's high-quality products. The United States focused on improvement in outcomes through measurement and involving the entire organization in its approach. In the 1980s and 1990s, healthcare rode the TQM wave and explored ways to apply TQM concepts to medical care. In 1987, the Malcolm Baldrige National Quality Program and Malcolm Baldrige National Quality Award were developed by the U.S. Congress. Now, in the twenty-first century, quality and TQM have matured and moved beyond manufacturing into all types of organizations including education, government agencies, healthcare, and medical practices.

The current phase of total quality upon us refers to customer satisfaction and cost control as the most advanced approach. Total quality control focuses on organization-wide cooperation to achieve shared goals and places technical and behavioral tools in the hands of all employees from the bottom of the medical practice to the top. In this concept, every individual takes direct responsibility for business excellence. The founder of this notion is the late W. Edwards Deming, who advocated that this approach is a way to obtain market leadership in the present market place. This three-stage evolution is seen as a cumulative aggregative concept proceeding from quality control to quality assurance to total quality.

The Concern for Quality in Today's Environment

There seems to be a virtual consensus that the American standard of living has decreased during the last several decades. While the U.S. economy is still the largest in the world and our lifestyles are still among the best worldwide, the manufacturing sector has experienced a substantial loss in market share. Industries that were developed and once controlled by American companies, such as automotive, electronic, semiconductors, and tools, are now under Asian and European domination. One of the underlying factors associated with this replacement of manufacturing supremacy has been attributed to the poor quality of products and services of American organizations.

The current record shows that quality has served as a successful business strategy, and companies that have used quality principles to improve their business performance are creating competitive advantages. Business research supports this assertion by concluding that quality and market share drive profitability. Low quality and low market share are associated with lower returns on investments.

The underlying principle driving results goes like this: As costs are driven down, prices are also reduced, which enables a company to increase its market share. With increased market share, the economy of scales is experienced, which causes a further reduction of costs. Growth and increased profits then seem to continue in a cyclical fashion. An example of this iteration is the Japanese automobile industry. Initially, Japanese auto manufacturers produced cheaper cars than their American counterparts. Over time, the Japanese developed a reputation for being reliable and cost efficient. As they became more profitable, they were able to reduce the cost of quality. The manufacturers moved to the high end of the market and used the same principles to reduce the cost of quality for more expensive cars. Today, we have the Acura, Infinity, and Lexus lines, which compete well in the luxury class of the automobile market.

The principle of quality-oriented business strategy places a focus on customer requirements. To implement this intention, manufacturers or service providers develop their outputs quickly and efficiently. They adopt "mass customization" production policies that enable them to dwell precisely on customer needs. Often, manufacturers use computer-aided design technology to reduce the period of time from design to delivery, which in turn leads to making smaller batches of a product, reducing inventories, and entering new markets. All of these business strategies involve improving processes so that waste is eliminated and the cycle time of production is reduced, largely as a result of having the entire medical practice focus on customer requirements and the perceived definition of quality. This philosophy is the opposite of planned obsolescence, which has been the driving force of many American manufacturers for decades and one of the causes of manufacturing quality problems today.

In healthcare, quality is one of the most talked about issues. This interest seems to have been fueled by the following forces:

■ The federal government, which assesses the quality of Medicare inpatient hospital visits through peer-review organization screens, annually reports hospital death rate statistics through the CMS, and funds research on methods of assessing ambulatory care quality

■ Numerous state governments that have recently created legislation mandating the collection and public dissemination of information related to quality

■ Consumer groups such as the People's Medical Society and the American Association of Retired Persons

■ Private businesses that have been joining coalitions that share healthcare quality and cost data

■ Professional organizations such as the American Medical Association and the American College of Physicians

■ Traditional accrediting bodies such as The Joint Commission (TJC)[15]

O'Connor and Lanning[16] also assert that this concern for quality is the result of three phenomena:

1. Efforts to help contain the escalating costs of healthcare have raised questions about their impact on quality. As reimbursement policies became more constrictive in the 1980s, many feared that some providers might respond by cutting corners to a point where substandard care was the norm. Thus, attention to healthcare quality is partially an outgrowth of these restrictive cost-containment measures.

2. Research findings show a variation in the rates and appropriateness of certain surgical procedures across small geographical areas. Because these variations do not appear to reflect the needed healthcare of the population and because 17 percent to 32 percent of selected surgical procedures are considered medically inappropriate, concern has been raised that physicians can differ widely on how to treat a patient. Thus, physicians may not always know or agree on what constitutes quality care.

3. The widespread interest in quality by all types of industries, including healthcare. As mentioned earlier, many American organizations have been jolted out of a false sense of competitive complacency by the effective quality initiatives implemented by foreign companies to gain a large share of many American markets. In this case, the emphasis is on quality as a competitive and market-driven response to the demands of consumers seeking value for their money.[17]

These trends have forced a movement toward a value orientation. Many advocate that purchasers of healthcare should "buy right" by supporting high-value providers who offer quality in a cost-effective fashion. And others have stated that healthcare organizations that are best able to manage and sell quality are the ones that will dominate the market.

VALUE-BASED PURCHASING AND HCAHPS

Quality is taking on a whole new look from the federal government through an effort called valued-based purchasing (VBP). Its relevance to medical groups is that hospitals and physicians are now being challenged to deliver quality care in a way that is specifically measured and rewarded based on the accomplishment of key metrics. This approach is both controversial and filled with numerous challenges for all providers. Regardless of how one feels about its effect, it is being implemented, and its efforts will continue to have a large impact on all healthcare providers in the future. The following information better describes how quality and finance are tied together through public policy to create a new paradigm shift for healthcare.

Value-Based Purchasing

According to the Issues Paper "Development of a Plan to Transition to a Medicare Value-Based Purchasing Program for Physician and Other Professional Services"[18] written on December 9, 2008, CMS communicated a healthcare quality vision — *the right care for every person every time* — and care that is safe, effective, timely, patient-centered, efficient, and equitable. Medicare's fee-for-service payment systems based on pay for quantity and consumption of resources didn't support this vision. VBP aligns payment more directly to quality and efficiency of care provided by rewarding providers for their measured performance across quality dimensions. Through a number of demonstration projects and pilot programs, CMS launched VBP initiatives for hospitals, professionals, nursing homes, home health agencies, and dialysis facilities. Congress enacted the Medicare Improvements for Patients and Providers Act of 2008 (MIPPA). Section 131(d) required the Secretary of the Department of Health and Human Services to develop a plan by 2010 to transition to a VBP program for Medicare payment for physician and other professional services. The workgroup was organized into subgroups to address four fundamental planning issues: (1) measures, (2) incentive methodology, (3) data strategy and infrastructure, and (4) public reporting.

According to a CMS fact sheet for the public distributed on April 29, 2011,[19] the Affordable Care Act includes policies to help physicians, hospitals, and other caregivers improve safety and quality of patient care and make healthcare more affordable. Starting in October 2012, Medicare rewards hospitals that provide high-quality care for their patients through the new Hospital Value-Based Purchasing Program. This program marks the beginning of an historic change in how Medicare pays healthcare providers and facilities: For the first time, hospitals are paid for inpatient acute care services based on care quality. This effort supports the goals of the Partnership for Patients, a new public-private partnership that helps improve the quality, safety, and affordability of healthcare.

Changing how Medicare pays for hospital inpatient acute care services is expected to foster higher-quality care for all hospital patients. In fiscal year 2013, the Hospital Value-Based Purchasing Program will distribute an estimated $850 million to hospitals based on their overall performance on a set of quality measures that have been linked to improved clinical processes of care and patient satisfaction. This will be taken from what Medicare otherwise would have spent for hospital stays, and the size of the fund will gradually increase over time, resulting in a shift from payments based on volume to payments based on performance. This redirection will encourage care quality improvement, which is intended to result in significant additional savings to Medicare, taxpayers, and enrollees over time.

The Hospital Value-Based Purchasing Program measures in fiscal year 2013 focus on how closely hospitals follow best clinical practices and how well hospitals enhance patients' experiences of care. Examples of the care processes included in the measures are:

- **How quickly do heart attack patients receive potentially life-saving surgery on their arteries?** Hospital Value-Based Purchasing will measure how quickly doctors perform procedures known as percutaneous coronary interventions (PCIs), which are among the most effective ways to open blocked blood vessels that cause heart attacks. Doctors may perform PCI or give medicine to open the blockage and, in some cases, may do both. Quick and effective PCI can prevent a heart attack from occurring or can prevent a heart attack from worsening or recurring. This leads to better outcomes for patients and lower healthcare costs.

■ **How satisfied are patients with their experience of care at the hospital?** Positive patient experiences mean that patients feel comfortable and safe while in the hospital and feel that they have the information they need to continue to heal after leaving the hospital. These measures reflect what thousands of patients have said on surveys about their perceptions of healthcare in thousands of hospitals across the country.

Hospitals will be scored based on their performance on each measure relative to other hospitals and on how their performance on each measure has improved over time. The higher of these scores on each measure will be used in determining incentive payments. By rewarding higher achievement or improvement on measures, Hospital Value-Based Purchasing gives hospitals the financial incentive to continually improve how they deliver care. In the future, CMS plans to add additional outcome measures that focus on improved patient outcomes and prevention of hospital-acquired conditions. Measures that have reached very high compliance scores would likely be replaced, continuing to raise the quality bar. Hospitals will continue to receive payments for care provided to Medicare patients based on the Medicare Inpatient Prospective Payment System, but those payments will be reduced across the board by 1 percent starting in fiscal year 2013 to create the funding for the new value-based payments. In federal fiscal year 2013, this amount is estimated to be $850 million, which will then be used for incentive payments.

The measures for fiscal year 2013 have been endorsed by national bodies of experts, including the National Quality Forum. CMS already posts information about how well America's hospitals are doing on a number of measures on the Hospital Compare Web site, which can be found at www.HealthCare.gov. All measures adopted for use in the Hospital Value-Based Purchasing Program are also included on the Hospital Compare site.

The Hospital Value-Based Purchasing initiative is just one part of a wide-ranging effort by the Obama administration to improve the quality of healthcare for all Americans, using important new tools provided by the Affordable Care Act. The National Quality Strategy will serve as a tool to better coordinate quality initiatives. Partnership for Patients is bringing together hospitals, doctors, nurses, pharmacists, employers, unions, and members of state and federal government committed to keeping patients from getting injured or sicker in the healthcare system and improving transitions between care settings. CMS intends to invest up to $1 billion to help drive these changes through the partnership. In addition, proposed rules allowing Medicare to pay new ACOs to improve coordination of patient care are also expected to result in better care and lower costs.

Through the Affordable Care Act, Medicare will link hospital payments with improving patient care in other ways. Beginning in 2013, hospitals will receive a payment reduction if they have excess 30-day readmissions for patients with heart attacks, heart failure, and pneumonia. By 2015, most hospitals will face reductions in their Medicare payments if they do not meaningfully use information technology to deliver better, safer, more coordinated care. In addition, beginning in 2015, hospitals with high rates of certain hospital-acquired conditions will receive further payment reductions from Medicare.

CMS will continue to administer the Quality Improvement Organization (QIO) Program in a manner that focuses on improving the quality of hospital care. To read a press release about the new Hospital Value-Based Purchasing Program, please visit www.hhs.gov/news/press/2011pres/04/20110429a.html. To learn more about Hospital Value-Based Purchasing, please visit www.cms.gov/ HospitalQualityInits.

HCAHPS

According to an HCAHPS Fact Sheet published by CMS,

> *The HCAHPS (Hospital Consumer Assessment of Healthcare Providers and Systems) survey is the first national, standardized, publicly reported survey of patients' perspectives of hospital care. HCAHPS (pronounced "H-caps"), also known as the CAHPS® Hospital Survey, is a survey instrument and data collection methodology for measuring patients' perceptions of their hospital experience. While many hospitals have collected information on patient satisfaction for their own internal use, until HCAHPS, there was no national standard for collecting and publicly reporting information about patient experience of care that allowed valid comparisons to be made across hospitals locally, regionally, and nationally.*
>
> *Three broad goals have shaped HCAHPS. First, the survey is designed to produce data about patients' perspectives of care that allow objective and meaningful comparisons of hospitals on topics that are important to consumers. Second, public reporting of the survey results creates new incentives for hospitals to improve quality of care. Third, public reporting serves to enhance accountability in healthcare by increasing transparency of the quality of hospital care provided in return for the public investment. With these goals in mind, CMS and the HCAHPS project team have taken substantial steps to ensure that the survey is credible, useful, and practical.[20]*

CMS implemented the HCAHPS survey in October 2006, and the first public reporting of HCAHPS results occurred in March 2008. The survey, its methodology, and the results it produces are in the public domain.

Hospitals implement HCAHPS under the auspices of the Hospital Quality Alliance (HQA), a private/public partnership that includes major hospital and medical associations, consumer groups, two measurement and accrediting bodies, government, and other groups that share an interest in improving hospital quality. Since July 2007, hospitals subject to the Inpatient Prospective Payment System (IPPS) annual payment update provisions (subsection (d) hospitals) must collect and submit HCAHPS data to receive their full IPPS annual payment update. IPPS hospitals that fail to publicly report the required quality measures, which include the HCAHPS survey, may receive an annual payment update that is reduced by two percentage points. The Patient Protection and Affordable Care Act of 2010 (P.L. 111-148) includes HCAHPS among the measures to be used to calculate value-based incentive payments in the Hospital Value-Based Purchasing Program, beginning with discharges in October 2012.

The HCAHPS survey asks discharged patients 27 questions about their recent hospital stay. The survey contains 18 core questions about critical aspects of patients' hospital experiences (communication with nurses and doctors, the responsiveness of hospital staff, the cleanliness and quietness of the hospital environment, pain management, communication about medicines, discharge information, overall hospital rating, and whether they would recommend the hospital). The survey also includes four items to direct patients to relevant questions, three items to adjust for the mix of patients across hospitals, and two items that support congressionally mandated reports.

The HCAHPS survey is administered to a random sample of adult patients across medical conditions between 48 hours and six weeks after discharge; the survey is not restricted to Medicare beneficiaries. Hospitals can use the HCAHPS survey alone, or include additional questions after the core HCAHPS items. Hospitals must survey patients throughout each month of the year. The survey and its protocols for sampling, data collection and coding, and file submission can be found in the HCAHPS *Quality Assurance Guidelines, Version 5.0,* which is available on the official HCAHPS Web site, www.hcahpsonline.org.

For each participating hospital, 10 HCAHPS measures (six summary measures, two individual items, and two global items) are publicly reported on the Hospital Compare Web site, www.hospitalcompare.hhs.gov. Each of the six summary measures, or composites, is constructed from two or three survey questions. Combining related questions into composites allows consumers to quickly review patient experience of care data and increases the statistical reliability of these measures. The six composites summarize how well nurses and doctors communicate with patients, how responsive hospital staff are to patients' needs, how well hospital staff help patients manage pain, how well the staff communicates with patients about medicines, and whether key information is provided at discharge. The two individual items address the cleanliness and quietness of patients' rooms, while the two global items report patients' overall ratings of the hospital and whether they would recommend the hospital to family and friends. The survey response rate and the number of completed surveys, in broad ranges, are also publicly reported.

Publicly reported HCAHPS results are based on four consecutive quarters of patient surveys. CMS publishes participating hospitals' HCAHPS results on the Hospital Compare Web site (www.hospitalcompare.hhs.gov) four times a year, with the oldest quarter of patient surveys rolling off as the most recent quarter rolls in. A downloadable version of HCAHPS results is also available through this Web site. To learn more about HCAHPS, please visit www.hcahpsonline.org.

TOTAL QUALITY MANAGEMENT

What does total quality healthcare mean? How can its principles be applied to the healthcare delivery environment? The process for accomplishing this is called total quality management (TQM).

What Is Total Quality Management?

TQM is a structured, systematic process for creating organization-wide participation in planning and implementing continuous improvements in quality. TQM is a means to an end — the end being the long-term success of an organization. In this sense, quality is defined as meeting or exceeding the customer's expectations of the product or service at a price that is considered reasonable to the customer. The logic of this concept dictates that if the entire medical practice is dedicated to meeting or surpassing customers' expectations, continuously looking for new ways to exceed these expectations, and delivering products or services at a competitive price, then success for the organization is virtually guaranteed.

TQM is a method to examine all processes within a system, establish key preference indicators, and continually improve on them. All employees should be involved to improve the processes. Everyone needs to be included because it is only through the empowerment of employees that any planned changes can be brought into reality. TQM combines a set of management principles with a set of tools and techniques that enable employees to carry out these management principles in their daily work activities. The principles of TQM by themselves are not especially complex. Implementing them (and all principles needed for TQM to work) is the real challenge.

In the TQM culture, quality is measured against the benchmark of customer satisfaction. Key indicators for improvement must be carefully selected for each department, among departments, and coordinated across functional areas. Techniques such as quality function deployment, benchmarking, and Pareto analysis can be used to match customer demands with the system responses, set standards, and identify problems for team quality circles to address. (Two of these techniques will be described in a later section.) Thus, improvements in one department reinforce and strengthen the operation of others. By applying TQM, the medical practice manages quality by strengthening horizontal communications; conducting concurrent evaluations; encouraging team interaction and collective accountability; and fostering the creation of internal, customer-validated standards.

Contrasting TQM and Traditional Quality Control Measures

Traditionally, high-quality medical care is thought to consist of a technical component and an interpersonal component that together enable a patient to attain the highest possible functioning state, both physically and psychologically. The quality control programs that practices followed included:

- Assessing or measuring performance
- Determining whether performance conformed to standards
- Improving performance when standards were not met

These measures are considered too limited in today's environment. These limitations relate to the following areas:[21]

- The traditional definition of quality is too narrow to meet the needs of modern healthcare providers. It refers to a patient's physical and psychological health only, but healthcare organizations are now increasingly being called upon to meet the needs of other individuals and groups, such as patients' families, referring physicians, and third parties.

- The traditional medical quality assurance features a static approach to quality with its goal of conformance to standards. This is distinguished from the professional ethic of physicians to continuously improve on existing practices. The old view implicitly assumes that some rate of poor outcomes is acceptable and that little useful information can be garnered from analyzing cases that met the standards. Furthermore, if standards are set too low, quality assurance programs may breed complacency and thus contribute to poor quality. If they are set unrealistically high, they may alienate or frustrate providers.

- The traditional way tends to focus on physician performance and to underemphasize the contributions of nonphysicians and organizational processes generally. For example, a quality control program might evaluate a physician's diagnostic skills and the choice of a certain drug. However, errors may occur at any step in the subsequent processes, and they, too, may cause the patient to receive suboptimal care. Also, traditional techniques for quality improvement in healthcare tend to focus on physicians and changing their behavior. But in today's world, quality improvement will require complex, simultaneous changes involving employees and professionals in other departments.

- The traditional way tends to emphasize certain aspects of a physician's performance: technical expertise and interpersonal competence. Other aspects of a physician's performance also have a bearing on quality, such as mobilizing a medical practice's resources to meet the needs of individual patients and the goals of the organization. For example, assume a physician accurately diagnosed and treated a patient's chest pain as an inpatient. But on succeeding days, assume the physician fails to order pain medication, overlooks the specification of an important test, and on the day of discharge, decides to refer the patient to another physician for an ancillary problem. Has high-quality care been rendered?

In contrast to the above characterization of quality assurance efforts currently being followed, TQM, as described earlier, involves a continuous effort by all members of a medical practice to meet the needs and expectations of the customer. The reference to "continuous effort" emphasizes the value of striving to exceed prevailing standards, rather than accepting them even temporarily as limits on preference. The term "all members of an organization" suggests an imperative for all staff members to study the organizational processes by which healthcare is produced and provided. Specifying "expectations" recognizes that patients' reports of their experiences and their assessments of results are valid indicators of quality, including some of its technical aspects. "Customers" are generally defined as the recipients of the medical services; but today, "customer" has taken on a new meaning.

Under TQM theory, medical practices have ascribed a new paradigm to the term *customer* with a much broader context. In healthcare, customers are defined as patients, payers, regulators, providers, and the government. Each of these entities has expectations of service satisfactions that confound the delivery of medical care in today's environment. To satisfy the customers, the medical practice must know who its customers are, what they expect, and how well these expectations are being met. And, furthermore, customer expectations change. What was once the unexpected becomes the expected shortly after it becomes available.

THE CUSTOMER FOCUS ON QUALITY CARE

As mentioned earlier, the definition of quality has largely been framed by physicians. However, in the TQM context, the perception of quality depends on which customer is defining it. Whetsell says that there are two sets of customers — an external and an internal group. The external customers are the patients, payers, other providers, regulators, and the government. In some respects, the clinical perspective is surpassed by a societal understanding of healthcare quality. The internal customers are any department, function, or employee that receives and relies on input from another part of the organization.[22]

The dilemma of meeting customer needs is compounded by the diversity of individuals and groups, each of which has a specific set of expectations that do not necessarily mesh in all aspects. And discovering what these expectations are can be a challenge. Surveys, focus groups, and other market research tools are often used to develop an understanding of external customers' expectations. Communications, both oral and written, and meetings among the medical groups' staff members can clarify the expectations of the internal cadre of customers.

A useful way to categorize the quality expectations of these diverse groups of healthcare customers is provided by O'Connor and Lanning.[23] Their classification uses three categories — structure, process, and outcomes — that have become widely accepted and used in TQM discussions. These categories help to grasp the nature of quality measures and provide some insights into how the perspective of the definer can influence the definition of quality.

Structure

Structural measures focus on how the medical practice or institution is organized to provide care. For example, does it use competent staff, modern equipment, and appropriate facilities? Accrediting bodies such as TJC, Medicare, state licensing commissions, and others require adherence to numerous standards that are largely structural in nature. These standards include professional staff qualifications, management credentials, age of the physical plant, licensure, available technology, staffing ratios, and institutional academic affiliations.

These measures are not directly associated with the quality of care provided by the medical practice. The assumption is that healthcare providers know what quality is when it comes to staff, organization, and technology and that the ability to deliver quality service increases when the desired structural features exist.

Process

Process measures deal with policies, procedures, training, and methodologies of the medical practice. They center on what is done to and for the patient. Often, process measures assess how well the providers' activities adhere to professionally specified standards and protocols. Specific process indicators include adherence to discharge planning procedures, follow-up on abnormal test results and medication errors, and following the procedures performed that meet specific criteria for medical necessity. A testimony as to how well professional activities are being carried out becomes even more important when coupled with measures of what differences the activities made to the patients.

Outcomes

Outcomes measures relate to the achievement of the highest possible functional and psychosocial state for the patient. They also examine the avoidance of injury or the complications caused by the care rendered. It is in the outcomes area that much of the current interest in quality care is being recast from the previous attention to structural and process-oriented measures. A flawless outcome measure ascertains whether specific changes in a patient's health or well-being can be directly and unambiguously linked to the actions or procedures performed on them. Because this determination is so difficult to evaluate in healthcare, most judgments of quality have by default centered on the structure and process categories.

CMS has been releasing diagnosis-specific hospital mortality data annually since 1986. Although not espoused as a true indicator of quality, the data have aroused a great deal of interest among consumers, businesses, insurers, researchers, providers, and governmental policymakers. Even though they do not directly and unambiguously denote the presence of adequate or inadequate care, mortality data are being viewed as outcome measures. Many commentators believe that for mortality rates to be useful, they must be adequately adjusted for the severity of illness, condition on admission to the hospital, and socioeconomic status. Because hospitals are being pressured into proving that their outcome quality is as good as or better than their competitors, they are obliged to choose a patient classification system. The following list describes the popular classification systems used for adjusting outcome awareness.

1. **APACHE II** (Acute Physiology and Chronic Health Evaluation II) is a severity-of-disease classification system for ICUs that uses easily collected lab results and other variables to evaluate the effectiveness of therapeutic treatments and risk of death in intensive care units.

2. **All Patient Refined DRGs** attempt to provide severity ratings by "refining" diagnosis-related groups (DRGs).

3. **Disease staging** models an individual illness from local disease to death in terms of levels of severity or "stages."

4. **MedisGroups (medical illness severity grouping system)** uses key clinical findings from the medical record to predict target organ.

5. **American Heart Association Classification of Stroke Outcome** is a valid and reliable global classification system that accurately summarizes the neurological impairments, disabilities, and handicaps that occur after stroke.

6. **Clinical Care Classification (CCC) System** is an American Nurses Association (ANA)-recognized comprehensive, coded nursing terminology standard accepted by the Department of Health and Human Services as the first national nursing terminology and determines care needs (resources), workload (productivity), and outcomes (quality).

CMS's peer review organizations have also been developing outcome measures for Medicare discharges. Some of the categories of outcomes include unexpected deaths, deaths during or following elective surgery, unscheduled returns to surgery, and trauma suffered in the hospital. They are also researching ambulatory care settings to develop indicators in the future. The JCAHO has an agenda for change that embraces a number of indicators for evaluating clinical outcomes, ranging from standard items such as certain infections to more patient-satisfaction measures.

And according to Cheryl Clark in *HealthLeaders Media*, by 2014, CMS will add mortality outcome measures for three health conditions, eight hospital-acquired condition measures, and nine Agency for Healthcare Research and Quality measures. The hospital-acquired condition measures include surgical foreign object retention, air embolism, blood incompatibility, pressure ulcer stages III and IV, falls and trauma such as burns or electrical shocks, catheter-associated urinary tract infections, and manifestations of poor glycemic control.[24] The regulations will apply to discharges at 3,000 acute care hospitals. All these hospitals will have their funding reduced, starting with 1 percent in fiscal year 2013 and rising to 2 percent by fiscal year 2017, but will have a chance to earn that money back, and perhaps more, under the incentives algorithm. In a statement, CMS director Don Berwick called the proposed regulations "a huge leap forward in improving the quality and safety of America's hospitals for both Medicare beneficiaries and all Americans. The hospital value-based purchasing program will reward hospitals for improving patients' experiences of care, while making care safer by reducing medical mistakes."[25] The new plans will revolutionize the Medicare payment system to one of rewarding improvements in quality and health outcomes over time.

In summary, these types of measures provide a starting point for sorting out the various imperfect measures of healthcare quality. Process measures focus on energy and effort expended but neglect effects achieved. Structural indicators do not assess work performed or effort expended but evaluate only the medical practice's capacity for work. Outcome measures have the advantage of focusing attention on changes produced and results achieved. Their drawbacks are that they do not in themselves provide evidence that can connect observed outcomes to the effects of performance.

Each constituent of the healthcare industry tends to favor a certain category of quality measurement over others. For example, healthcare managers frequently endorse the structural category because they understand these measures and have a fair degree of influence over them. Clinical professionals tend to view quality in terms of process measures because they are most familiar and comfortable with the standards and protocols that affect patient care. Finally, patients, purchasers, and society tend to emphasize outcomes with their overriding interest in health restoration, costs, and satisfaction. Outcome measures will continue to become more important as purchasers demand better value for their money and as consumers become partners in defining healthcare quality.

THE PRINCIPLES OF TOTAL QUALITY MANAGEMENT

The principles of TQM are based on the ideas and writings of the late W. Edwards Deming, physicist, statistician, management consultant, and author. Deming's efforts helped shape the Japanese working culture after World War II. Essentially, Deming was concerned with the flow of activities from the original state of materials to the finished product in the manufacturing process, keeping in mind the needs of the customers throughout. Even though his principles were directed at manufacturing industries, they can be transferred to the medical practice environment, especially to administrative procedures.

Deming outlined five beliefs that he asserted were the underlying foundation for all quality efforts:

1. Build quality into the process. Do not rely on inspections to catch errors; eliminate errors altogether.
2. Foster teamwork and remove the barriers that divide departments. Make people cooperate rather than compete.
3. Establish long-term, mutually beneficial relationships with employees, suppliers, and customers.
4. Provide managers and workers with all the training they need to participate fully in the improvement process.
5. Top management must be in the effort for the long haul. You cannot turn quality on and off like a faucet. Remember, it's a process rather than an event.[26]

Deming laid out a series of 14 management points that can lead to making quality an integral part of the service business. The following summary contains an adaptation of Deming's basic points to the healthcare setting.

Create Constancy of Purpose for the Improvement of Service

This means total dedication to quality, productivity, and service — today and tomorrow. To maintain constancy of purpose, medical groups must concentrate on the interplay of three basic elements:

1. Unit cost, which must be kept as low as possible while maintaining the objectives of accuracy and timeliness

2. Patients' needs, wants, and satisfaction

3. Employees, who must understand the medical practice's mission and then be properly trained and given the tools necessary to fulfill the mission

Constancy of purpose to the medical group requires that the practice stay competitive with an unshakable commitment to quality. This might entail even the most minor items. For example, if the patient registration form is cluttered, change it. If the group's patients are elderly, use big print. Update the office equipment and the computer software.

Adopt a Total Quality Philosophy

To maintain the viability of the medical group in the local marketplace, a complete transformation of management philosophy must be made. Quality must become the preeminent concern. Errors and poor service must be eliminated throughout all stages of patient care. There should be a focus on the process of rendering care, on the team and how it performs, and on the system that will naturally produce long-term quality results. All members of the group must be oriented to treating patients as their best friends. The staff must know what to do, how to do it, and do it efficiently and effectively.

Cease Dependence on Mass Inspection

This point flows from the premise that you cannot inspect quality into any product or service. When a producer throws out or reworks a defective item, quality improvement is not being addressed (nor is unit cost). Thus, producers must stop relying on mass inspections of the final result of a process to achieve quality of output but should concentrate on improving the process itself so that errors will be prevented from occurring. If errors are made, correct them as they happen instead of relying on a final inspection to catch the defective item. Quality should be measured and ensured at each stage of service rendering. Thus, if all patients are treated in a professional manner and with a touch of quality awareness at each phase of the process, the patients' perception of the quality of their visits will be positive.

End the Practice of Awarding Business on Price Tag Alone

The lowest bid for any purchase of goods or services is rarely the most cost efficient. Using too many suppliers decreases effective communication and economies of scale. Groups should concentrate on a group of suppliers and continue to build a business relationship with them. This, in turn, can result in a spirit of mutual trust and cooperation that leads to the achievement of high quality and lower costs. Standards and requirements for every item or service purchased from vendors should be established and then adhered to closely. Managers must insist on compliance with these arrangements; otherwise, the inefficient supplier will be replaced by another who will abide by the requirements of the purchaser.

Health maintenance organizations (HMOs) and other prospective payers are being challenged by their members to balance costs with quality. Even though this point focuses on suppliers, medical groups should recognize that they are suppliers of medical care. One way to attract and keep long-term arrangements is to offer a quality product that sets consistently high standards, not only in terms of medical care but also in terms of freedom from administrative nightmares. Since groups demand the best from their suppliers, they should offer the best service to their customers — the patients.

Improve Constantly and Forever the System of Production and Service

When quality improvements are first initiated, major gains in accuracy, timeliness, and productivity are fairly easy to realize. Gradually, the primary causes of errors are eliminated, and the process is brought into statistical control. However, there are still errors. The real work for continuous improvement begins at this point. Group management must lead the way toward continual progress in quality- and cost-improvement systems. The basic statistics of customer satisfaction and employee productivity must be constantly measured and communicated at all levels. All members of the medical group must subscribe to constant improvement. A few indicators will be evident if you look back to conditions a few years ago and compare them with the present. Do patients seem more satisfied? Have complaints decreased? Do employees seem to take more pride in their tasks, and has their performance improved? Are there fewer billing mistakes?

Institute Training and Retraining

Medical group employees cannot learn solely from instruction manuals and other workers. Also, frequently, workers learn their jobs from other employees who are poorly trained themselves. Many employees do not know what constitutes a good job or a bad job. Thus, training in quality, cost effectiveness, and skill must come from managers. It must be a planned part of the system or process. Quality service cannot be delivered if all staff members do not have the proper understanding about what and how they should perform their responsibilities. Besides on-the-job training (which is probably the most effective method to develop people's skills), opportunities for training programs outside the group exist in abundance. If necessary, contact MGMA for a catalog of course offerings. These programs are tailored to the needs of professional staff members (physicians and nonphysicians) of medical groups.

Teach and Institute Leadership

There are two aspects to this point. First, it is important for managers, especially the financial managers of medical groups, to develop their management skills, both on a one-on-one basis and in leading groups of employees. Basic management skills — delegating, coaching, communicating, planning, counseling, and decision making — must be acquired by all managers. And managers must work at developing these skills in other people in the office.

The second element is becoming a leader. Frequently, managers are so concerned with their own tasks that they forget to lead others. Being an effective leader is one of the most difficult traits for managers to acquire. While some training in leadership can assist in developing leadership skills, the best method for inculcating this asset is through observing effective leaders and what they do to get followers to embrace them as the head of a group or medical practice. Then experimenting with actions and behaviors that individuals believe will bring them followers should be practiced and evaluated.

Drive out Fear

One of the emotions prevalent in the workplace that is not often mentioned is fear. There seems to be a great deal of fear, such as fear of asking questions, fear of expressing ideas, fear of asking for further instructions, fear of mentioning that the equipment is not working properly, and fear of raising issues about working conditions. Deming says that the cost of fear in business is appalling.

The response to fear is to eliminate it by creating an office environment where trust and understanding are the common prevailing attitudes. Managers can help establish this kind of climate by trusting others and treating each individual fairly and openly. With a managerial model that provides an example of proper behavior and decorum, employees will feel comfortable in freely bringing their concerns and fears to the attention of management where they can be discussed and dealt with in an open manner. Employees should be encouraged to challenge old ways of doing certain activities and use their initiative to set up new ways of performing certain tasks. Innovation should also be rewarded so that others can emulate the new example set.

Break Down Barriers between Departments

A frequently overlooked cause of inefficiencies or errors is a work groups or department's lack of awareness of the responsibilities of other groups or departments in the medical practice. Everyone should have an adequate understanding of the major activities of each of the group's operations. For example, a nurse may be upset because she was not informed about some changes in the physicians' operating schedule. The data-entry person is frustrated because certain information was not completed by the admissions employees. The radiology technologist can't find the patient order to perform the test. Every medical office experiences its share of workflow breakdowns because of various inefficiencies. It is the managers' job to create a cooperative system in which all employees participate in a common goal — quality patient service.

Eliminate Slogans, Exhortations, and Targets for the Workforce

This point raises a contradictory issue in that many believe that slogans are effective in rallying individual efforts to productive accomplishments. Deming espouses the elimination of the exhortations of posting weekly targets, zero-defects programs, and having people sign their work. All these efforts are aimed at getting people to work faster and produce more. Actually, many believe these actions have a negative impact on productivity and quality. Implicit in these slogans is the supposition that everyone can do better if they would only try. This offends rather than inspires team members. It often signals that management does not understand the real problems. Quality is a process, and it is the manager's job to ensure that the process achieves the end result to the satisfaction of the customer.

Eliminate Work Standards That Prescribe Numerical Quotas

Theoretically, productivity standards are set for the workforce so that management meets its output goals. Standards are usually based on averages, which means that half of the people fail to reach the standard. Furthermore, there is the emphasis on meeting a certain quantitative goal, and attempting to do so can result in shoddy performance and poor service. Not everyone can move at the same rate and still create quality. The key to productivity and quality improvement is to look for differences in performance and to create an atmosphere of receptivity to new ideas and recognition. An effective productivity standard should be developed and communicated so that everyone knows the acceptable standards of quality. Allowing employee teams to establish productivity targets that work best for the medical group and for the team itself is the best course to follow.

Remove Barriers That Rob People of Their Right to Pride of Workmanship

A fact often disregarded is that managers forget that front-line employees know more about their jobs than managers might give them credit for. Most employees realize that their improvements in quality also lead to increased productivity. But management frequently places roadblocks in the way of such improvement. Managers must take time to discover what hinders the workflow of staff members. This might require asking certain questions of staff, such as, Do you understand what your job entails and what level of work is acceptable? Is the equipment in use in good condition? Are you getting enough assistance from me and others to do your job? Is there a better way to do your job? If so, make the needed changes. Managers must understand that most people want to do a good job. Two-way communication between manager and subordinates and the elimination of de-motivators are critical.

Institute a Vigorous Program of Education and Self-Improvement

As a medical practice makes progress in quality and productivity improvement, two types of training needs will arise. First, as productivity improves, the number of employees required to provide services will likely decline or extra hours will be available for individual workers. Training can be given to these individuals for new roles in the medical practice. Secondly, there is a need to train certain individuals in the fundamentals of statistical quality control. Techniques, such as Pareto analysis, allow one to discover the most common errors in a certain procedure, such as billing. Without employees who have a thorough understanding of statistical techniques, control charts, and Pareto analysis, further improvement will be limited.

Take Action to Accomplish the Transformation

Top management of the medical group must have a clear plan of action to carry out the quality mission. Quality must be given equal status with all other operations and goals in the medical practice. Without senior management involvement and support, improvement efforts will fail. Beyond top management commitment, group resources must also be allocated to carry out quality improvement activities. Physicians and the management group must serve as quality spokespersons and make the commitment to quality clear to all staff members. Then quality must be managed with the same degree of emphasis that financial management receives.

THE PROCESS OF IMPROVING QUALITY

In this section, we will present the basic process that medical practices are using to examine and improve the quality of their services and products. The process described will be representative of the approach advocated by followers of TQM. In fact, this process has been referred to as total quality improvement.

What Is a Process?

A process is how people, materials, methods, machines, and the environment combine to add value to a product or service. It includes all phases of an operation, which take various forms of inputs and convert them into a product or service desired by a user. For example, performing a surgical procedure is a process. The major phases include the following:

- Physician's diagnosis of the surgical procedure needed
- Scheduling of patient's surgery at the facility based on physician, patient, and facility availability
- Having patient obtain preadmission testing including possible labs
- Admission to a hospital or ASC
- Planning for the procedure by the physician and supporting clinical staff and obtaining appropriate equipment, tools, and medications to be used

■ Preparing patient for surgery (e.g., using a time-out procedure to verify appropriate services and surgical location)

■ Performing the surgical procedure(s)

■ Providing postoperative care by the physician and nursing staff

■ Providing supportive services such as meals, medications, and personal care

■ Dictating physicians' care

■ Transcribing the physicians' notations

■ Billing the patient's insurance company for services by the hospital and physician

■ Returning for subsequent office visits as part of the global surgery service provided

There are probably several other steps in the total process that can be added, but the point is that all phases in any process include a multitude of different activities and participants, which encompass individuals, physicians, nonphysicians, third-party reimbursers, and regulators, among others. Also involved are suppliers, other patients, and subprocesses that interrelate in some way with the surgical procedure described above.

How to Improve a Process

As stated previously, every product or service is produced through a series of related work activities involving people, methods, materials, and equipment. TQM focuses on the understanding and improvement of the process used to produce the product or service. A key TQM axiom is that the quality of the output is determined by the quality of the production process, and that improvements in quality result primarily from improvements in the process. In the TQM approach, quality is improved by systematically documenting a process, analyzing its operating characteristics, and identifying ways to improve it. In essence, TQM is fairly simple because it focuses on the process of creating a product or performing a service. It implies that setting quotas, offering incentives, or trying to motivate employees through slogans will have little impact on quality; it is the process that determines the quality of outputs, not the workers.

Most businesses, including hospitals and medical groups, have several layers of management, formal policies and procedures, and well-defined boundaries of responsibility. However, the process of producing products and services does not follow the organizational hierarchy but cuts across various segments of the medical practice. In delivering patient services, a series of supplier-customer interfaces are created between functions or departments of the medical practice. Often the most promising opportunities for improving a process are at these interface points. TQM addresses this issue through cross-functional teams, comprised of representatives of all of the functions and departments involved in a process, working together to improve the process.

TQM recognizes that employees directly involved in the current process are the "experts" in the process and are the best source of information on weaknesses and areas for improvement. Employees participate in identifying and implementing improvements in the total process. The complexity of the services is recognized, and it is noted that one person seldom has sufficient knowledge to deal with all aspects of a process. For this reason, TQM uses teams, called quality improvement teams (QITs). Through this team approach, the prospects of identifying and implementing improvements are greatly enhanced. Establishing QITs often requires managers to change their management style, as well as their relationship with workers. Under TQM, managers are expected to be leaders rather than administrators.

Continuous Improvement and the PDCA Cycle

The essence of TQM requires continuous improvement with the assumption that every process can be improved regardless of its present status or condition. The goal is to have every employee continuously looking for process improvements. Traditionally, management was interested only in innovative breakthroughs — dramatic new inventions, technologies, or automation. TQM is in the opposite position on a continuum of change in that it focuses on finding small, incremental improvements by applying the Plan-Do-Check-Act cycle (PDCA cycle) to every process used to produce products and services. Although innovative breakthroughs are welcome, TQM has demonstrated that the gains from continuous improvements will equal or exceed the gains from innovation.

The PDCA Cycle

The PDCA cycle is a road map for continuous process improvement. Originally developed by Walter Shewhart and popularized by Deming, it is a systematic approach to finding and eliminating the root cause of an adverse condition through the following steps:

▪ **Plan** — The process improvement is planned in this step. It includes determining which process will be improved, establishing targets for improvement, reviewing data to establish what improvements will be made, establishing what units will be used to measure the improvement, and determining who will be involved in the improvement effort.

▪ **Do** — In this step, the plan is implemented and the process improvement is made. Actions taken include collecting data to determine the condition of the process before implementing the improvement, making the improvement (often as a trial run), and continuing to collect data on the performance of the process.

▪ **Check** — This step is conducted to determine the results of the process improvement efforts as compared to the established goals. The phases of this step include:

– Reviewing the data collected on the process before the improvement was made and comparing them to the current data

– Assessing whether the root cause of the problem was corrected

The correct data would also be compared to the target established for the plan step.

■ **Act** — The analysis of the check step is used to make the improvement permanent. The action taken in this step depends on the results. If the process improvement reached its target, the improvement would be standardized to "hold the gains." If the process improvement did not reach its target, the root cause was not corrected, or if room for additional improvements exists, the PDCA cycle would begin again. Determining the root causes helps to focus on where to apply changes that will create process improvement. When going through a complete PDCA cycle does not result in the expected improvements, the process may be repeated in the next cycle iteration and attention placed on different stages of the process.

The continuous nature of the PDCA cycle is obvious since, regardless of the result, the cycle starts again. If there is no satisfaction with the results of the process improvement, the PDCA cycle will be repeated. If there is satisfaction with the results of the process improvement, the PDCA cycle will be used to improve another process.

Even though quotas and numerical standards are not compatible with TQM, standardization of the process of improving processes is needed. The standardization principle states that at any point in time, the best way for a process to work should be known, and everyone involved in the process should be using the best approach. Combining continuous improvement with standardization is one of the more difficult concepts of TQM to understand and implement. Through continuous improvement efforts, QITs look repeatedly for better ways to carry out the process; thus, standardization means a never-ending search for higher levels of performance through a continuous pursuit of ways to improve implementation of all phases of the medical care service continuum.

The process of continuous improvement includes a set of process-analysis tools that support the PDCA cycle. These tools are based on the premise that "a picture is worth a thousand words." Consequently, all of the tools provide visual outputs.

TOOLS AND TECHNIQUES OF QUALITY IMPROVEMENT

There are eight basic tools used as analytical and problem-solving tools in TQM and in the collection of data for use in quality improvement efforts:

1. Flow charts
2. Tally sheets
3. Cause-and-effect diagrams
4. Pareto charts
5. Histograms
6. Scatter diagrams
7. Run charts
8. Control charts

Flow Charts

A flow chart is a graphical or symbolic representation of a process where each step in the process is represented by a symbol with a brief description. The flow chart symbols are linked together with arrows showing the direction of the process flow.

The flow chart describes what major operations are performed during a certain process. It shows the flow of the work through various departments and who performs what tasks to complete the work necessary to reach the conclusion of the process. Flow charts are powerful tools for defining the current process; facilitating group consensus on what the current process is; and identifying delays, redundancies, and bottlenecks inherent in the process.

Tally Sheets

According to the 1998 *Guide for Managing Quality* from Management Sciences for Health, a tally sheet is a simple data collection form for observing how frequently something occurs used by an individual to easily and efficiently collect and organize data.[27] It is used to collect data on the frequency of events — that is, after the causes of a problem have been analyzed and selected, it acts as a first step of the Pareto analysis. In using the form, it is important to review the process, or the causes of the problem to observe.

1. Make a list of examples to observe. Only information intended to use should be included in this list.

2. Decide on the time interval for observing the events (e.g., number of days, number of claims).

3. Use external observation of the process to measure frequencies, or ask staff to use tally sheets during their daily work. An observation of the event is registered by a check in the corresponding cell of the sheet each time the event occurs.

4. The frequency is calculated by adding up the number of events in the last column. The data will serve as the basis for the creation of a Pareto graph.

5. It is necessary to make sure that staffers interpret the categories in the same way, using agreed-upon operational definitions.

6. Separate tally sheets should be kept for different days and different people. In that way, one can look for patterns related to those factors.

Cause-and-Effect Diagram

A cause-and-effect diagram is used to identify, explore, and display the possible causes for variation. It is frequently called a fishbone diagram because of its shape, or an Ishikawa diagram after its developer, Kaoru Ishikawa. To construct a cause-and-effect diagram, develop a clear problem statement and place it in a box on the right side of the diagram as the effect. To illustrate further, this statement might then be the focus of a brainstorming session by a team to identify the cause(s) of the problem. The diagram facilitates the process by repeatedly asking the question "Why?" The "why" responses are inserted on the diagram under one of the four cause categories — methods, people, material, and equipment — as a branch of the main stem. Every problem has many possible causes. Those written on the diagram are only possible causes; the data collected later will point to the actual cause(s). It helps identify the root cause(s), provides a picture of what affects the process, educates the participants, and promotes teamwork.

Pareto Charts

The Pareto chart is a bar chart that displays the relative importance or frequency of collected data that may indicate the causes of problems. As used in process improvement, the Pareto principle says that 80 percent of the effects come from 20 percent of the causes. Joseph M. Juran, a leading quality expert, calls the 20 percent the "vital few" and the rest of the causes the "useful many."[28] Although the percentages will never be exact, the Pareto chart draws our attention to the "vital few" factors where the payback to remediation is likely to be the greatest.

To construct a Pareto chart, data from tally sheets will likely be used. After comparing the frequency of each category on which data are collected, the categories are listed from left to right in descending order. The actual number is recorded on the left vertical axis and the percentage scale on the right vertical axis. A line is then added that starts at the top of the first bar and moves upward from left to right. This line represents the cumulative frequency.

Histograms

A histogram is a bar chart that displays quality and other performance measurements associated with a process. It presents the distribution and variation of the data within a process. As a snapshot of a process, a histogram shows the spread of measurements and how many of each measurement occur. It is prepared after data have been gathered and the appropriate classes are determined for display in bar chart form.

Histograms might be used to compare one process with another or to measure conformance to one's expectations. For example, histograms might be prepared to document the range of current performance levels and by segmenting the data (by physician, machine, day-of-week, month, etc.) to help pinpoint problems. They are also helpful in assessing the impact of process improvements.

Scatter Diagrams

A scatter diagram is a graphic presentation of the relationship between two variables. To develop one, points are plotted on x- and y-axes. The pattern of the points tells whether there is a relationship between the two points and the strength of that relationship. For example, assume management was interested in determining whether working overtime by the staff contributed to payroll errors. Data about hours of overtime would be plotted on the x-axis, and data on payroll errors would be plotted on the y-axis. The pattern might indicate that as overtime hours increase, errors also increase. The direction and closeness of the points would reflect a fairly strong, positive relationship. Thus, the scatter diagram may confirm management's initial hunch that there was a relationship between overtime and payroll errors. Note that this correlation does not mean that overtime caused the errors. The diagram only confirms the relationship between the two variables. Causative factors would have to be discovered with further analysis.

Run Charts

Run charts are visual presentations of data over time. Data is collected sequentially, and the data points are plotted on the run chart. The points are connected to form a line graph. The graph provides a visual tool for highlighting trends that might suggest that the process has changed. In preparing run charts, the data must be plotted in the order in which the event(s) occurred; otherwise, the run chart is meaningless.

Control Charts

A control chart is the primary tool used in SPC. It helps to determine whether the variation of the process is normal or abnormal. (Additional comments on variation appear in a later section.) A control chart is a run chart with statistically calculated control limits. Upper and lower control limits are calculated by taking data collected from the process and using statistical formulas to arrive at the limit amounts. Additional data are then collected and plotted on the control chart. If the data points plotted are within the control limits and do not exhibit any special patterns, the control chart indicates that the variation in the process is due to normal sources. In this case, the process is said to be "in statistical control." If a data point falls outside the control limits or has one of a number of unusual patterns, an abnormal variation has been introduced into the process. In this case, the process is considered "out of statistical control."

Being in or out of statistical control is important because the approach to improving the process depends on the source of the variation. When using control charts, it is probably a good practice to seek the assistance of a statistician. Also, remember that control charts only show that something has changed; they do not indicate what it is that has changed. Additional analysis is needed to determine the cause. Being in control merely means that the process is stable and predictable. It does not necessarily mean that the process is meeting the customer's needs. A process may be in control but providing a great disservice to patients.

Variation and the Use of Statistics

TQM recognizes that variation is an inherent part of any process. It is the result of the combination of a process's five elements: (1) people, (2) machines,

(3) methods, (4) materials, and (5) the environment. For example, the time required to perform an activity, even when performed exactly the same way, will vary each time it is performed. Thus, the quality of process outputs also varies, even when the process is performed in an identical or standardized manner every time.

There are statistical characteristics of the variation that can be measured. While variation cannot be eliminated, it can be reduced through improvements in the production process. As variation is reduced, delays and waste due to poor quality are also reduced, and this can result in lower costs. Thus, the concept of variation is important because as variation is reduced, processes are improved.

Through the use of statistical tools, the range of variation in a process can be calculated and analyzed to gain insight into the ways to improve the process. Using control charts, two types of variation can be identified:

- **Normal variation** is always present and can never be completely eliminated. Called *common cause variation,* it results from the everyday combination of people, machines, material, methods, and the environment. Each factor contributes a small amount to the total variation. Normal variation is also chronic since it has been in the process for a long time or recurs frequently. For these reasons, it is predictable within limits.
- **Abnormal variation** is not always present and can be eliminated in most business processes. Called *special cause variation,* it is the result of an extraordinary event and represents variation over and above what is inherent in the system. Abnormal variation is sporadic and unpredictable.

The concepts of normal variation, or common causes, and abnormal variation, or special causes, are important because they help focus improvement efforts. To improve processes where the source of the variation is normal, the entire process must be examined. To reduce this type of variation requires changing the process. To improve processes where abnormal variation has been introduced, the extraordinary event must be isolated and eliminated (if bad) or standardized (if good). Thus, since abnormal variations are caused by factors that are independent of the process, they can only be reduced by eliminating the cause.

In summary, TQM focuses on reducing variation due to common causes and improving quality by improving the production process while simultaneously looking for ways to eliminate the special causes of variation.

PUTTING THE STEPS TOGETHER

Medical practices that have implemented TQM have developed specific problem-solving methodologies that they follow to improve processes or solve problems. Regardless of their approach, they all have one common element — they are based on the PDCA cycle. An application of this cycle is presented in the following summary to capture the essence of the total quality improvement process:

In the new model of quality improvement, a great effort is made to establish the process of care as it happens. All participants of a care team meet and construct a flow chart representing their best understanding of the care process. The team verifies the flow chart of the process of care by observing the process to determine if it happens as they collectively thought. Once the flow of the process is verified, the team develops a data collection plan and collects the data on the process using the various tools and techniques. The data are analyzed to discover the greatest source of variation within the process. Using time-series statistics in the analysis of the care process, the team distinguishes variation inherent in the process (common causes) from variation occurring as a result of extraordinary events (special causes). Using the PDCA cycle, the team will select an improvement, plan the change in the process, implement it, and continue to collect data to determine whether the anticipated change achieved improved results. In this manner, a cause-and-effect relationship between process and results has been systematically established. Variation has been studied, and hypotheses about the variation are tested scientifically. The end results are improvements in the processes of providing patient care that will satisfy customer needs.[29]

In another summary view of the TQM process, healthcare providers must learn to perceive themselves as suppliers to many more customers in addition to the patient. As indicated previously, customers are all parties — internal and external — to the total medical care service being provided and go beyond the familiar customers (patient, care provider, purchaser of care, and external regulator). The continuous process improvement involves the placement of customers in each step of the process. Customers are asked to supply information about what is most important to them in the care process. Customers evaluate the care and provide input to the design, provision, monitoring, and revision of the healthcare system to provide better care. All system outputs are judged against the customers' explicit needs and expectations about the outcome. Design and monitoring are enclosed into a continuous loop of process improvement (like the PDCA cycle). In this way, providers of care have explicit, organized input from their customers so they can objectively evaluate the efficiency of care provided.

A dramatic contrast is apparent when traditional healthcare quality concepts are compared with a quality model that is driven by customer needs — continuously improving and internal to the system of healthcare itself. Under the new paradigm, the opportunities to consider new relationships among the major interest groups in healthcare are numerous and revolutionary.

Information Systems Support

All phases of the TQM cycle for a typical project require a great deal of data and statistical analysis. Unfortunately, most of the data required for TQM are neither part of nor captured by the current operational/transaction-processing healthcare information systems. For example, to capture the service/procedure performance indicators would necessitate setting up point-of-service workstations or devices throughout the medical practice to obtain the details of the actual service events in real time. Also, it would be necessary to capture customer satisfaction with the individual service events, such as patient satisfaction surveying.[30]

Because so little of the TQM-type outcomes and performance data are available online, most TQM studies use specially designed data-entry forms unique to each quality improvement project.[31] Usually the data collection is added subsequently as an additional step in the service event. Some of the data collection is for all patients during a limited time interval; other studies involve statistical sampling on an ongoing basis.

TQM has fostered a new language of terms. The ability to apply its concepts depends on a thorough understanding of their meanings.

To the Point

- Benchmarking is the search for and implementation of an organization's best operating practices that lead to exceptional performance.

- To be successful, benchmarking needs strong management commitment, complete understanding of the medical group's operations, openness to change and new ideas, willingness to share information with benchmarking partners, and a dedication to continuous benchmarking efforts.

- Three categories of benchmarking are competitive benchmarking, cooperative benchmarking, and collaborative benchmarking.

- The benchmarking process includes several steps within six distinct phases. They are:
  - Planning
  - Analysis
  - Integration
  - Action
  - Maturity
  - Quality

■ Total quality management (TQM) is a structured, systematic process for creating organization-wide participation in planning and implementing continuous improvements in quality. Thus, quality means meeting or exceeding the customer's expectations of the product or service at a price considered reasonable to the customer. TQM is a method to examine all processes within a system, establish key preference indicators, and continually improve on them. Quality is measured against the benchmark of customer satisfaction.

■ Seen as too limited today, traditional quality control measures included assessing or measuring performance, determining whether performance conformed to standards, and improving performance when standards were not met.

■ Today, quality refers not only to a patient's physical and psychological health, but also includes patients' families, referring physicians, and third parties' perspectives.

■ The old TQM approach underemphasized the contributions of nonphysicians and organizational processes, but the new model places them in positions of equal importance. The traditional way addressed physicians' technical expertise and interpersonal competence. The new model embraces broader aspects such as the ability to mobilize the medical group's resources to meet the patients' needs and to meet the group's goals.

■ Customers under TQM include both external and internal groups.

■ The customer classes in the TQM process help define the nature of quality measures from three dimensions:

  – Structure

  – Process

  – Outcomes

■ TQM principles are largely based on the ideas and writings of the late W. Edwards Deming. He was concerned with the flow of activities from the original state of materials to the finished product in the manufacturing setting. His 14 principles have been adapted to the healthcare setting.

■ In TQM, the quality of the output is determined by the quality of production processes and quality results from process improvements. Quality is improved by systematically documenting the process, analyzing its operating characteristics, and identifying ways to improve it. The essence of TQM requires continuous improvement, and every employee continuously looks for process improvements.

■ Value-based purchasing (VBP) is an important new process that impacts all providers in the provision of quality, and HCAHPS is the nationally recognized measurement tool used to determine patient satisfaction on the inpatient basis.

■ The Plan-Do-Check-Act (PDCA) cycle is a road map for continuous process improvement.

■ There are eight basic tools used as analytical and problem-solving tools in TQM:

1. Flow charts
2. Tally sheets
3. Cause-and-effect diagrams
4. Pareto charts
5. Histograms
6. Scatter diagrams
7. Run charts
8. Control charts

■ Statistical variation is inherent in any process and results from the combination of people, machines, methods, materials, and environment. Variation is separated into two types: normal, or common cause variation, and abnormal, or special cause variation.

■ In the data analysis to improve processes, TQM focuses on reducing variation due to common causes and improving quality by refining the production process while looking for ways to eliminate the special causes of variation.

■ The methodologies used to improve processes under TQM approaches are based on the PDCA cycle.

■ The support and integration of information systems are crucial to a successful TQM program.

BIBLIOGRAPHY

Berwick, D. M., James, B., and Coye, M. J. 2003. "Connections between Quality Measurement and Improvement." *Medical Care, 41.* Philadelphia, PA: Lippincott Williams and Wilkins.

Brassard, M. 1988. *The Memory Jogger: A Pocket Guide of Tools for Continuous Improvement.* Methuen, MA: GOAL/QPC.

Brent, J. 2002. "Quality Improvement Opportunities in Health Care — Making It Easy to Do It Right." *Journal of Managed Care Pharmacy*, 8(5): 394–405. Alexandria, VA: Academy of Managed Care Pharmacy.

Frontiers of Health Services Management. 1991. "The Quest for Quality and Productivity in Health Services," *Frontiers of Health Services Management*, 7(4): 2–55.

Healthcare Executive. 2009, January/February. "The Triple Aim: Optimizing Health, Care, and Cost." *Healthcare Executive, 64–66.*

James, B. 1989. *Quality Management in Healthcare Delivery.* Chicago, IL: Hospital Research and Educational Trust of the American Hospital Association. pp. 1–73.

James, B. 1992. "Good Enough? Standards and Measurement in Continuous Quality Improvement." *National Quality of Care Forum on Bridging the Gap between Theory and Practice: Exploring Continuous Quality Improvement.* Chicago, IL: Hospital Research and Educational Trust.

James, B. C. 1993. "Implementing Practice Guidelines through Clinical Quality Improvement." *Frontiers of Health Services Management*, 10(1): 3–37. Chicago, IL: Health Administration Press.

Martin, L. A., Neumann C. W., Mountford, J., Bisognano, M., and Nolan, T. W. 2009. *Increasing Efficiency and Enhancing Value in Health Care: Ways to Achieve Savings in Operating Costs Per Year.* IHI Innovation Series White Paper. Cambridge, MA: Institute for Healthcare Improvement.

Reinersten, J. L., Gosfield, A. G., Rubb, W., and Whittington, J. W. 2007. *Engaging Physicians in a Shared Quality Agenda.* IHA Innovation Series White Paper. Cambridge, MA: Institute for Healthcare Improvement.

Stremikis, K., Davis, K. and Guterman, S. 2010, October. "Health Care Opinion Leaders' Views on Transparency and Pricing." *Data Brief, Pub. 1451, 102.* New York: The Commonwealth Fund.

REFERENCES

1. "Benchmarking." *Wikipedia.* Retrieved from http://en.wikipedia.org/wiki/Benchmarking. Accessed September 26, 2012.

2. Camp, R. C. 1989. *Benchmarking: The Search for Industry Best Practices That Lead to Superior Performance.* Milwaukee, WI: American Society for Quality Control.

3. Info-Line. 1992. "Understanding Benchmarking: The Search for Best Practice." *American Society for Training and Development, 9207,* 5–6.

4. Camp, R. C. 1989. *Benchmarking: The Search for Industry Best Practices That Lead to Superior Performance.* Milwaukee, WI: American Society for Quality Control, 9–12.

5. Hyden, M. 2012, January 31. "How Better-Performing Practices Use Their EHRs." *MGMA In Practice Blog.* Retrieved from http://www.mgma.com/blog/How-better-performing-practices-use-their-EHRs. Accessed September 27, 2012.

6. Cooke, D. J., and Iannacchino, K. L. 1991. "The Deming Method for Problem Solving in Group Practice." *Medical Group Management Journal*, 52.

7. Kaiser, L. R. 1984. "Winning Medical Groups." *Medical Group Management Journal*, 14.

8. "Quality." *BusinessDictionary.com.* Retrieved from http://www.businessdictionary.com/definition/quality.html. Accessed September 27, 2012.

9. "Quality." *Merriam-Webster.com.* Retrieved from http://www.merriam-webster.com/dictionary/quality. Accessed September 27, 2012.

10. ASQ Statistics Division. 1983. *Glossary & Tables for Statistical Quality Control.*

11. Ibid.

12. Ibid.

13. Info-Line. 1991. "Fundamentals of Quality." *American Society of Training and Development, 119*, 1.

14. Ibid.

15. O'Connor, S. J. and Lanning, J. A. 1991. "The New Health-Care Quality: Value, Outcomes, and Continuous Improvement." *Clinical Laboratory Management Review*, 221.

16. Ibid.

17. Ibid., p. 222.

18. U.S. Department of Health and Human Services. 2008, December 9. "Development of a Plan to Transition to a Medicare Value-Based Purchasing Program for Physician and Other Professional Services." Issues Paper. Retrieved from http://www.cms.gov/Medicare/Medicare-Fee-for-Service-Payment/PhysicianFeeSched/downloads/PhysicianVBP-Plan-Issues-Paper.pdf. Accessed September 27, 2012.

19. Centers for Medicare and Medicaid Services. "Administration Implements New Health Reform Provision to Improve Care Quality, Lower Costs." Fact Sheet. Retrieved from http://www.healthcare.gov/news/factsheets/2011/04/valuebasedpurchasing04292011a.html. Accessed September 27, 2012.

20. Centers for Medicare and Medicaid Services. n.d. "HCAHPS: Patients' Perspectives of Care Survey." *CMS.gov*. Retrieved from http://www.cms.gov/Medicare/Quality-Initiatives-Patient-Assessment-Instruments/HospitalQualityInits/HospitalHCAHPS.html. Accessed September 27, 2012.

21. These ideas are excerpted from Laffel, G., and Blumenthal, D. 1989, November 24. "The Case for Using Industrial Quality Management Science in Health Care Organizations." *Journal of the American Medical Association*, 2869–2870.

22. Whetsell, G. W. 1991. "Total Quality Management." *Topics in Health Care Financing*, 12–20.

23. O'Connor, S. J. and Lanning, J. A. 1991. "The New Health-Care Quality: Value, Outcomes, and Continuous Improvement." *Clinical Laboratory Management Review*, 228.

24. Clark, C. 2011, January 11. "CMS Releases Value-Based Purchasing Incentive Plan." *Health-Leaders Media*. Retrieved from http://www.healthleadersmedia.com/content/HEP-261211/CMS-Releases-ValueBased-Purchasing-Incentive-Plan##. Accessed September 27, 2012.

25. Ibid.

26. Info-Line, 1991. "Fundamentals of Quality." *American Society of Training and Development, 119*, 10.

27. Management Sciences for Health. 1998. *Guide for Managing Quality*. Arlington, VA: MSH and UNICEF.

28. Wood, M. C., and Wood, J. C. 2005. *Joseph Juran: Critical Evaluations in Business and Management*. New York, NY: Routledge (Taylor and Francis Group).

29. McEachern, J. E., Makens, P. K., Buchanan, E. D., and Schiff, L. 1991. "Quality Improvement: An Imperative for Medical Care." *Journal of Occupational Medicine*, 366–367.

30. Patrick, M. S. 1992. "Benchmarking — Targeting 'Best Practices.'" *Health Care Forum Journal*, 72.

31. Belman, M. J., Payne-Simon, L., Tom, E., and Rideout, J. 1999. "Using a Quality Scorecard to Measure and Improve Medical Groups' Performance." *Journal on Quality Improvement, 25*, 239–251.

CHAPTER 14

Evaluating Short- and Long-Range Investment Alternatives

Edited by Lee Ann Webster, MA, CPA, FACMPE

After completing this chapter, you will be able to:

- Describe the nature of short-range investment decisions and the steps to follow in analyzing various related situations.

- Identify the relevant costs and benefits of various short-term problem analyses, and apply the appropriate data in choosing a course of action.

- Describe the nature of long-range investment decisions and the kinds of expenditures that they typically cover.

- Use the basic concepts of the time value of money, both future and present values, in the evaluation of investment proposals dealing with long-range investment opportunities.

- Explain the important variables and information needed to carry out investment analysis and apply this knowledge in the four techniques usually followed in the capital budgeting process.

A medical group's governing body and financial manager are faced with many investment decisions, some with long-range implications and others impacting the immediate future. Usually, the approach involves measuring the benefits to be achieved from an alternative and comparing those with the costs of pursuing that course of action. A crucial element, then, is to identify, measure, and compare benefits and costs attributable to each kind of decision. As such, we can envision most of these decisions within an investment context and treat them as an evaluation process that compares alternative avenues for placing some of a group's assets into ventures to achieve some amount of return.

There are two general classifications of these investment alternatives. Each type requires considerably different information for analysis. The first type — long range — involves the acquisition or replacement of capacity and requires a long period of time before the benefits are fully realized. These investments normally entail acquiring buildings, equipment, and to some extent, key people. The second type of investment alternative — short range — embodies the use of capacity, usually within a short period of time. It relates to decisions about the volume and mix of services to offer and the fees to charge.

In this chapter, we will cover the approaches used to accumulate relevant financial information and analyze both long-term and short-term investment alternatives, starting with the latter. Our discussion will provide examples of the typical situations in which these investment evaluations are made and how they can be accomplished. Readers who need some introduction to the basic mathematics of finance will find some material on the time value of money and how to use compound interest tables. In some areas, our discussion will be somewhat generic for comprehension reasons, but in most respects, it will focus on the healthcare setting.

SHORT-RANGE INVESTMENT DECISIONS

Short-range decisions differ from long-range decisions in three primary areas. First, short-range decisions relate to short periods of time. Although the time value of money is important for long-range decisions, it is not critical in short-range decisions and is generally not considered in the analysis. The *time value of money* is a term meaning that a unit of money — the dollar — is worth more today by having it "in hand" than it is worth at some point in the future because of the need to consider the interest factor or a return for the use of money. This is true because short-term decisions usually involve a limited investment in and a quick recovery of cash. Second, short-range decisions usually involve repetitive activities, while long-range choices may not. Because the immediate future will likely be similar to the recent past, accounting measurements of revenue and costs are relevant for short-term analysis. Although past data may be adjusted to reflect expected price and other changes, the historical record in the accounting system will provide most of the data for short-range decision analysis. A third difference is the setting of the decisions. Short-range decisions relate to the types, amounts, and prices of services that will be performed with the existing capacity of the organization, while long-range decisions embrace a change in the size of the capacity to provide goods or services.

ALTERNATIVE CHOICE PROBLEMS

We have described short-range investment decision making as situations for deciding on alternatives. In an alternative choice problem, the manager seeks the alternative that will most likely accomplish the objectives of the organization. Those objectives will most likely include a profit element and may also entail nonfinancial gains. To choose the best alternative, the analysis should involve these steps:

1. Define the problem. Be careful not to assume that symptoms are the "problem."

2. Select possible alternative solutions.

3. Measure and evaluate for each selected alternative those consequences that can be expressed in quantitative terms.

4. Identify those consequences that cannot be expressed in quantitative terms and evaluate them against each other and against the measured consequences.

5. Reach a decision.

We will now mostly focus on quantitative information (Step 3) but will mention all the other steps briefly.

Steps 1 and 2: Define the Problem and Select Alternative Solutions

To compile the relevant quantitative data for analysis, the problem must be defined clearly and precisely. In many situations, this is the most difficult part of the entire process. Moreover, even after the problem has been identified, the possible alternative solutions may not be obvious.

> **Example:** *A medical group uses an outside laboratory for tests needed in patient diagnoses. The group has become dissatisfied with the lab's recent testing services. It is faced with the problem of what to do about the declining performance of the outside entity. It has identified three alternatives: (1) Set up its own laboratory inside the group and carry out its own testing; (2) seek another outside laboratory and move its business to this new firm; or (3) meet with the management of the present laboratory and determine whether changes can be made to improve the services.*

The more alternatives considered, the more complex the analysis becomes. For this reason, once all possible alternatives have been identified, those that are clearly unsuitable should be eliminated on a judgmental basis. As in most cases, one alternative is to continue what is currently being done. This status quo alternative, called the base case, is used as a benchmark against which other alternatives are measured.

Step 3: Measure the Quantitative Factors

With each alternative, there are usually many advantages and disadvantages. The decision maker's task is to evaluate each relevant factor and decide, after careful consideration, which alternative has the largest net advantage. If the factors or variables are expressed solely in words, such an evaluation is a very difficult task.

> **Example:** *Assume the financial manager of a medical practice states: "If we add another physician, our revenue will increase but so will our costs, and the malpractice insurance premiums will also go up." Such a statement provides no basis to weigh the relative importance of each element of revenue and cost that will change unless these items are quantified. Alternatively, the manager might say, "The addition of another physician will add $500,000 revenue to our total, increase our operating costs by $210,000, and cause our insurance premiums to go up by $20,000."*

The latter statement is a much clearer way to express the likely outcome and provides data to use in arriving at a decision.

Step 4: Identify the Unmeasured Factors

Many problems involve important factors that cannot be easily measured. The final decision must take into account both measurable and immeasurable differences between the alternatives. This process is using one's judgment in evaluating the pros and cons of each choice. It is easy to overlook the nonquantifiable factors. Often the numerical calculations require some hard work and give the appearance of being definite, precise, and even obvious. Yet all the factors that influence the final number may be collectively less important than a simple factor that cannot be measured.

Nevertheless, to the extent that calculations can be made to determine the quantitative net effect of many factors, this effort should be completed. These calculations serve to reduce the number of factors that must be considered separately in the final judgment process. However, numerical data do not eliminate the necessity for tempering quantitative analysis with qualitative judgments.

Step 5: Reach a Decision

After completing the first four steps, the decision maker has two choices: (1) Seek additional information or (2) make a decision and take action. Many decisions could be improved by gathering more data, if that is possible. However, obtaining this information always entails effort (which means cost) and time. There comes a time when the manager will conclude that it is better to take action than to defer a decision until more data have been collected.

DIFFERENT INFORMATION FOR DIFFERENT DECISIONS

To make any decision, the decision maker needs to know the relevant benefits and costs of each alternative being considered. A relevant benefit is the change in revenue directly attributable to a decision. A relevant cost is the change in costs directly attributable to a decision. Most importantly, benefits and costs relevant to one decision will not necessarily be relevant to another decision. Once the relevant benefits and costs have been identified, the analysis then becomes one of concentrating on differences between the relevant benefits and costs for each alternative, resulting in short-range analysis, which is also called differential analysis.

Fixed and Variable Costs

In many alternative choice decisions, such as those involving the volume and mix of services, the practice must know which costs will change with changes in activity levels. Here, the concept of fixed and variable costs is important. As stated previously, variable costs are costs that change as activity goes up and down and include such items as supply costs and laboratory costs. On the other hand, fixed costs are costs that do not change as activity moves up and down. Often called capacity costs, fixed costs include such expenses as rent, insurance, property taxes, and administrative salaries.

Since both revenues and variable costs change as activity levels go up and down, a simple measure of the change in profit as activity changes is called the contribution margin. The contribution margin is the difference between revenue and variable costs. Thus, for those decisions involving a change in activity levels, the measurement of contribution margin provides a criterion for evaluating these decisions. Assuming that fixed costs do not change, management should select the alternative that will maximize contribution margin.

Avoidable Costs

Another classification of costs relevant to some short-range investment decisions is avoidable costs. An avoidable cost can be defined as a cost that can be eliminated as a result of choosing one alternative over another.

Assume a medical group is considering the elimination of its own laboratory within the group and purchasing its laboratory services from an outside source. If the equipment for the in-house laboratory is rented on a cancelable lease, the equipment rent expenses would be avoided and, thus, would be a relevant cost to consider in making the decision. However, the rental cost of the space occupied by the laboratory within the group's office would not be eliminated (since rent for the group's office facility would continue to be paid). This rental cost would not be an avoidable cost. It will be referred to as an unavoidable cost. Thus, a key element in sorting out costs relevant to the analysis of short-range investment decisions is the determination of costs that are avoidable under each alternative and those that continue or are considered to be unavoidable.

Full Costs

In chapter 7, the process of determining the full cost of a responsibility center or a procedure was explained and illustrated. The full cost of a procedure includes both the direct costs traceable to the procedure, such as lab services, and a fair share of all indirect costs that cannot be traced, and therefore, must be allocated to the procedure. The full cost of a procedure is useful as an aid in setting fees.

ILLUSTRATIONS OF SHORT-RANGE DECISIONS

Let's examine several situations that apply the concepts of short-term analysis. The situations cited are not intended to fully encompass all short-term decisions but rather provide illustrations of different types that are common to many practices. They are:

- Break-even analysis
- Adding a physician
- Dropping an activity

The first, break-even analysis, can be the focus of short-term analysis itself or it could be used in conjunction with other methods as a means of evaluating that alternative further.

Break-Even Analysis

Break-even analysis was covered in some depth in chapter 11. It deals with the relationships between variable and fixed costs, volume of business, and the resulting impact on net income for periods of usually one year. The example in chapter 11 showed the application of determining how many tests were necessary in a laboratory to break even — the point at which total revenue of the laboratory equaled total expenses. Additional analyses could be carried out by varying any of the key elements of the break-even formula to see what impact changes in the elements would have on the break-even point and on profit. Thus, break-even analyses make it possible to test the impact of anticipated changes in costs or fees on the volume of business necessary to achieve management objectives. It is also especially useful in assessing the volume of services needed to cover the incremental costs of going prepaid.

Adding a Physician

Another area in which break-even analysis (or cost-volume-profit analysis) is applied is in the decision to add a new physician to avoid outside referrals for services to prepaid patients. If additional facilities and equipment are required, the decision should be evaluated by long-range decision techniques that include considering the time value of money as well as incremental revenues and costs. If facilities and equipment are not a factor, analysis can focus on the differential revenues and costs involved in adding the new physician.

To illustrate this application, assume that Coastal Medical Center wants to determine when to add a general surgeon to the group. Before the financial implications of this decision can be considered, there are several policy questions that must be answered. These deal with such issues as: Does the group wish to remain a primary care group? Will any new physician serve FFS patients as well as prepaid patients? What impact will the addition of specialists, such as surgeons, have on the income distribution formula? After these basic policy issues are answered, or perhaps coincident with these policy considerations, the group will examine the financial implications.

The critical data in this type of analysis include the incremental revenues and costs from the expanded capability of providing services. These amounts are determined from the membership and utilization projections. The group must then determine the point at which capitation revenue for general surgery will exceed the cost of maintaining a general surgeon. Assuming the following costs, the break-even point for adding a surgeon will be reached between the twelfth and fifteenth months, as indicated in Exhibit 14.2.

Using data in Exhibit 14.1, the flexible budget formula for the cost of a general surgeon is determined to be $44,000 per month plus $11.25 per patient visit. The revenue for the general surgeon will be the portion of the monthly capitation payment for general surgery. Assume that $6.60 of the monthly capitation payment per-member is for surgery.

EXHIBIT 14.1 ■ Data-Determining Incremental Costs

Costs of General Surgery		
Salary and benefits	$30,000.00	per month
Support staff and benefits	$8,500.00	per month
Equipment rental	$1,500.00	per month
Professional liability	$1,800.00	per month
Space (1,500 sq. ft. x $1.467 per month)	$2,200.00	per month
Total fixed costs	$44,000.00	per month
Supplies and other variable expenses	$11.25	per patient visit

EXHIBIT 14.2 ■ Analysis of When to Add a Doctor — Coastal Medical Center

Month	Surgery Enrolled Members	Patient Visits	Fixed Costs	Incremental		
				Variable Costs	Total Costs	Revenues
1	175	3	$44,000.00	$33.75	$44,033.75	$1,155.00
3	472	6	$44,000.00	$67.50	$44,067.50	$3,115.20
6	2,669	30	$44,000.00	$337.50	$44,337.50	$17,615.40
9	3,266	37	$44,000.00	$416.25	$44,416.25	$21,555.60
12	5,221	57	$44,000.00	$641.25	$44,641.25	$34,458.60
15	7,777	82	$44,000.00	$922.50	$44,922.50	$51,328.20

Enrollment projections, surgery patient visits (now being referred out), incremental costs, and incremental revenues are presented for selected months in Exhibit 14.2.

The incremental revenues will cover the incremental costs in about the fourteenth month. This conclusion is based on a number of assumptions including: There will be no change in the "gatekeeper" role of the primary care physician, utilization rates will continue as projected, and enrollment projections will be reached.

For this decision, break-even analysis provided the decision framework. While the reader might argue with the specific numbers in the illustration, the framework is sound. The importance of accurate planning and projections cannot be overemphasized.

Dropping an Activity

Another setting involving short-range considerations relates to dropping a particular line of service or activity. In the following example, it is assumed that the medical group opened a satellite office in anticipation of member growth in a particular geographic area. Also, we assume that the satellite location has been unprofitable, and the group is now asking, "How much will we save by eliminating the unprofitable satellite office?"

The most recent operating statement for the satellite office is presented in Exhibit 14.3. The satellite office has shown a loss since it was opened. The combination of increased competition from other medical groups, a downturn in the economy in the area, and the inability to provide proper supervision of the office all contributed to the loss. It is doubtful that the satellite office could produce additional revenue without substantial additional resources.

Although the concept of variable and fixed costs is useful in this situation, an additional factor is necessary. The group must know which costs will be avoided if the satellite office is closed and which costs will continue.

EXHIBIT 14.3 ■ **Operating Statement for Satellite Clinic**

Current Month		
Revenues		$36,200
Operating expenses:		
Associate physician's salary	$13,000	
Associate physician's benefits	$1,500	
Staff salaries	$11,000	
Staff benefits	$2,500	
Lab and X-ray services	$4,000	
Supplies	$2,200	
Occupancy	$4,200	
Administrative service for main clinic	$5,000	
Total operating expenses		$43,400
Net loss		($7,200)

To make these determinations, assume the associate physician is on a contract that is dependent on the continuation of the satellite office. The staff is assumed to be working on an hourly basis, only as needed. Space is rented on a five-year noncancellable lease. The best the group can do with the space is to sublease it for $3,500 per month, thereby losing $700 per month in rent. The administrative services represent allocated costs from the main office. Closing the satellite office will have little, if any, effect on administrative costs. Exhibit 14.4 identifies the avoidable and unavoidable costs of closing

EXHIBIT 14.4 ■ **Illustration of Avoidable and Unavoidable Costs of Closing Satellite Clinic**

Type of Expense	Fixed or Variable	Monthly Costs	Avoidable Costs	Unavoidable Costs
Associate physician's salary	Fixed	$13,000	$13,000	
Associate physician's benefits	Fixed	$1,500	$1,500	
Staff salaries	Variable	$11,000	$11,000	
Staff benefits	Variable	$2,500	$2,500	
Lab and X-ray services	Variable	$4,000	$4,000	
Supplies	Variable	$2,200	$2,200	
Occupancy	Fixed	$4,200	$3,500	$700
Administrative service for main clinic	Fixed	$5,000	–	$5,000
Total operating expenses		$43,400	$37,700	$5,700

the satellite office. The exhibit shows that $37,700 of the $43,400 in costs are avoidable and $5,700 would still need to be paid out if the satellite office is closed.

The effect of closing the satellite office can now be determined as follows:

Decrease in revenue.......................... $36,200
Decrease in operating costs................... $37,700
Savings by closing satellite office $1,500

At this level of activity, the group will save $1,500 per month by closing the office. The group now knows that continuing the office is costing at least $7,200 per month. The $5,700 of unavoidable costs will continue regardless of what the group decides to do with the satellite office.

The relevant data in this example are revenues, variable costs, and avoidable fixed costs. Variable costs should always be avoidable in a decision of this nature. The occupancy and administrative costs that continue are unavoidable and, therefore, are irrelevant to this decision.

The data in this example may suggest other possible decisions, such as reducing costs or changing staff. These alternatives require other cost concepts besides avoidable and unavoidable costs. However, the analysis still focuses on differential costs; for example, the cost of continuing the satellite operations as is versus the cost of operating it with the changes envisioned.

LONG-RANGE INVESTMENT DECISIONS

Long-range investments are commitments of funds to acquire an asset that will provide benefits over a long period of time. Such investments for a medical group pertain to acquiring buildings, purchasing equipment, and leasing facilities or equipment. In all these cases, there is an addition to or a replacement of the capacity of the group in the form of long-lived assets to render medical services.

Nature of Investments

When an organization purchases a long-lived asset, it makes an investment similar to that made by a bank when it lends money. The essential characteristic of both types of transactions is that cash is committed today in the expectation of recovering that cash plus some additional amount in the future. That additional amount is called a return on investment.

In the case of a bank loan, the return on investment is the inflow of interest payments received over the life of the loan. In the case of the long-lived asset, both the return of investment and the return on investment are in the form of cash earnings generated by use of the asset. If, over the life of the investment, the inflows of cash earnings exceed the initial investment outlays (cost), then we know that the original investment was recovered (return of investment) and that some profit was earned (positive return on investment). Thus, an investment is the purchase of an expected future stream of cash flows.

When an organization considers whether to purchase a new long-lived asset, the key question is: Will the future cash inflows likely be large enough to justify making the investment? The consideration of these purchases is always framed in the form of a proposal, supported by detailed analysis that contains projections of the streams of expected cash inflows and an evaluation as to whether these inflows will warrant the initial expenditure. Some of the kinds of proposals typically developed pertain to:

- **Replacement** — Should the organization replace existing equipment with more efficient equipment? The future expected cash inflows would be the cost savings resulting from lower operating costs or the profits from the additional volume produced by the new equipment or both.

- **Expansion** — Should the practice build or otherwise acquire a new facility? The future expected cash inflows on this investment are the cash profits from the goods and services produced in the new facility.

- **Cost reduction** — Should the medical group buy equipment to perform an operation or activity now done manually? That is, should it spend money to save money? The expected future cash inflows are the savings resulting from lower operating costs.

- **Choice of equipment** — Which of several proposed equipment items should be purchased for a given purpose? The choice often depends on which item is expected to provide the largest return on the investment made in it.

- **New product or service** — Should a new product or a new service be added to the existing line? The choice depends on whether the expected future cash inflows from the sale of the product or service are large enough to warrant the investment in equipment, additional working capital, and the costs required to make or develop and introduce the new product or service.

- **Lease or buy** — Having decided that the group needs a building or a new piece of equipment, should it be leased or bought? The choice in this case depends on whether the investment required to purchase the asset will earn an adequate return because of the cash inflows that will result from avoiding the lease payments. In this instance, avoiding a cash outflow is equivalent to receiving a cash inflow.

Traditionally, long-range decisions for medical practices have been made on the basis of medical need. If economic considerations were taken into account at all, usually simple techniques were employed that did not embrace expected future cash inflows or the return on giving up cash today for a larger amount in the future. As we have discussed, a long-range decision involves an investment of cash in an asset that yields its return over an extended period of time. The accounting measurements of income and historical cost are appropriate for performance evaluation and for providing the relevant information to make short-range decisions. However, because of the long period of time involved in long-range decisions, it is important to consider the time value of money. We will discuss this concept next.

TIME VALUE OF MONEY

As noted before, the time value of money is a concept recognizing that a dollar of cash in hand today is worth more than a dollar of cash to be received at any time in the future. The difference is called the time value of money. This concept can be explained by using the principle of compound interest. Suppose we invest $1,000 in a savings account that pays interest of 10 percent annually. (Interest is always stated as an annual rate; thus, "10 percent" means 10 percent per year.) Compounded annually means that interest earned in the first year is retained in the account and, along with the $1,000, earns interest in the second year and so on for future years. If we make no withdrawals from this account, over time the account balance will grow as shown:

	Investment at Beginning of Year	Interest Earned	Investment at End of Year
Year 1	$1,000	$100	$1,100
Year 2	$1,100	$110	$1,210
Year 3	$1,210	$121	$1,331

Based on this table, we can say: "With $1,000 invested today at 10 percent interest, compounded annually, it will accumulate to $1,331 after three years." An equivalent statement is that the future value of $1,000 invested for three years at 10 percent interest is $1,331.

Future Value and Present Value

There are two concepts that are important in explaining the time value of money: future value and present value. As just stated, future value is the amount to which a given amount of cash invested will grow at the end of a given period of time when compounded at a given rate of interest. Thus, in the example, the future value of $1,000, compounded at 10 percent, is $1,100 at the end of one year; $1,210 at the end of two years; and $1,331 at the end of three years. If a person is satisfied to earn 10 percent on his or her money, ignoring inflation and other variables, there should be no difference among the following: receiving $1,000 now; $1,100 one year from now; $1,210 two years from now; or $1,331 three years from now.

The second concept, present value, is the reverse of the future-value concept. The reverse of interest compounding is called discounting. For example, if the future value of $1,000 at 10 percent interest for 10 years is $2,593.74, then we can say that the present value of $2,593.74 discounted at 10 percent for 10 years is $1,000. The interest rate (10 percent in the example) in present-value problems is commonly referred to as the discount rate or the rate of return. This illustration leads to a more formal definition of present value:

The present value of an amount expected to be received at a specified time in the future is the amount that, if invested today at a designated rate of return, would accumulate to the specified amount.

Thus, assuming a 10 percent rate of return, the present value of $2,593.74 to be received 10 years hence is $1,000 because if $1,000 is invested today at 10 percent, it would accumulate to $2,593.74 after 10 years.

Referring to our earlier table of the $1,000 investment for three years, we can say: The present value of $1,100 to be received at the end of year one, compounded at 10 percent, is $1,000; the present value of $1,210 to be received at the end of two years, compounded at 10 percent, is also $1,000; and, the present value of $1,331 to be received at the end of three years, compounded at 10 percent, is also $1,000. A person satisfied with earning 10 percent on his or her money should not care whether $1,000 would be received now; $1,100 at the end of one year; $1,210 at the end of two years; or $1,331 at the end of three years.

The tools of time value of money allow the comparison of any two or more dollar amounts of cash paid or received at different points of time. The two amounts can be measured in terms of future value — what they will be worth at some future time — or they can be measured in terms of present value — what they are worth today. Either approach will provide similar results. Because an investment is being made today, it is much easier to understand and to work with present values than to deal in future values.

Present Value Tables

For the concept of present value to be useful, a way of computing the present value of cash at any future point in time is needed. There are mathematical formulas that can be used for this purpose; however, these are quite complex and cumbersome to put into practice. Rather, present value tables have been developed that show the present value of $1 at different rates of interest and at different points in time. These present value factors may then be multiplied by any given amount for any point in time to provide the amount of present value. The present value factor of $1 may be computed by dividing each present value by its future value. For example, in our previous illustration, the future value of $1,000 was computed at the end of each of three periods using a 10 percent rate of interest. The present value factor of $1 compounded at 10 percent may be computed as follows:

Period of Time	Present Value/Future Value	Present Value Factor
1 year	$1,000/$1,100	0.909
2 years	$1,000/$1,210	0.826
3 years	$1,000/$1,331	0.751

A full table could be developed showing the present value of $1 at any interest rate and for any number of time periods chosen. Present value tables for selected rates of interest and selected time periods are presented in Exhibits 14.5.

EXHIBIT 14.5 ▪ Present Value of $1 $\left(PV = \dfrac{1}{(1 + r)^n}\right)$

Period	2%	4%	6%	8%	10%	12%	14%	16%
1	0.980	0.962	0.943	0.926	0.909	0.893	0.877	0.862
2	0.961	0.925	0.890	0.857	0.826	0.797	0.769	0.743
3	0.942	0.889	0.840	0.794	0.751	0.712	0.675	0.641
4	0.924	0.855	0.792	0.735	0.683	0.636	0.592	0.552
5	0.906	0.822	0.747	0.681	0.621	0.567	0.519	0.476
6	0.888	0.790	0.705	0.630	0.564	0.507	0.456	0.410
7	0.871	0.760	0.665	0.583	0.513	0.452	0.400	0.354
8	0.853	0.731	0.627	0.540	0.467	0.404	0.351	0.305
9	0.837	0.703	0.592	0.500	0.424	0.361	0.308	0.263
10	0.820	0.676	0.558	0.463	0.386	0.322	0.270	0.227
11	0.804	0.650	0.527	0.429	0.350	0.287	0.237	0.195
12	0.788	0.625	0.497	0.397	0.319	0.257	0.208	0.168
13	0.773	0.601	0.469	0.368	0.290	0.229	0.182	0.145
14	0.758	0.577	0.442	0.340	0.236	0.205	0.160	0.125
15	0.743	0.555	0.417	0.315	0.239	0.183	0.140	0.108
16	0.728	0.534	0.394	0.292	0.218	0.163	0.123	0.093
17	0.714	0.513	0.371	0.270	0.198	0.146	0.108	0.080
18	0.700	0.494	0.350	0.250	0.180	0.130	0.095	0.069
19	0.686	0.475	0.331	0.232	0.164	0.116	0.083	0.060
20	0.673	0.456	0.312	0.215	0.149	0.104	0.073	0.051
21	0.660	0.439	0.294	0.199	0.135	0.093	0.064	0.044
22	0.647	0.422	0.278	0.184	0.123	0.083	0.056	0.038
23	0.634	0.406	0.262	0.170	0.112	0.074	0.049	0.033
24	0.622	0.390	0.247	0.158	0.102	0.066	0.043	0.028
25	0.610	0.375	0.233	0.146	0.092	0.059	0.036	0.024
30	0.552	0.308	0.174	0.099	0.057	0.033	0.020	0.012
35	0.500	0.253	0.130	0.068	0.036	0.019	0.010	0.006
40	0.453	0.280	0.097	0.046	0.022	0.011	0.005	0.003
45	0.410	0.171	0.073	0.031	0.014	0.006	0.003	0.001
50	0.372	0.141	0.054	0.021	0.009	0.003	0.001	0.001

18%	20%	22%	24%	26%	28%	30%	35%	40%	45%	50%
0.847	0.833	0.820	0.806	0.794	0.781	0.769	0.741	0.714	0.690	0.667
0.718	0.694	0.672	0.650	0.630	0.610	0.592	0.549	0.510	0.476	0.444
0.609	0.579	0.551	0.524	0.500	0.477	0.455	0.406	0.364	0.328	0.296
0.516	0.482	0.451	0.423	0.397	0.373	0.350	0.301	0.260	0.226	0.198
0.437	0.402	0.370	0.341	0.315	0.291	0.269	0.223	0.188	0.156	0.132
0.370	0.335	0.303	0.275	0.250	0.227	0.207	0.165	0.133	0.108	0.088
0.314	0.279	0.249	0.222	0.198	0.178	0.159	0.122	0.095	0.074	0.059
0.266	0.233	0.204	0.179	0.157	0.139	0.123	0.091	0.068	0.051	0.039
0.225	0.194	0.167	0.144	0.125	0.108	0.094	0.067	0.046	0.035	0.026
0.191	0.162	0.137	0.116	0.099	0.085	0.073	0.050	0.035	0.024	0.017
0.162	0.135	0.112	0.094	0.079	0.066	0.056	0.037	0.025	0.017	0.012
0.137	0.112	0.092	0.076	0.062	0.052	0.043	0.027	0.018	0.012	0.008
0.116	0.093	0.075	0.061	0.500	0.040	0.033	0.020	0.013	0.008	0.005
0.099	0.078	0.062	0.049	0.039	0.032	0.025	0.015	0.009	0.006	0.003
0.984	0.065	0.051	0.040	0.031	0.025	0.020	0.011	0.009	0.004	0.002
0.071	0.054	0.042	0.032	0.025	0.019	0.015	0.008	0.005	0.003	0.002
0.060	0.045	0.034	0.026	0.020	0.015	0.012	0.006	0.003	0.002	0.001
0.051	0.038	0.028	0.031	0.016	0.012	0.009	0.005	0.002	0.001	0.001
0.043	0.031	0.023	0.017	0.012	0.008	0.007	0.003	0.002	0.001	
0.037	0.026	0.019	0.014	0.010	0.007	0.005	0.002	0.001	0.001	
0.031	0.022	0.015	0.011	0.008	0.006	0.004	0.002	0.001		
0.026	0.018	0.013	0.009	0.006	0.004	0.003	0.001	0.001		
0.022	0.015	0.010	0.007	0.005	0.003	0.002	0.001			
0.019	0.013	0.008	0.006	0.004	0.003	0.002	0.001			
0.016	0.010	0.007	0.005	0.003	0.002	0.001	0.001			
0.007	0.004	0.003	0.002	0.001	0.001					
0.003	0.002	0.001	0.001							
0.002	0.001	0.001								
0.001										

Application of Present Value in Decision Making

Now let's apply the concept of present value in a long-range investment decision. Assuming the desired rate of return on the investment is 10 percent, which of the following investments is acceptable?

1. Invest $1,000 now and receive $1,200 at the end of two years.
2. Invest $1,000 now and receive $600 at the end of one year, $400 at the end of two years, and $200 at the end of three years.
3. Invest $1,000 now and receive $200 at the end of one year, $400 at the end of two years, and $600 at the end of three years.

All three investments involve $1,000 of initial cash outflow and $1,200 of cash inflows. Timing of the cash inflows, however, is different in each alternative. The present value of cash outflows, in each case, is $1,000 because the cash is paid now. A dollar today is worth $1. The present value of the cash inflows is determined by multiplying each cash inflow amount by its appropriate present value factor. The present values of the $1,000 cash outflow and the $1,200 cash inflow for each investment alternative are computed as follows (note that cash outflows or payments are shown in parenthesis):

Investment A	**Present Value**
Present value of cash outflows......................	$(1,000)
Present value of cash inflows:	
Year 2 − $1,200 × 0.826............................	$991

Conclusion: The present value of future cash inflows is only $991. If any amount above $991 is paid for an investment that will pay $1,200 at the end of the second year, the investment will earn less than 10 percent. Based on a desired rate of return of 10 percent, Investment A should be rejected.

Investment B	**Present Value**
Present value of cash outflows......................	$(1,000)
Present value of cash inflows:	
Year 1 − $600 × 0.909 = $545	
Year 2 − $400 × 0.826 = $330	
Year 3 − $200 × 0.751 = $150.....................	$1,025

Conclusion: The present value of future cash inflows is $1,025. By paying only $1,000 for an investment with a present value of $1,025, more than 10 percent will be earned on the investment. As much as $1,025 could be paid for this investment to earn the desired rate of return of 10 percent. Therefore, based on a desired rate of return of 10 percent, Investment B should be accepted.

Investment C	**Present Value**

Present value of cash outflows. . . . . $(1,000)

Present value of cash inflows:
 Year 1 — $200 × 0.909 = $182
 Year 2 — $400 × 0.826 = $330
 Year 3 — $600 × 0.751 = $451. . . . . $963

Conclusion: With a required rate of return of 10 percent, Investment C should be rejected since the present value of cash inflows, $963, is less than the cash outflow of $1,000. An investment greater than $963 in exchange for the future cash flows in this example will *not* earn 10 percent.

This process in which amounts to be received or paid in the future are discounted to their present value is called *discounted cash flow analysis*. It is the method we will use in developing quantitative data for evaluating various alternative long-range investments.

Long-Range Decision Rule

We can now formulate a long-range decision rule as follows:

> *A long-range decision is favorable if the incremental discounted cash inflows attributable to the proposed investment are equal to or greater than the incremental discounted cash outflows attributable to the investment.*

The decision rule requires that every future cash flow be discounted back to its present value using the desired rate of return. In this way, discounted benefits can be compared with discounted costs.

In applying this long-range decision to Investments A, B, and C in the earlier illustration, only Investment B satisfies this rule. For Investment A, an investment of $1,000 now will produce discounted benefits of only $991. Investment B, however, also requires $1,000 now but will produce future cash inflows with a present value of $1,025. Investment C, on the other hand, requires the same $1,000 now but will produce cash inflows with a present value of only $963.

A further look at Investments B and C reveals that each involves total cash inflows of $1,200 over three years and cash outflows now of $1,000. Note that in Year 1, Investment B had cash inflows of $600, whereas Investment C had cash inflows of $200. In Year 2, each had cash inflows of $400. In Year 3, Investment B had cash inflows of $200, whereas Investment C had cash inflows of $600. Note that the cash inflows in Investment B are just reversed from those of Investment C. Investment B receives most of its cash early, whereas Investment C receives most of its cash return later. This difference in timing of cash inflows produces considerably different present value figures for cash inflows. Because Investment B will allow reinvestment of cash early, it is a much better investment than Investment C.

Would Investments A and C be acceptable if the practice were satisfied with an 8 percent return on its investment? Referring to Exhibit 14.5, the present value factors for 8 percent are as follows:

Year	Present Value Factor
1	0.926
2	0.857
3	0.794

The present value of cash flows for Investments A and C when discounted at 8 percent are as follows:

Investment A	Present Value

Present value of cash outflows. . . . . $(1,000)

Present value of cash inflows:

Year 2 − $1,200 × 0.857 . . . .$1,028

Conclusion: The present value of cash inflows exceeds the present value of cash outflows. Based on an 8 percent return, Investment A is now acceptable.

Investment C	Present Value

Present value of cash outflows. . . . . $(1,000)

Present value of cash inflows:

Year 1 − $200 × 0.926 = $185
Year 2 − $400 × 0.857 = $343
Year 3 − $600 × 0.794 = $476. . . . .$1,004

Conclusion: The present value of cash inflows exceeds the present value of cash outflows, indicating an acceptable investment. Investment C will earn slightly more than the new required rate of return of 8 percent.

Present Value of an Annuity

In the preceding illustrations, the present value for single amounts has been computed. When the future cash flows are not equal (e.g., $600 in Year 1, $400 in Year 2, and $200 in Year 3), the present value of each amount must be computed and then summed to arrive at the present value of the stream of cash flows. There is an easier calculation possible when the stream of future cash flows is equal. An annuity is an equal stream of cash flows at equal intervals of time. For example, assume that Investment D required an investment of $1,000 and provided cash inflows of $400 each year for three years.

The present value of an annuity of cash inflows may be computed in one of two ways. First, using the present value factors in Exhibit 14.5, compute the present value of each amount and sum the present values.

Investment D **Present Value**

Present value of cash inflows (assuming 10%)
Year 1 — $400 × 0.909 = $364
Year 2 — $400 × 0.826 = $330
Year 3 — $400 × 0.751 = $300...................... $994

Second, to compute the present value of an annuity, multiply the appropriate present value factor from Exhibit 14.6 by one periodic amount in the annuity.

Investment D **Present Value**

Present value of an annuity of $400 for three years at 10 percent:
$400 × 2.486 =.................................... $994

The present value factors in Exhibit 14.6 are determined by accumulating the present value factors in Exhibit 14.5. For example, the present value of an annuity of $1 at 10 percent follows:

Year	Present Value of $1	Present Value of an Annuity of $1
1	0.909	0.909
2	0.826	1.735 (0.909 + 0.826)
3	0.751	2.486 (1.735 + 0.751)

Exhibit 14.6 allows the present value of an annuity at selected discount rates for any number of years to be computed in one calculation.

The time value of money is a concept that allows the comparison of the present value of any two or more cash payments or receipts. Present value is the amount that must be invested now to accumulate to a given amount, at some given point in time, when compounded at a given rate of interest.

INFORMATION RELEVANT TO LONG-RANGE DECISIONS

To carry out investment analysis, we need to know when cash is invested and, therefore, not available for other purposes, as well as when cash is recovered and, therefore, available for other purposes. Furthermore, we need to know both the amount and timing of cash flows, which must be estimated as accurately as possible.

The conventional accounting measurement of income for a particular time period, even on a modified cash basis, includes some allocations of cost, such as depreciation, that do not involve cash. As we mentioned earlier, the accrual basis of income measurement requires the assignment of several costs to a particular period. For the evaluation of current operating performance, the accrual basis of accounting provides us with useful tools for measurement.

EXHIBIT 14.6 ■ Present Value of an Annuity of $1

Period	2%	4%	6%	8%	10%	12%	14%	16%	18%
1	0.980	0.962	0.943	0.926	0.909	0.893	0.877	0.862	0.847
2	1.942	1.882	1.833	1.783	1.736	1.690	1.647	1.605	1.566
3	2.884	2.775	2.673	2.577	2.486	2.402	2.322	2.246	2.174
4	3.808	3.630	3.465	3.312	3.170	3.037	2.914	2.914	2.798
5	4.713	4.452	4.212	3.992	3.791	3.605	3.433	3.274	3.127
6	5.601	5.242	4.917	4.623	4.355	4.111	3.889	3.685	3.498
7	6.472	6.002	5.582	5.206	4.868	4.564	4.288	4.039	3.812
8	7.325	6.733	6.210	5.747	5.759	4.968	4.639	4.344	4.078
9	8.162	7.435	6.082	6.247	6.145	5.328	4.946	4.607	4.303
10	8.983	8.111	7.360	6.710	6.495	5.650	5.216	4.833	4.494
11	9.787	8.760	7.887	7.139	6.814	5.938	5.453	5.029	4.656
12	10.575	9.385	8.384	7.536	7.103	6.194	5.660	5.197	4.793
13	11.348	9.986	8.853	7.904	7.367	6.424	5.842	5.342	4.910
14	12.106	10.563	9.295	8.244	7.357	6.628	6.002	5.468	5.008
15	12.849	11.118	9.712	8.559	7.606	6.811	6.142	5.575	5.092
16	13.578	11.652	10.106	8.851	7.824	6.974	6.265	5.668	5.162
17	14.292	12.166	10.477	9.122	8.022	7.120	6.373	5.749	5.222
18	14.992	12.659	10.828	9.372	8.201	7.250	6.467	5.818	5.273
19	15.678	13.134	11.158	9.604	8.365	7.366	6.550	5.877	5.316
20	16.351	13.590	11.470	9.818	8.514	7.469	6.623	5.929	5.353
21	17.011	14.029	11.764	10.017	8.649	7.562	6.687	5.973	5.384
22	17.658	14.451	12.042	10.201	8.772	7.645	6.743	6.011	5.410
23	18.292	14.857	12.303	10.371	8.883	7.718	6.792	6.044	5.432
24	18.914	15.247	12.550	10.529	8.965	7.784	6.835	6.073	5.451
25	19.523	15.622	12.783	10.675	9.077	7.843	6.873	6.097	5.467
30	22.396	17.292	13.765	11.258	9.427	8.055	7.003	6.177	5.517
35	24.999	18.665	14.498	11.655	9.644	8.176	7.070	6.215	5.539
40	27.355	19.793	15.046	11.925	9.779	8.244	7.105	6.233	5.548
45	24.490	20.720	15.456	12.108	9.863	8.283	7.123	6.242	5.552
50	31.424	21.482	15.762	12.233	9.915	8.304	7133	6.246	5.554

20%	22%	24%	26%	28%	30%	35%	40%	45%	50%
0.833	0.820	0.806	0.794	0.781	0.769	0.714	0.714	0.690	0.667
1.528	1.492	1.457	1.424	1.392	1.316	1.289	1.224	1.165	1.111
2.106	2.042	2.981	1.923	1.868	1.816	1.696	1.589	1.493	1.407
2.690	2.589	2.494	2.404	2.320	2.166	1.997	1.849	1.720	1.605
2.991	2.864	2.745	2.635	2.532	2.436	2.220	2.035	1.876	1.737
3.326	3.167	3.020	2.885	2.759	2.643	2.385	2.168	1.983	1.824
3.605	3.416	3.242	3.083	2.937	2.802	2.508	2.263	2.057	1.883
3.837	6.619	3.421	3.241	3.076	2.925	2.598	2.331	2.109	1.922
4.031	3.786	3.566	3.366	3.184	3.019	2.665	2.379	2.114	1.948
4.192	3.923	3.682	3.465	3.269	3.092	2.715	2.414	2.168	1.965
4.327	4.035	3.776	3.543	3.335	3.147	2.752	2.438	2.185	1.977
4.439	4.127	3.851	3.606	3.387	3.190	2.779	2.456	2.196	1.965
4.533	4.203	3.912	3.656	3.427	3.223	2.799	2.469	2.204	1.990
4.611	4.265	3.962	3.695	3.459	3.249	2.814	2.478	2.210	1.993
4.675	4.315	4.001	3.726	3.483	3.268	2.425	2.484	2.214	1.995
4.730	4.367	4.033	3.751	3.503	3.283	2.834	2.489	2.216	1.997
4.775	4.391	4.059	3.771	3.518	3.295	2.840	2.492	2.218	1.998
4.812	4.419	4.080	3.786	3.529	3.304	2.844	2.494	2.219	1.999
4.843	4.442	4.097	3.799	3.539	3.311	2.848	2.496	2.220	1.999
4.870	4.460	4.110	3.808	3.546	3.316	2.850	2.497	2.221	1.999
4.891	4.476	4.121	3.816	3.551	3.320	2.852	2.498	2.221	2.000
4.909	4.488	4.130	3.822	3.556	3.323	2.853	2.498	2.222	2.000
4.925	4.499	4.137	3.827	3.559	3.325	2.854	2.499	2.222	2.000
4.937	4.507	4.143	3.831	3.562	3.327	2.855	2.499	2.222	2.000
4.948	4.514	4.147	3.834	3.564	3.329	2.856	2.499	2.222	2.000
4.979	4.534	4.160	3.842	3.569	3.332	2.857	2.500	2.222	2.000
4.992	4.541	4.164	3.845	3.571	3.333	2.857	2.500	2.222	2.000
4.997	4.544	4.166	3.846	3.571	3.333	2.857	2.500	2.222	2.000
4.999	4.545	4.166	3.846	3.571	3.333	2.857	2.500	2.222	2.000
4.999	4.545	4.167	3.846	3.571	3.333	2.857	2.500	2.222	2.000

However, for long-range investment decisions, a projection of cash flows is more relevant data for use than accrual income measures.

The important variables and information needed to carry out this investment analysis include:

- Required rate of return or the discount rate used to measure the time value of money
- Economic life or the number of years for which cash inflows are anticipated
- Amount and timing of cash outflows
- Amount and timing of cash inflows

Each of these will be discussed in the next section.

Required Rate of Return

The required rate of return indicates the desired rate that a particular medical practice expects to achieve from any investment it makes. A rate of return to any investor is comprised of three elements: (1) a risk-free or real rate of return, (2) a recovery of any inflationary loss, and (3) a portion to cover the risk of losing the principal amount. If inflation is deemed to be a serious factor, future cash flows must be adjusted for this element. The possibility of losing all or a portion of the principal amount invested is gauged by an evaluation of the business risk surrounding the investment. This risk varies among types of investments and must be considered. We will have more to say about risk in a later section.

Managers use two methods to determine the appropriate discount rate for measuring the present value of future cash flows. The first approach involves the determination of the cost of capital; the second approach pertains to the opportunity cost of the funds to be invested.

The cost of capital relates to the minimum rate of return on a particular investment that an organization needs to achieve in order to cover the cost of acquiring and maintaining the entity's capital resources. The cost of capital (from the standpoint of the user of the funds) is determined by the general formula:

$$\text{Cost of capital} = \frac{\text{Annual payment to investor}}{\text{Market value of security}}$$

The annual payment to investor might, for example, be the amount of interest paid (received) from a debt instrument. The market value of security represents the current market price of the debt or equity security.

Each source of capital has a different cost. The commercial banker, the mortgage banker, and the physician have different expectations of how much he or she should earn on the investment in the medical group. The cost of capital approach would probably set a lower desired rate of return if the group were able to borrow all or a majority of the money for an investment in facilities and equipment than if the physician provided the funds. Owners of any business, particularly physician owners, seek a higher return than creditors seek.

The general formula for computing cost of capital applies to profit-making corporations. The cost of each source of capital is calculated, and a weighted average cost of capital is computed. This example illustrates this calculation:

> **Example:** *Assume a company in which the cost of debt capital (e.g., bonds) is 7 percent, the cost of equity capital (e.g., common stock) is 18 percent, 40 percent of the total capital is debt, and 60 percent of capital is equity. The cost of capital is calculated as follows:*

Capital		Weighted	
Type	Cost	Weight	Cost
Debt (bonds)	7%	0.4	2.8%
Equity (stock)	18%	0.6	10.8%
Total		1.0	13.6%

Thus, the cost of capital is 13.6 percent, rounded to 14 percent.

The cost of capital approach is difficult to apply in practice and involves careful reflection and estimates of future market conditions and personal preferences. For example, should a medical group seek to earn a reasonable rate of return on all assets employed? Should a medical group seek merely to recover the cost of its investment in facilities and equipment and compensate the physician out of charges for his or her professional services?

The second approach to determining the proper discount rate is an opportunity cost approach. This entails answering the question: What is the next best opportunity for obtaining a return for investing its funds? One of the best possible uses of cash is to make distributions to the physicians rather than retaining it in the practice and investing in some long-lived asset. The group should earn a rate of return not less than the next best opportunity for investing.

In the final analysis, the required rate of return will ultimately be decided by the group's management. Generally, the return demanded for an investment varies with the investment's risk. Thus, the required rate of return for an individual investment project of greater-than-average risk should be higher than the average rate of return on all projects. Conversely, a project with below-average risk should have a lower required rate.

There is another set of investment opportunities — called nondiscretionary projects — about which decisions will be made based on necessity rather than on the project's profitability. Examples include pollution-control equipment and installation of devices to protect employees from injury. These investments use capital but provide no demonstrable cash inflows. Thus, if the other discretionary investments had a present value of zero when discounted at cost of capital, the company would not recover all of its capital costs. In effect, the discretionary projects not only must stand on their own feet, but also must carry the capital-cost burden of the nondiscretionary (i.e., necessity) projects. For this reason, many companies use a required rate of return that is higher than the cost of capital.

Economic Life

The economic life of an investment is the number of years over which cash inflows are expected from the investment. When a proposed project involves the purchase of equipment or a facility, the economic life of the investment corresponds to the estimated service life of the equipment or facility to the user. When thinking about service life, one usually relates it to physical life — the number of years until the equipment wears out. Although the physical life can be considered an upper limit, in most cases, it is the economic life of the equipment that is considerably shorter than its physical life. One reason is that technological progress makes equipment obsolete, and the investment in the equipment will cease to earn a return when it is replaced by even better equipment.

The end of the period selected for the economic life is called the investment horizon. This suggests that beyond this time, cash inflows are not visible. Economic life can rarely be estimated exactly. Nevertheless, it is important that the best possible estimate be made because economic life has a significant effect on the calculations. In view of the uncertainties associated with the operation of an organization, most managers are conservative in estimating what the economic life of a proposed investment will be.

Amount and Timing of Cash Outflows

The relevant cash outflows are incremental cash outflows directly traceable to the investment. For most investment decisions, there will be a large initial cash outflow for the acquisition or construction of the asset, such as the purchase cost and shipping, installation, and training costs for a piece of equipment. In addition, all cash outflows relevant to the investment project must be identified. For equipment, this will include maintenance and repair costs, property taxes, and other cash outflows directly related to the asset. All additional resources that are related to the investment item and needed to support the higher level of activity such as an increase in working capital (e.g., increased accounts receivable and supplies inventory) must be included as cash outflows. When this working capital is recovered (usually at the end of the economic life), these amounts will be treated as cash inflows.

The present value of all relevant cash flows is being measured regardless of what they are called. A thousand dollars invested in working capital, in equipment, in maintenance, or in training personnel to operate the equipment are all relevant cash outflows.

Amount and Timing of Cash Inflows

Like cash outflows, the relevant cash inflows are the incremental cash inflows to be received in the future that are directly related to the investment decision. It does not matter what the particular cash inflow item is. A dollar of cost savings is as much a cash inflow as an additional dollar of cash collected for patient visits. Usually, most cash inflows emanate from the investment's earnings or the cost savings that result from putting the new investment into use. If the purchase of a new asset results in the sale of an existing asset, the net proceeds from the sale are treated as an element of cash inflow. The net proceeds from the existing asset are its selling price less any costs incurred in selling it and in dismantling and removing it.

IMPACT OF TAXES ON CASH FLOWS

As long as medical practices have the goal of not paying income taxes, taxes are not relevant to any decision. But any income taxes paid by a group must be considered as a cash outflow and taken into account in the analysis. Income taxes are based on taxable income of the entity, regardless of how it is measured. Even on the cash basis, the practice must use some accrual measurements for tax purposes such as depreciation. Thus, the amount of income taxes paid in a given year will be affected by depreciation of long-lived assets, as well as by operating cash inflows and cash outflows. Depreciation is the annual deduction allowed for recovery of an expenditure for fixed assets.

The tax code is very complex. The Modified Accelerated Cost Recovery System (MACRS) in the Tax Reform Act of 1986 applies to all tangible property in service after 1986. The amount of depreciation depends on three factors:

1. **Depreciation method** — The group may use a specified schedule (based on the declining balance method) or the straight-line method (equal amounts per year over the life of the asset).

2. **Recovery period** — A period of time is specified for each property class.

3. **First-year convention** — The group may choose to treat property as having been placed in service mid-year (half-year convention) or as having been placed in service in the middle of the quarter in which the property was acquired (mid-quarter convention).

Each item of property is assigned to one of eight property classes. Each class has a specific asset depreciation range (ADR). The most commonly used classes by medical groups are:

- **Five-year property** — includes automobiles, trucks, property used in research or experimentation, computers, and peripheral equipment and office machinery

- **Seven-year property** — includes office furniture and fixtures and any property that does not have a specifically designated class life and has not been defined by law as belonging to another class

- **Nonresidential real property** — this property is depreciated over 39 years

Exhibit 14.7 presents the depreciation percentage allowances permitted by the U.S. tax code for a piece of equipment with an asset class of five years that was purchased on the first day of the year. Note that the five-year class actually extends over six years. If the asset is held less than six years, the depreciation for the year of disposal should be prorated by multiplying the full year depreciation by the applicable percentage for the applicable convention (i.e., half year, mid-year, or mid-month).

Instead of claiming a depreciation deduction, the group may expense up to a certain amount per year of the cost of most tangible personal property and some real property. This amount is often referred to as a "Section 179" deduction after the tax code that governs the applicable rules. The limitation as to the amount and type of property eligible for this treatment varies by year. For example, the limit for 2011 was $500,000, with a limit of $250,000 for qualified real estate additions; these limits would be reduced for taxpayers with additions in excess of $2 million.

This description about income taxes is not intended to be a comprehensive discussion of medical practice tax issues. It is presented to demonstrate the impact of taxes on important decisions. Depending on the group's tax strategy, it is necessary to determine whether to expense up to the allowable amount of depreciable assets or depreciate them over a period of years or to use straight-line depreciation or an accelerated method, such as MACRS. In some cases, leasing may be more advantageous than buying. We will comment on the lease-or-buy decision in a later section.

Exhibit 14.8 shows the tax impact on the acquisition of a piece of equipment. Assume the equipment costs $100,000. Although the equipment has a five-year life for tax purposes, the group expects it to be replaced at the end of three years. The new equipment will reduce annual operating costs by $16,000 per year over three years. Any salvage or residual value is expected to be equal to the removal. The remaining undepreciated cost (or book value) of the equipment will be recognized as a loss at the time of disposal. Assume a 38 percent blended federal and state income tax rate for a professional service corporation. Exhibit 14.8 presents, first, the before-tax cash flows, and second, the after-tax cash flows.

EXHIBIT 14.7 ■ Asset Recovery Allowances for Tax Return — Five-Year Assets Class

Year	Half-Year Convention	Quarterly Convention (1st quarter)	Straight Line
1	20.00%	35.00%	10.00%
2	32.00%	26.00%	20.00%
3	19.20%	15.60%	20.00%
4	11.52%	11.01%	20.00%
5	11.52%	11.01%	20.00%
6	5.76%	1.38%	10.00%

EXHIBIT 14.8 ▪ Impact of Income Taxes on Cash Flows

	0 (Now)	Year 1	Year 2	Year 3
Before-tax cash flows				
Cash outflows:				
1. Payment of $100,000 for equipment	$(100,000)	$—	$—	$—
Cash inflows:				
2. Annual cost savings		$16,000	$16,000	$16,000
3. Additional patient billings	$—	$35,000	$35,000	$35,000
Total cash flows by year	$(100,000)	$51,000	$51,000	$51,000
After-tax cash flows				
Cash outflows:				
1. Payment of $100,000 for equipment	$(100,000)			
2. (Payment) refund of income taxes		$(6,080)	$(9,500)	$(4,560)
Cash inflows:				
3. Annual cost savings		$16,000	$16,000	$16,000
4. Additional patient billings	$—	$35,000	$35,000	$35,000
Total cash flows by year	$(100,000)	$44,920	$41,500	$46,440
Computation of income taxes:				
Additional patient billings		$35,000	$35,000	$35,000
Annual cost savings		$16,000	$16,000	$16,000
Total		$51,000	$51,000	$51,000
Less: Depreciation				
Year 1: $100,000 × 35%		$(35,000)		
Year 2: $100,000 × 26%			$(26,000)	
Year 3: $100,000 × 15.6%				$(15,600)
Loss on disposal of asset		$—	$—	$(23,400)
Taxable income (loss)		$16,000	$25,000	$12,000
Income tax payment (refund) 38%		$6,080	$9,500	$4,560

The before-tax cash flows are the investment of $100,000 now and cash inflows of $51,000 in each of the three years ($35,000 additional patient billings and $16,000 cost savings). The after-tax cash flows result in tax payments of $6,080 in Year 1; $9,500 in Year 2; and $4,560 in Year 3.

Different depreciation strategies would result in different cash flows. Exhibit 14.9 uses the same facts used in Exhibit 14.8, except that it uses Section 179 to expense the entire $100,000 cost of the equipment in Year 1, rather than using the applicable MACRS five-year property rates. For the purposes of this illustration, we are assuming that the amount spent for this piece of equipment combined with all other eligible assets added during the year of acquisition do not exceed the Section 179 limitation. Thus, the practice can expense the entire $100,000 cost of the equipment during the first year of the asset's life.

In comparing the cash flows in Exhibit 14.8 with those in Exhibit 14.9, notice that the before-tax cash flows are the same; however, the different deprecation methods create different tax situations, which in turn lead to different timing of cash flows. The Year 1 depreciation deduction of $100,000 is so large that

EXHIBIT 14.9 ■ Impact of Income Taxes on Cash Flows (Using Section 179 Depreciation)

	0 (Now)	Year 1	Year 2	Year 3
Before-tax cash flows				
Cash outflows:				
1. Payment of $100,000 for equipment	$(100,000)	$—	$—	$—
Cash inflows:				
2. Annual cost savings		$ 16,000	$16,000	$16,000
3. Additional patient billings	$—	$ 35,000	$ 35,000	$35,000
Total cash flows by year	$(100,000)	$51,000	$51,000	$51,000
After-tax cash flows				
Cash outflows:				
1. Payment of $100,000 for equipment	$(100,000)			
2. (Payment) refund of income taxes		$ 18,620	$ (19,380)	$(19,380)
Cash inflows:				
3. Annual cost savings		$ 16,000	$16,000	$16,000
4. Additional patient billings	$—	$ 35,000	$ 35,000	$35,000
Total cash flows by year	$(100,000)	$69,620	$31,620	$31,620
Computation of income taxes:				
Additional patient billings		$35,000	$35,000	$35,000
Annual cost savings		$16,000	$16,000	$16,000
Total		$51,000	$51,000	$51,000
Less: Depreciation				
Year 1: $100,000 × 35%		$(100,000)		
Year 2: $100,000 × 26%			$—	
Year 3: $100,000 × 15.6%				$—
Loss on disposal of asset		$—	$—	$—
Taxable income (loss)		$(49,000)	$51,000	$51,000
Income tax payment (refund) 38%		$(18,620)	$19,380	$19,380

EXHIBIT 14.10 ■ Computation of Present Values of Before-Tax Cash Flows for Investment

End of Year	Cash Inflows	×	Present Value Factor	=	Present Value
1	$51,000		0.893		$45,543
2	$51,000		0.797		$40,647
3	$51,000		0.712		$36,312
Total present value of cash inflows					$122,502
Less: Total present value of cash outflows					$100,000
Excess present value of cash inflows over present value of cash outflows					$22,502

Conclusion: The present value of cash inflows exceeds the present value of cash outflows; therefore, the investment project should be accepted.

it creates a taxable loss of $49,000, a tax refund of $18,620, and after-tax cash flows of $69,620. This is as compared to the MACRS depreciation taken in Exhibit 14.8 leading to Year 1 taxable income of $16,000, income tax expense of $6,080, and after-tax cash flows of $44,920. The situation reverses in Years 2 and 3. Because the Section 179 Deprecation Method used in Exhibit 14.9 took all the depreciation expense in Year 1, the practice gets no depreciation deduction in Years 2 or 3, and no loss on disposal of the equipment in Year 3. This leads to greater taxable income, great income tax expense, and lower after-tax cash flows in Years 2 and 3 for the Section 179 depreciation example in Exhibit 14.9.

Exhibit 14.10 applies the long-range decision rule to the before-tax cash flows from Exhibits 14.8 and 14.9 using an interest rate of 12 percent. Note that the before-tax cash flows were the same for both examples. Because discounted cash inflows exceed discounted cash outflows, the project is favorable and should be accepted.

Exhibit 14.11 applies the long-range decision rule to the after-tax cash flows from the examples in Exhibits 14.8 and 14.9. Although smaller than before considering taxes, the excess of discounted cash inflows over discounted cash outflows for both examples indicates a favorable project. Expensing the entire equipment cost of $100,000 in the first year provides a higher after-tax return because the practice gets the tax benefits at an earlier point in the project's life. Any postponement of cash outflows or advancements of cash inflows will increase the present value of the project and make it more favorable.

As you will note, determining the tax effect on an investment project is very complex. In addition to the tax provisions introduced in this section, there are many such provisions to be considered. Our presentation is intended to show that taxes affect cash flows and must be considered in the analysis.

EXHIBIT 14.11 ■ Computation of Present Values of After-Tax Cash Flows for Investments (Using MACRS Depreciation)

End of Year	Cash Inflows	×	Present Value Factor	=	Present Value
1	$44,920		0.893		$40,114
2	$41,500		0.797		$33,076
3	$46,440		0.712		$33,065

Total present value of cash inflows	$106,255
Less: Total present value of cash outflows	$100,000
Excess present value of cash inflows over present value of cash outflows	$6,255

Conclusion: The present value of cash inflows exceeds the present value of cash outflows; therefore, the investment project should be accepted.

Using Section 179 First-Year Expensing (from Exhibit 14.9)

End of Year	Cash Inflows	×	Present Value Factor	=	Present Value
1	$69,620		0.893		$62,171
2	$31,620		0.797		$25,201
3	$31,620		0.712		$22,513

Total present value of cash inflows	$109,885
Less: Total present value of cash outflows	$100,000
Excess present value of cash inflows over present value of cash outflows	$9,885

Conclusion: The present value of cash inflows exceeds the present value of cash outflows; therefore, the investment project should be accepted.

IMPACT OF INFLATION ON INFORMATION FOR LONG-RANGE DECISIONS

When prices are increasing at a 2 percent or less annual rate, one could safely ignore any impact of inflation on most decisions. However, double-digit inflation requires consideration when doing analyses about investment proposals.

As we have stated, the long-range decision rule requires the projection of cash flows over the life of the investment project and the selection of an appropriate discount rate. A common practice of projecting cash flows is to estimate the first year's cash flows and use those estimates over the life of the project. These estimates, however, must be adjusted for the impact of anticipated price changes. Because there are several cash flows, a single rate of inflation should not be used. Salaries, supplies, maintenance, fees charged to patients, and rent are expected to change at different rates. The appropriate rate of price changes should be applied to each cash flow.

For example, assume that costs are expected to increase by 10 percent per year and that fees to patients are expected to increase by only 5 percent per year. How will this affect the example used above? If it is assumed that the first-year projections are correct, the cash flows for Years 2 and 3 would be adjusted as follows:

Cost savings:
Year 1......................................$16,000
Year 2 — $16,000 × 110 percent.............17,600
Year 3 — $17,600 × 110 percent.............19,360

Additional patient billings:
Year 1...................................... $35,000
Year 2 — $35,000 × 105 percent.............36,750
Year 3 — $36,750 × 105 percent.............38,587

Because the cost savings and additional billings to patients are changed, additional taxes arising from the investment will also change. Depreciation amounts, however, will not change. The new taxes for the project originally introduced in Exhibit 14.8 are determined as follows:

	Year 1	Year 2	Year 3
Computation of income taxes:			
Additional patient billings	$35,000	$36,750	$38,587
Annual cost savings	$16,000	$17,600	$19,360
Total	$51,000	$54,350	$57,947
Less: Depreciation			
Year 1: $100,000 x 35%	$(35,000)		
Year 2: $100,000 x 26%		$(26,000)	
Year 3: $100,000 x 15.6%			$(15,600)
Loss on disposal of asset	$—	$—	$(23,400)
Taxable income (loss)	$16,000	$28,350	$18,947
Income tax payment (38%)	$6,080	$10,773	$7,200

The after-tax cash flows for the investment project are as follows:

	0 (Now)	Year 1	Year 2	Year 3
After-tax cash flows				
Cash outflows:				
1. Payment of $100,000 for equipment	$(100,000)			
2. (Payment) refund of income taxes		$(6,080)	$(10,773)	$(7,200)
Cash inflows				
3. Annual cost savings		$16,000	$17,600	$19,360
4. Additional patient bills	$—	$35,000	$36,750	$38,587
Total cash flows by year	$100,000	$44,920	$43,577	$50,747

EXHIBIT 14.12 ■ **Computation of Present Values of After-Tax Cash Flows for Investments Adjusted for Inflation**

End of Year	Cash Inflows	×	Present Value Factor	=	Present Value
1	$44,920		0.893		$40,114
2	$43,577		0.797		$34,731
3	$50,747		0.712		$36,132

Total present value of cash inflows	$110,977
Less: Total present value of cash outflows	$100,000
Excess present value of cash inflows over present value of cash outflows	$10,977

Conclusion: The present value of cash inflows exceeds the present value of cash outflows; therefore, the investment project should be accepted.

The discount rate, if properly determined, will reflect investors' expectations, and thus, already consider inflation. As the rate of inflation increases, investors will increase their expected returns, and the cost of capital will reflect these changed expectations.

Exhibit 14.12 applies the long-range decision rules to the after-tax cash flows adjusted for inflation. Adjusting the project for inflation has made it more attractive because the cash inflows were increased (as well as the tax effect). The cash outflow, however, was not increased. In other examples, both cash inflows and cash outflows may change. The results will not always improve the desirability of the project.

RISK AND UNCERTAINTY IN LONG-RANGE DECISIONS

In addition to the general lack of consideration of the time value of money in long-range investment decisions, medical practices do not always consider risk or uncertainty. Both of these factors concern the variability of future cash flows. Uncertainty relates to a lack of knowledge about future cash flows, but may be reduced through additional research. Additional information can usually be gathered but at a cost. The difficult point is determining when the added cost will be warranted. Risk, however, concerns factors over which the practice has no control. To accommodate these two factors, some analysts do not prepare a single estimate of cash flows for a given period for a particular project. Rather, they prepare a range of cash flows with an estimate of the probability of each occurring. For example, rather than a single project of additional billings of $35,000 in Year 3 in the previous illustration, the practice may determine an optimistic projection, a best estimate projection, and a pessimistic projection along with the probability of the likelihood for each to occur. To illustrate, assume the following range of estimates for additional billings for Year 3:

	Projection	Probability	Computation
Optimistic	$45,000	0.20	$9,000
Best estimate	$35,000	0.50	$17,500
Pessimistic	$25,000	0.30	$7,500
Weighted probability estimate			$34,000

By multiplying each project by its probability and totaling the three, a projection of $34,000 is reached. The heavier weighting of the pessimistic estimate reduced the single projection of $35,000 to a weighted probability estimate of $34,000.

In addition to using a range of values for each projection, two other ways of adjusting for risk are commonly used. First, you can increase the discount rate whereby the present values of the cash inflows decline because the practice is placing less reliance on the later projections that have both greater uncertainty and greater risk. To demonstrate this point, examine Exhibit 14.5 for 10 percent and 20 percent rates over a five-year period and note the lower present value factors for the 20 percent rates.

The second method of adjusting for risk involves the use of two decision criteria discussed later. The project should not only meet the long-range decision rule but should also pay back the investment over a short period of time. In this way, the group recovers its investment in the early years when uncertainty and risk are lower but also earns the desired rate of return.

For any investment project, the analyst should ask a number of "what if" questions. In doing so, the analyst will develop an estimate of the sensitivity of the project to errors in estimates. If the project involves a replacement of existing equipment with newer equipment where there are few unknowns, the estimates will be very reliable. However, when acquiring a new technology that is untried, future cash flows will be subject to a great deal of variability. Much of decision making is learning to deal with uncertainty and risk.

TECHNIQUES OF CAPITAL BUDGETING

Since long-range investment decisions are some of the most important decisions that group management makes, a system for evaluating, planning, and controlling these investments must be carefully developed and implemented. The system is referred to as a *capital budgeting process* and usually involves some formalities in larger groups. There may be written proposals developed for each potential long-term investment opportunity that include a description of the nature of the project, the benefits to be expected, and the costs involved. The system will also have a designated flow of proposal preparation and documentation, a review procedure for each proposal, and a final approval process by the governing body.

There are several techniques used to evaluate capital investment proposals, and they can be grouped into two general categories: (1) techniques that satisfy the long-range decision rule and (2) techniques that do not satisfy this rule. The characteristic that distinguishes one category from the other is the way in which the concept of the time value of money is treated. As stated earlier, the long-range-decision rule embodies the use of the time value of money by employing present value calculations.

The techniques that satisfy the long-range decision rule are (1) the net present value method and (2) the internal rate of return method, sometimes called the adjusted rate of return method. The two techniques that do not satisfy the long-range decision rule are (1) the payback period method and (2) the average rate of return method, sometimes called the unadjusted rate of return method or the accounting rate of return.

In many companies and in some medical groups, management will use some combination of the four methods in evaluating various aspects of the long-range investment proposals. Each of the methods has advantages and limitations, and some of the computations can become rather complex. With the use of a computer, however, the calculations can be performed easily and quickly. More importantly, the computer can be used to develop models that track changes in key factors of the long-range investment proposals. We will discuss each of these methods next.

Net Present Value Method

As pointed out in our previous illustrations, an investment in equipment or a facility may be viewed as the acquisition of a series of future net cash inflows that are composed of two elements: (1) the recovery of the initial investment and (2) income. The period of time over which these net cash inflows will be received may be an important factor in determining the value of the investment.

The net present value method uses present value concepts to compute the net present value of the cash flows expected from a proposal. The long-range decision rule is stated in terms of the net present value method. It requires that the discounted cash inflows be at least equal to the discounted cash outflows. Discounted cash outflows are deducted from discounted cash inflows to measure the net present value. A zero net present value indicates that exactly the desired rate of return will be earned from those particular cash flows. If the net present value is positive (i.e., discounted cash inflows exceed discounted cash outflows), more than the desired rate of return is being earned. If the net present value is negative — the discounted cash outflows exceed the discounted cash inflows — the desired rate of return is not being achieved. For example, assume that a piece of equipment may be purchased for $3,170. This equipment will generate cost savings of $1,000 each year for four years. If taxes are ignored, and a desired rate of return of 10 percent is assumed, is this a good investment?

> Present value of cash outflows................. $(3,170)
> Present value of cash inflows ($1,000 × 3.170) = 3,170
> Net present value $0

The zero net present value indicates that the investment will generate exactly 10 percent.

To prove that 10 percent will be earned, examine the return from investment and the recovery of the initial investment over the four periods in Exhibit 14.13. Note that a portion of each $1,000 cash inflow represents recovery of the investment. In Year 1, $317 was earned, a 10 percent return on an investment of $3,170. The balance of the Year 1 cash inflow ($683 of the $1,000) reduced the investment from $3,170 to $2,487. The final cash inflow of $1,000 in Year 4 included income of $91 and reduced the investment to zero (actually a $1 balance remains, due to rounding).

EXHIBIT 14.13 ▪ Illustration of Recovery of an Investment

Year	Investment at Beginning of Year	10% Return on Beginning Balance	Balance of $1,000 Annual Cash Inflow	Investment at End of Year
1	$3,170	$317	$683	$2,487
2	$2,487	$249	$751	$1,736
3	$1,786	$174	$826	$910
4	$910	$91	$909	$1*

* Rounding error

Let's review the four investments introduced earlier. It should be noted that each investment involved a $1,000 cash outflow and a total of $1,200 cash inflow. The only difference among the investments is the timing of cash inflows:

Investment	Initial Investment Amount	Cash Inflows by Year 1	2	3
A	$1,000		$1,200	
B	$1,000	$600	$400	$200
C	$1,000	$200	$400	$600
D	$1,000	$400	$400	$400

The net present value of each investment, assuming a desired rate of return of 10 percent, follows. The details of the calculations are not repeated; refer to the earlier illustrations for the specific calculations.

Investment	Present Value of Cash Outflows	Present Value of Cash Inflows	Net Present Value
A	$(1,000)	$991	$(9)
B	$(1,000)	$1,025	$25
C	$(1,000)	$963	$(37)
D	$(1,000)	$994	$(6)

In no case was the net present value exactly zero; therefore, none of the investments earned exactly 10 percent. If it is assumed that 10 percent is the cutoff rate for investing or not investing, only Investment B should be accepted. Although Investment D is earning close to 10 percent, it is still below 10 percent.

The net present value technique has distinct advantages over all other techniques. It is simple and does not involve repeated calculations that may be necessary in the internal or adjusted rate of return method. The net present value method can be applied in any situation, regardless of whether cash inflows are equal or unequal and in cases where competing projects have unequal lives.

The net present value method is perceived to be the easier of the two methods. As it incorporates the time value of money and is superior to the methods not using time value of money principles, the following summarizes its use:

Step 1. Select a required rate of return for all investment proposals. This rate applies to projects deemed to be of average risk and may be adjusted for a specific proposal where risk is felt to be well above or below average.

Step 2. Estimate the economic life of the proposed project.

Step 3. Estimate the net cash inflows for each year during the economic life.

Step 4. Find the net investment or net cash outflows pertaining to the proposed project.

Step 5. Find the present value of all the cash inflows identified in Step 3 by discounting them at the required rate of return, using the table in Exhibit 14.5 (for single annual amounts) or the table in Exhibit 14.6 (for a series of equal annual amounts).

Step 6. Find the net present value by subtracting the present value of the net cash outflows from the present value of the net cash inflows. If the net present value is zero or positive, the proposal is acceptable insofar as the monetary factors are concerned.

Step 7. Consider the nonmonetary factors related to the proposal before a final decision is reached. (This part of the process is at least as important as all other parts and should not be omitted.) More will be said about this aspect in a later section.

Internal Rate of Return or Adjusted Rate of Return Method

When the net present value method is used, the required rate of return must be selected in advance of making the calculations because this rate is used to discount the cash inflows in each year. As mentioned earlier, the choice of an appropriate rate of return is a difficult matter. While this required rate of return still needs to be determined, it is not used in making the calculations of present value in the internal or adjusted rate of return method. This method computes the rate of return that equates the present value of the cash inflows with the amount of net investment or the present value of the cash outflows, that is, the rate that makes the net present value equal zero. This rate is called the internal rate of return or the adjusted rate of return.

After this adjusted rate of return is calculated, it is then compared to the required rate of return, sometimes called a cutoff rate. The decision rule: Any investment project earning less than the cutoff rate should be rejected; any investment project earning at or above the cutoff rate should be accepted. The cutoff rate may be increased or decreased to reflect the availability of funds and other factors such as risk.

The adjusted rate of return is computed in two ways depending on the nature of the cash flows. If the cash outflow is a single amount at the beginning of the project and the cash inflows are in a stream of equal receipts (an annuity), the adjusted rate of return may be determined by the use of present value tables. For example, what is the adjusted rate of return for a piece of equipment with an initial cost of $32,740 and annual cash inflows of $10,000 for five years?

This approach involves two steps. First, determine the present value factor (PVF) that equates the initial cash outflow and the stream of cash inflows. Second, find the PVF computed in the first step in Exhibit 14.6. In the example, the PVF that equates the cash inflows and cash outflows is 3.274, determined as follows:

$$\$32,740 = \$10,000 \times PVF$$

$$PVF = \frac{\$32,740}{\$10,000}$$

$$PVF = 3.274$$

For the next step, find the PVF nearest 3.274 in the five-year row (remember the project had a five-year life). The PVF in the 16 percent column of the five-year row is 3.274, indicating an adjusted rate of return of 16 percent. If the computed PVF falls between two values in the table, it will be necessary to estimate the actual rate by interpolating between the two columns in the table.

Now return to Investments A, B, C, and D. The actual rates of return for Investments A and D may be determined from the present value tables. Investment A involves a single receipt of $1,200; therefore, it will be necessary to use Exhibit 14.5. The PVF that equates the two cash flows is 0.833, determined as follows:

$$\$1,000 = \$1,200 \times PVF$$

$$PVF = \frac{\$1,000}{\$1,200} = 0.833$$

In the two-year row of Exhibit 14.5, 0.833 falls between the 8 percent and 10 percent columns. By interpolation, the actual rate is found to be 9.54 percent:

$$ARR = 8\% + 2\% [(0.857 - 0.833)/(0.857 - 0.826)]$$
$$= 8\% + 2\% (0.77)$$
$$= 9.54\%$$

Investment D involves a $1,000 investment and an annuity of $400 for three years. The PVF that equates the two cash flows is 2.500, determined as follows:

$$\$1,000 = \$400 \times \text{PVF}$$

$$\text{PVF} = \frac{\$1,000}{\$400} = 2.500$$

In the three-year row of Exhibit 14.6, the PVF of 2.500 also falls between the 8 percent and 10 percent columns. The actual rate of return is found by interpolation:

$$\text{ARR} = 8\% + 2\% \, [(2.577 - 2.500)/(2.577 - 2.486)]$$
$$= 8\% + 2\% \, (0.85)$$
$$= 9.70\%$$

If the cash inflows over the lifetime of the investment are not equal, a trial-and-error method must be used. Remember that if the desired rate of return on investment is attained, the net present value of cash flows is zero. This approach involves computing the net present value of the cash flows at different rates until a zero net present value is achieved. From earlier calculations, it is known that Investment B will have an actual rate of return above 10 percent, and Investment C will have an actual rate below 10 percent. As a second trial for Investment B, 12 percent is used as follows:

Present value of cash outflows. . . . . $(1,000)

Present value of cash inflows:

   Year 1 — $600 × 0.893 = $536

   Year 2 — $400 × 0.797 = $319

   Year 3 — $200 × 0.712 = $142 . . . . $997

Net present value . . . . $(3)

Because the net present value is so near to zero, the practice will accept 12 percent as the adjusted rate of return. Similarly, the actual rate of return for Investment C may be determined by computing the net present value at 8 percent:

Present value of cash outflows. . . . . $ (1,000)

Present value of cash inflows:

   Year 1 — $200 × 0.926 = $185

   Year 2 — $400 × 0.857 = $343

   Year 3 — $600 × 0.794 = $476 . . . . $1,004

Net present value $4

The net present value for Investment C is so near zero that an actual rate of 8 percent may be accepted. The actual adjusted rates of return for the four investments are:

Investment	Actual Adjusted Rate of Return
A	9.54%
B	12.00%
C	8.00%
D	9.70%

If the cutoff rate is 10 percent, only Investment B is acceptable. Note the decision under the adjusted rate of return method is exactly the same as that reached under the net present value method.

The Payback Period Method

Of all the techniques of investment analysis, the payback period method is the simplest and the most widely used by medical groups. The payback period method, as the name implies, calculates the payback period or the number of years over which the investment outlay will be recovered or paid back from the cash inflows, assuming the estimates made turn out to be correct. The decision rule: If the payback period is more than, equal to, or slightly less than the economic life of the project, then the proposal is clearly unacceptable. If the payback period is considerably less than the economic life, then the project begins to look attractive.

Calculation of the payback period for the four investment projects examined earlier shows a range from one and five-sixth years to two and two-thirds years, as shown in the following calculation:

Investment	Invested Amount	Period 1	Period 2	Period 3	Payback Period
A	$1,000	$0	$1,200	$0	$1\frac{5}{6}$ years
B	$1,000	$600	$400	$200	2 years
C	$1,000	$200	$400	$600	$2\frac{2}{3}$ years
D	$1,000	$400	$400	$400	$2\frac{1}{2}$ years

If the cutoff time period for the return of the initial investment is less than two years, only Investment A would be acceptable. The decision maker may stretch it to approve Investment B but would reject Investments C and D. It is interesting to note that the investment evaluated as the most profitable when using the net present value or the adjusted rate of return methods is rejected if less than a two-year payback period is used as the decision criterion. In the illustration, however, an investment found unacceptable by the net present value method is evaluated as the best proposed under the payback period method.

The major deficiency in the payback period method is that neither the profitability nor the life of the investment beyond the payback period is considered. For example, the following two investments have the same payback period but substantially different rates of return:

	Investment X	Investment Y
Initial investment	$10,000	$5,000
Annual cash inflow	$5,000	$2,500
Estimated useful life	2 years	5 years
Payback period	2 years	2 years

The payback period method provides an excellent supplement to the net present value or adjusted rate of return methods. This is true when there is a high degree of risk associated with the investment or when the rate of obsolescence is high. In these cases, the better investment will be the one that pays back its investment first.

Average or Unadjusted Rate of Return Method

In this method (also sometimes called the accounting rate of return), cash flows are not used to compute a rate of return for a particular investment. Rather, accounting income or the income amount derived by the application of generally accepted accounting principles is employed in the calculation, as follows:

$$\frac{\text{Accounting or unadjusted}}{\text{rate of return}} = \frac{\text{Average annual accounting income}}{\text{Initial investment}}$$

Because average accounting income is used, all investments with equal lives, equal total income, and equal initial investments will be evaluated the same, regardless of when the cash is recovered. To illustrate this point, the accounting or unadjusted rates of return are computed for four investments as shown:

Investment	Average Inflows	Straight-Line Depreciation	Annual Income	Initial Investment	Adjusted Rate of Return
A	$600	$500	$100	$1,000	10.0%
B	$400	$333	$67	$1,000	6.7%
C	$400	$333	$67	$1,000	6.7%
D	$400	$333	$67	$1,000	6.7%

Like the payback method, the unadjusted rate of return method evaluated in Investment A is highest because of its shorter life. Note that Investments B, C, and D have identical unadjusted rates of return because total cash revenues and total costs for the three-year period are the same.

The accounting or unadjusted rate of return uses accounting measurements; thus, it is consistent with the accounting records. Those practices that use this method do so because it is easily understood and consistent with the accounting records. Conceptually, though, this method does not provide the best way to evaluate new investment proposals.

Nonmonetary Considerations

The quantitative information just illustrated does not provide the complete picture of the variables to be considered in deciding on long-range investment proposals. The quantitative data encompass only those elements that can be reduced to numbers. As was true in our discussion about short-range investment opportunities, full consideration of all short- and long-range proposals involves evaluating the nonmonetary factors, as well. For example, assume a group used a net present value calculation to evaluate the likely profitability of purchasing a new scanner, and the analysis clearly indicated that the investment is highly desirable from a quantitative basis. However, assume a possibility exists that new governmental regulations, arising from a national healthcare program, may establish controls over the number of these scanners that may be permitted in the geographical region of the medical group. This potential dampening effect on the use of the scanner may become the overriding factor in causing a negative decision on the acquisition. Qualitative factors like these that do not have any reasonable quantitative base must be considered with equal weight with the numbers in reaching a final decision on the investment proposals.

LONG-RANGE DECISIONS — SOME SUMMARY COMMENTS

In this chapter, we portray a riskless world of certainty. In each of the examples, the amounts to be paid and received are certain. In reality, financial managers are faced with both risk and uncertainty. Uncertainty involves a lack of knowledge. With more thorough research and modeling of a situation, however, uncertainty can be brought into manageable proportions. Risk, on the other hand, involves an inability to control the outcome of given actions. Many managers are at the mercy of conditions or events that are beyond their control. Investment decisions often involve a tendency to compensate for risk and uncertainty by insisting that the investment be recovered early and that greater return be achieved on the investment.

The decision rules and the techniques developed in this chapter are to be used to determine which of a number of proposals for acquiring capacity are economically feasible. It must be remembered that the tools presented do not replace the judgment of a medical group's financial manager and governing body. Intangible factors often outweigh economic logic; however, a decision maker using these techniques will be aware of the costs to the practice that relate to noneconomic criteria.

To the Point

- Short-range investment decisions relate to short periods of time; usually involve repetitive activities; and pertain to the kinds, amounts, and prices of services that will be performed with the existing capacity of the organization.

▪ To make short-range investment decisions, the process involves choosing the best alternative after defining the problem, selecting possible alternative solutions, identifying and measuring consequences of each, and making a decision.

▪ Short-range decision making can be called differential analysis in that the process entails comparing relevant benefits (changes in revenue directly attributable to the decision) with relevant costs (changes in costs directly attributable to the decision).

▪ In determining relevant costs in short-run analysis, the concepts of fixed and variable costs, avoidable costs, and full costs are used.

▪ Typical applications of relevant costs and benefits in short-term decision making include break-even analysis for helping to decide whether to add another physician or drop an activity from the practice.

▪ Long-range investments are commitments of funds to acquire an asset that will provide benefits over a long period of time.

▪ Time value of money is a concept that recognizes that a dollar of cash today is worth more than a dollar of cash in the future because of the interest factor. There are two directions for using time value of money concepts: Future value is the amount to which a given amount of cash invested now will grow at the end of a specific period of time when compounded at a designated rate of interest. Present value of an amount expected to be received at a specified time in the future is the amount that, if invested today at a designated rate of return, would cumulate to the specified amount.

▪ Using the time value of money, the long-range decision rule is: A long-range decision is favorable if the incremental discounted cash inflows attributable to the investment proposal are equal to or greater than the incremental discounted cash outflows attributable to the investment.

▪ The important variables and information needed to carry out discounted cash flow analysis are:

　— Required rate of return or the discount rate used to measure the time value of money

- Economic life or the number of years for which cash inflows are anticipated
- Amount and timing of cash outflows
- Amount and timing of cash inflows

◼ Risk and uncertainty are crucial variables that require special consideration in the evaluation of the quantitative data.

◼ There are two general categories of capital budgeting techniques. Techniques satisfying the long-range decision rule are (1) the net present value method and (2) the internal or adjusted rate of return method. Techniques that do not satisfy this rule are (1) the payback period method and (2) the average or unadjusted rate of return method.

◼ The net present value method finds the net present value of a project by subtracting the present value of the net cash outflows from the present value of the net cash inflows. If the net present value is zero or positive, the proposal is acceptable as far as the monetary factors are concerned.

◼ The adjusted rate of return method computes the rate of return implicit in the net cash inflows that equates the present value of the net cash inflows with the amount of the net investment. This rate is compared with the desired rate of return or cutoff rate. If the project earns less than the cutoff rate, the project is rejected. If it earns more, the project is accepted.

◼ The payback period method calculates the payback period or the number of years over which the investment outlay will be recovered or paid back from the cash inflows. If the payback period is more than, equal to, or slightly less than the economic life of the project, then the proposal is clearly unacceptable. If the payback period is considerably less than the economic life, then the project begins to look attractive.

◼ The unadjusted rate of return method calculates a return using accounting measurements of the average annual accounting income divided by the initial investment. This method is not used very widely because it does not use cash flows and does not consider the timing of the cash flows.

◼ Nonmonetary factors need to be considered along with the quantitative data before a final decision is made on all short- and long-range investment proposals.

CHAPTER 15

Assessing Capital Needs and Evaluating Sources of Capital

Edited by James D. Barrett, MS, FACMPE

After completing this chapter, you will be able to:

- Understand why physicians and medical groups need capital.

- Be able to relate capital needs to the type of medical group.

- Know about the various sources of financing for medical groups.

- Understand how financing relates to strategic planning.

- Evaluate potential capital partners.

- Develop a financially oriented capital business plan.

Capital Needs of Medical Group Practices

Joseph Hutts, CEO of Phycor, the first large physician practice management company (PPMC), said that his experience indicates that medical groups need capital for four primary reasons. He said, "The most important is to build critical mass, primarily through the expansion of primary care. Information system development is often the second most important requirement, followed by the needs of managed care and maintaining state-of-the-art equipment."

Keith Korenchuk, a healthcare attorney with Davis Wright Tremaine, LLP, looks at the financial needs of medical groups a little differently. "The first funding need is practice rationalization, including the addition of specialties and satellite offices. Secondly, there is often a need to internalize ancillaries. Third, there are the long-term readiness needs such as information system and improving patterns of care." He added, "Some groups may also need capital to get into the disease management business."

In considering the opinions of Hutts and Korenchuk, along with others in medical groups and the investment community, we find that the most common requirements for funding fall into the 10 categories discussed in the paragraphs that follow. Not every medical group has capital needs for all 10; many focus on just two or three. Exhibit 15.1 provides a list of common needs for capital.

Capital Requirement #1: Growing and Optimizing the Existing Practice

Many physician practices have the opportunity to increase their revenues but are hindered by the lack of available funding. One physician leader of a multispecialty clinic with a strong primary care component told us, "The docs in our clinic aren't real excited about retaining earnings for network development or information systems. They need to pay their taxes, and when this is done, there isn't much left over."

EXHIBIT 15.1   ■   Common Needs for Capital

1. Growing and optimizing the existing practice
2. Adding primary care physicians and sites
3. Investing in new profit centers
4. Adding next-generation facilities and equipment
5. Adding next-generation information systems
6. Developing single-specialty networks
7. Accepting and managing medical risk
8. Providing an exit strategy for older physicians
9. Covering cash flow shortages
10. Insulating against risk

For most multispecialty clinics, initiatives that enhance revenues and patient growth are part of their business strategy. None of these types of groups is satisfied with the status quo. Of course, implementing a growth strategy takes capital to hire physicians, build practices, develop new practice locations, contract with health plans, and market to consumers.

The reality is that growth involves an element of risk. The larger the risk in proportion to the operating base of the existing organization, the stronger the argument for outside capital. By outside capital, we are referring to bank loans or leasing or funds from hospitals, PPMCs, and other sources.

Capital Requirement #2: Adding Primary Care Physicians and Sites

Primary care network development continues to be one of the more controversial, more prevalent, and most necessary uses of funds. Large multispecialty groups add locations and build their own primary care bases. The need to acquire primary care practices is often important for multispecialty clinics that use these practices to support insurance contracts that will generate referrals to specialists or to serve health plan subscribers. Many multispecialty clinics have significant primary care networks. Although some sites are built from scratch, many are acquired from physicians with established practices. For example:

- Marshfield Clinic in central Wisconsin has 30 primary care locations. The majority of these practices were acquired.
- Carle Clinic in Urbana, Illinois, has 15 primary care sites.
- Meritcare in Fargo has 32 locations in eastern North Dakota and western Minnesota.
- Park Nicollet, part of HealthSystem Minnesota, has 19 sites in Minneapolis.
- Scott & White Clinic in Temple, Texas, has 19 locations covering a broad geographic area between Dallas and Ft. Worth to the north and Austin to the south.

Although acquisition of primary care practices may not generate positive direct returns, it is an excellent strategy, especially for multispecialty clinics and integrated healthcare systems. In certain situations, it is also a reasonable strategy for hospitals and health plans. There are ample opportunities to structure primary care investments in such a way that they do not incur significant losses, even on a direct accounting basis.

Capital Requirement #3: Investing in New Profit Centers

Physicians often have the opportunity to invest in new ventures. These include outpatient surgery centers, provider-owned health plans, medical office buildings, or a piece of medical equipment (e.g., cath lab). These investments tend to be risky, capital-intensive endeavors. However, for many medical groups, the upside potential more than justifies the risk.

The following are examples of situations in which new profit centers might be identified:

■ A practice internalizes its diagnostic equipment.

■ A group practice, its PPMC, and its hospital affiliate jointly develop an ambulatory surgery center. (By PPMCs, we are referring to for-profit entities that manage physician practices. About 30 PPMCs are publicly traded on stock exchanges and another 300 are in the venture capital stage.)

■ A physician MSO buys a former hospital and converts it into a diagnostic center.

■ A practice and its PPMC develop their own hospital.

In these four examples, the medical practices required outside capital to meet their strategic goals. Although in many ways disparate, the examples have certain common characteristics:

1. The funding requirements and risks are large enough for the medical group to believe that it has a need for outside capital to supplement what it can raise from more conventional sources.

2. The upside potential is substantial, more than enough to provide an incentive for outside investors to become involved.

3. The implications for physicians go beyond the new profit centers themselves. The strategic implications often redefine the business purpose of the medical group.

Capital Requirement #4: Adding Next-Generation Facilities and Equipment

Compared with several of the emerging needs for funding, such as primary care network development and the acquisition of clinical information systems, the need for capital to build new offices and purchase equipment seems mundane. However, it is not. These requirements continue, and with rapid technology advances in medical equipment, there is no easy solution at hand.

New locations — In addition to the requisites for modernized and expanded facilities, many clinics need to move to new locations, either adjacent to a hospital or into growth areas. Many hospitals and integrated systems and physician networks are finding that the practices are not in optimal locations for meeting consumer demands. Like banks and supermarkets, the growth of many metropolitan areas is forcing medical groups to move farther out into the suburbs.

Construction costs — With construction costs running well over $250 per square foot for clinic space plus furnishings and equipment, a group of physicians can quickly find themselves in a multimillion dollar building with huge debt service payments.

Hospitals have traditionally been a source of financial assistance in these kinds of situations, often using off-balance sheet financing. Even when physicians join a PPMC, they may find that the PPMC does not want to purchase fixed assets. However, most PPMCs will assist in finding financial resources for real estate-oriented financial needs.

Capital Requirement #5: Adding Next-Generation Information Systems

Of all the reasons that medical groups need capital, adding next-generation information systems may be the most important. Every medical group is considering what it needs to do to improve its clinical and management information systems. These systems are essential for contracting managed care, controlling costs, developing clinical guidelines, measuring medical outcomes, and managing the group practice. Further information on information systems is provided in chapter 4. The development of information systems can be costly but needs to be done.

In regard to medical groups that become part of a PPMC, Doug Williams, a partner with Arthur Andersen in Dallas, said that the cost of information system development depends on the structure of the organization in terms of a practice's geographic location. He added, "A company with 65 physicians in one building will spend a lot less than one with 100 primary care sites." Physician practices will need to invest dollars in information management and link all clinics through new software.

The information system advantage of PPMCs — Some of the organizations providing capital for medical groups also offer access to information systems as part of the package. In other words, being part of an established PPMC can mean that a medical group can avoid the full cost of information system development. Furthermore, participating groups can gain access to the experience of these PPMCs with a variety of approaches to information system development at the practice level.

Capital Requirement #6: Developing Single-Specialty Networks

The movement toward medical groups acquiring or merging with other practices has progressed well beyond multispecialty groups. Single-specialty groups are getting together, not only in the same market, but also across markets.

In specialty after specialty — cardiology, neonatology, ophthalmology, oncology, orthopedics, and podiatry — medical practices are exploring opportunities to come together. Their interest in larger single-specialty networking is stimulated in part by the chance to invest in new profit centers related to their specialty (see Capital Requirement #3); however, it is also related to the longer-term potential to provide a better form of care by focusing on specific diseases and the infrastructure, data, and management systems that would optimize their treatment.

The development of national single-specialty networks, or the acquisition of specialty groups by either multispecialty clinics or other single-specialty clinics, also requires significant capital resources. As groups of oncologists, orthopedists, cardiologists, and other specialists consolidate their practices, the accumulation of assets and the costs of clinical and administrative integration often require capital to fund new infrastructure development. In cases involving successful specialists, the capital has tended to be internally generated. However, these specialty groups often turn to PPMCs and other external financial sources.

Capital Requirement #7: Accepting and Managing Medical Risk

Much of the consolidation of physician practices and their need for capital goes back to the early growth of managed care. One healthcare consultant observed, "This is what triggered the recognition on the part of many doctors that in order to compete and meet patients' needs, they were going to have to consolidate and work together with the managed care plans." Indeed, there appears to be a correlation between the medical groups recognizing that they need capital and the growth of managed care in their markets.

Infrastructure development needs — One of the authors facilitated a meeting between the top managers of a large health plan and a number of tightly organized medical groups. One of the key issues: Did the groups have the capability to pay physician and hospital claims and manage medical costs? All responded that they did have these capabilities and thought, "Let us at those capitated dollars, and see what we can do!" In other words, physicians want to have access to capitated payment because they think they can make more money this way than on fee-for-service. This would normally be the attitude of a well-organized primary care group.

But paying claims is only part of it. Medical groups also have to demonstrate the capabilities to perform medical management. This includes developing and implementing clinical guidelines and finding innovative ways to deliver care in more cost-effective ways. Developing this infrastructure will require capital. (More recent research indicates that paying claims and performing medical management functions have often proven more difficult than anticipated, and many primary care groups have pulled back from accepting global capitation.)

Market clout — Related to dealing with health plans in a managed care environment, one of the reasons that physicians seek a capital partner is to grow and gain market power. Practices that position themselves as critical to any network development by a managed care organization have developed market clout.

In practice, it is often difficult for single-specialty groups to exercise market clout. With the huge surpluses of specialists in many areas, payers often have a multitude of choices. The reality is that market power probably doesn't exist, at least in a meaningful sense.

Capital Requirement #8: Providing an Exit Strategy for Older Physicians

One of the reasons physicians and medical groups are interested in external funding is that it represents a once-in-a-lifetime opportunity to sell their interest in the practice at a substantially higher price than might otherwise be possible. In other words, finding a capital partner is a way to accomplish a difficult task — converting an equity interest in a closely held small business, namely a physician practice — into cash.

In the past, retiring physicians typically recruited doctors right out of residency who would be expected to take over the practice as the founder(s) retired. The sale price would normally be based on book value plus a small premium for "goodwill." A decade ago, most of the literature on buying and selling medical groups or a solo practice focused on how to estimate goodwill — the "premium" that the practice was worth beyond tangible assets such as accounts receivable and equipment. In some cases, this was referred to as the value of the medical records or the patient base that had been built up by the founders over several decades.

However, with the growth in managed care and pressures to consolidate, solo practices often have little or no intrinsic value. It has become virtually impossible for a retiring physician to find a recent graduate to purchase a practice. Therefore, many of these traditional types of physicians face the prospect of closing down their practices at retirement with no opportunity to realize significant financial returns (other than the cash flow they generated) from their lifetime of work.

For many older physicians, the market pressures to consolidate plus the availability of financing, initially from hospitals and more recently from PPMCs, have been a godsend. It often meant that a practice built up over 30 or 40 years had economic value and someone willing to pay for it, often at a price well beyond expectations.

In effect, the traditional exit strategy for older physicians requires a significant investment from younger physicians. Most arrangements that involve selling a practice or some or all of the practice's assets to a third party also have the effect of reducing the buy-in of entering physicians. "We will be more competitive in recruiting," argues the leader of a large Kansas multispecialty group that is considering selling its assets. While this is true, it may also limit the upside potential for the new physicians. Their buy-in will be lower, but they will have to share future practice revenues with an outside investor in a way that their predecessors never experienced.

Capital Requirement #9: Covering Cash Flow Shortages

Typical activities within medical group practices include hiring new providers, moving to new offices, adding equipment, and developing new networks. If undertaken by an existing group without adequate capital, they are all likely to lead to short-term reductions in cash flow.

Most medical group administrators work hard to avoid disenchanting their physicians by causing their take-home pay to decline in the pay period after new strategies have been initiated. It has become commonplace in financial transactions to recognize the need for protection against short-term cash flow problems.

Fluctuations in cash flow are very much a part of doing business as a medical group. When special expenses are added on top of the normal cash-flow ups and downs, the probabilities of an occasional monthly shortfall increase dramatically. Making sure that the medical group has an adequate base of working capital (usually short-term lines of credit from commercial banks) is one way to guard against these circumstances.

Capital Requirement #10: Insulating against Risk

As one medical group administrator said, "It is almost impossible to plan even six months down the road. We know that reimbursement rates are going to drop, and that competition will become more intense. It's going to take deep pockets to weather the storm."

In discussing why the Dreyer Medical Clinic, a 103-physician multispecialty group in Aurora, Illinois, 35 miles west of Chicago, decided to affiliate with Advocate Health System, clinic president John Potter said that he did not think the clinic could grow fast enough or keep up with competition on its own.

Many healthcare organizations, including hospitals and medical groups, long for the "deep pockets" of a financial partner. Part of this is in response to the financial resources of several large health plans; hospital systems (both for profit and not for profit); and during the mid- to late 1990s, Wall Street-backed PPMCs. There is a sense of security about the future when physicians have access to capital, and this is another of the factors driving physician practices to seek capital partners.

DIFFERENT GROUPS, DIFFERENT NEEDS: FOUR INVESTMENT PHILOSOPHIES

How is it that two medical groups can be similar and face comparable circumstances and yet make such different choices on business strategies and capital partners? Just as the personalities of physicians differ, so do the personalities and cultures of medical groups. Just as the investment patterns of individuals differ, so do those of physician practices.

There are at least four different investment philosophies at work among medical groups: (1) aggressive long-term investors, (2) aggressive short-term investors, (3) cautiously optimistic investors, and (4) defensive investors. Each philosophy is briefly described in the following paragraphs.

Aggressive long-term investors — The medical groups most responsible for driving change in medicine today are aggressive and good at deferring immediate financial gratification. They are constantly seeking ways to better themselves in their market. They are trying to look at least one step beyond current market conditions to position themselves for the next turn of events.

The Lipscomb Clinic was advocating multiple sites for sports medicine before they became popular, and it was an early developer of close relationships with a network of trainers. In the Nashville area, the clinic was ahead of the market in developing alliances with multiple small rural hospitals surrounding the metropolitan area. This was not a medical practice that was likely to sit back and view changing events in healthcare and in its market area while holding a pat hand.

These are the types of groups that are fueling change. The impetus for change is not just in the opportunities presented by the marketplace, nor solely among potential capital partners. It is in the groups themselves and the individuals who lead them.

Aggressive short-term investors — These groups are also changing the landscape in medical practice. They are driven by a sense of timing. They recognize that early investors often take more risk, but they often gain more in terms of financial rewards and control. We continually work with physician medical groups who are aggressive, short-term investors who recognize that their practices represent a valuable asset, and that one way to get the value out is to find a way to capitalize future earnings. This is often done by joining a PPMC.

Cautiously optimistic investors — There is a group of physician practices that are proceeding but at a much slower pace. Many of these groups are led by relatively young physicians. Many have been and continue to be highly successful. A number of the practices attribute their past success, in part, to the culture and/or management style of their leaders, and they are concerned that this could be lost. They are receptive to change, but they are equally concerned with maintaining the success they have already achieved. This group of physicians is probably not a candidate for partnership with a PPMC; it may look more favorably on obtaining capital from a health plan or hospital system. This type of group would also attempt to borrow to meet some of its financial needs.

Defensive investors — The final group of physicians and medical practices is making decisions based almost entirely on what it will take to retain patients and financial performance and hold the competitive position it has today. The capital requirements of this kind of physician practice are minimal and can probably be met with leasing and a limited amount of borrowing.

Right Medical Group, Right Strategy, Right Partner

Not surprisingly, at this point in the movement toward consolidating medical groups, those practices that have been most active have come from the long-term investor segment. Aggressive long-term investors see a need for large amounts of capital, and they give more careful consideration to the pros rather than the cons of various options for capital partners. However, this does not mean that other types of medical groups should not seek outside financing.

Regardless of the type of group and its perceived need for capital, medical groups are well advised to understand their investment preferences and how much risk they are willing to accept. In some cases, medical groups may need to consider a change in their financing approach if they recognize that it is well aligned with their overall strategies. Capital partners also certainly need to recognize whom they are dealing with. It is unrealistic, for example, to expect a defensive physician group to partner with a PPMC that has ambitious growth and earnings expectations. On the other hand, a local commercial bank may be more compatible with this kind of conservative physician practice.

Acting on Capital Needs Assessment

Exhibit 15.2 illustrates the thinking of many successful practices that see a need to move their group to the next level of sophistication. By the "next level," they often refer to an ability to demonstrate superior medical outcomes, success in managed care contracting, lower costs than their competitors, excellent patient feedback, and a growing reputation in the community. They say that the primary "big picture" motive for accessing and investing outside capital is to achieve a competitive advantage, one that simply cannot be realized by continuing with "business as usual." These practices usually do not make just

EXHIBIT 15.2 ■ **The Strong Get Stronger: Combinations of Investment by Aggressive Long-Term Investor Medical Groups**

Growing and Optimizing the Practice	Investing in New Ventures	Positioning for the Future
Uses of funds	**Uses of funds**	**Uses of funds**
■ Adding, renovating office; expanding the service area	■ Adding, internalizing ancillaries	■ Better, more integrated information systems
■ Adding specialties	■ Adding other new services or profit centers	■ Protocols, patterns of care, benchmarking
■ Augmenting the management team		■ Improved patient and work flows
■ Reducing, spreading overhead		■ Disease management
■ Cash flow protection during growth		
Benefits	**Benefits**	**Benefits**
■ Greater market share	■ Improved financial performance	■ Better performance under capitated or risk-sharing contracts
■ More negotiating leverage	■ More negotiating leverage	■ More negotiating leverage
■ Readiness for other investments	■ Readiness for other investments	■ Readiness for other investments
		■ Quality, service improvements

one investment; they make several. Even though they may space out their new initiatives over time, they are trying to think several steps ahead. They think in terms of combinations of investments. These practices are likely to say that each successful investment gives them not only a leg up on the competition, but also affords them the opportunity to make another investment.

Obtaining adequate capital for a successful practice is a major initiative — one that is seldom taken lightly because it can change a medical group for a long time to come. For this reason, changing or expanding the capital structure is a step that will not be taken by all medical groups. The most common medical practice that recapitalizes is one that is (a) aggressive and (b) sees itself being in the business for the long term.

Medical practices that think in terms of the power curve "moving to the next level" generally believe that the strong practices are going to get stronger and that the distance between strong and weak practices will widen. They expect to be among the strong. This includes their plan to rationalize and optimize their existing practices — for example, by adding new practice locations, adding more primary care physicians, and filling in specialties that complement their existing areas of expertise. In some cases, optimizing the practice also means developing or bringing new expertise to the management team.

These groups also frequently add new profit centers — for example, internalizing diagnostic capabilities currently provided by others. They also add new capabilities for the longer term, such as new information systems that will enable them to practice more easily from multiple sites and to manage capitated contracts and accept medical risk.

They take these steps to change their place in the market — to gain market share, to become more competitive for payers or others that choose providers, to become more attractive to physicians considering joining their group, and to make more money.

The capital required — The potential investment needs of an aggressive group are enough to get a physician's or an investor's attention. Exhibit 15.3 provides one illustration of the potential magnitude.

It becomes clear that the very aggressive medical group almost always has to consider outside capital sources. Given the potential payback, this can indeed be a place where "opportunity" and "motive" meet for both the physician practice and the investor.

DISTINGUISHING BETWEEN FUNDING SOURCE AND STRATEGY

"What do you think? Should we work with one of these three hospitals, or should we go with a capital partner?" asked one staff surgeon. Following this shareholder meeting, the leaders of this 130-physician multispecialty clinic hoped to make a preliminary decision as to whether to enter further discussions with either Phycor or another PPMC. After a pause, the physician chairing the meeting said, "We could do both." Right answer!

EXHIBIT 15.3 ■ Magnitude of Investment Requirements for Aggressive 100-Physician Group, Six-Year Time Horizon

Investment Requirements	Dollars in Millions
Adding, renovating office; expanding, filling in the service area	$3.9
Adding specialties, improving the mix of specialties	$0.39
Augmenting the management team	$0.91
Reducing, spreading overhead	($1.04)
Cash flow protection during growth	$1.3
Adding, internalizing ancillaries	$13.0
Adding new services or profit centers	$5.2
Better, more integrated information systems	$6.5
Protocols, patterns of care, benchmarking	$0.52
Improved patient and work flows	$0.13
Total	**$30.81**

The dual approach proposed by the surgeon — simultaneously partnering with one of the hospitals in the community and selecting a PPMC — was not the group's strategy; it was a means of implementing strategy. To be sure, the decision as to which PPMC to select was critical. And it was definitely important to have discussions with the CEOs of the community hospitals to find out which one would be the most interested in providing capital to further the clinic's plans.

The strongest determinant of the medical group's capital needs is its strategy. Following are some guidelines about finding and using capital to position physicians for the future. This includes how much capital a medical group requires to gain competitive advantage and the cost, as well as how much capital should come from outside the financial resources of physicians in the group. As suggested earlier, different medical groups approach these questions in different ways.

CAPITAL SOURCES: THE ALTERNATIVES

As with any business, medical groups have financing sources such as retained earnings, borrowing, and leasing available to them. However, medical groups now have several additional alternatives that are not available to other businesses. These include selling all or a portion of the practice or entering into some other kind of arrangement with a hospital. They can also think about partnering with a health plan. Or they can be part of a PPMC that is either in its formative (pre-IPO) stages or publicly traded.

Here are the seven broad options for accessing capital available to medical groups:

1. Retained earnings

2. Borrowing, usually from a commercial bank or other financial institution

3. Leasing

4. Hospitals and multihospital systems

5. Integrated healthcare systems

6. Health plans

7. PPMCs

Retained Earnings

Retained earnings are great for the long term but difficult to accumulate. The result of keeping a portion of net income in the practice and not distributing it to the physicians is called retained earnings. These earnings originate from the annual cash flows that are generated from collections of patient revenue. Many of the most spectacular financial successes among multispecialty groups — Marshfield, Fallon, Scott & White, Dakota Clinic in Fargo — have been at least partially funded with retained earnings. But these are exceptions rather than the rule.

The principal advantage of financing through retained earnings is that it does not require any authorization to fund this way other than the support of physicians/owners, stockholders, or managers of the practice. However, retaining earnings from the practice is difficult to achieve, especially in a professional partnership or an unincorporated entity because the physicians/partners/owners will be taxed on their personal tax returns on income that they never received. Even in the case of a professional corporation structure, corporate income taxes will be paid on earnings not classified as salaries if profits are reported. Thus use of accumulated earnings as a source of internal financing involves a reflective exercise by management to trade off current taxation of retained earnings as a cost of funds with the cost of other alternative sources of financing. In addition, many medical group administrators who have tried to implement this approach have been unable to stand up against the pressures of not pursuing the policy exerted by physicians and their outside accountant.

Borrowing

Physicians and medical groups have traditionally experienced difficulty in borrowing from financial institutions, mainly because practices often do not have assets representing adequate collateral for a loan. When a small medical practice has been able to borrow, it has often pledged its accounts receivable, or individual physicians have personally guaranteed loans.

Selecting a financial institution — In general, the selection process can be broken down into three phases:

1. Research potential funding sources.
2. Interview bank officials who will service the medical group's account.
3. Evaluate acceptable candidates.

To determine which banks might accommodate the needs of a medical group, it is important to survey local banks and to obtain information about their policies and experience handling medical practice accounts. One way is to ask other physicians and groups which banks they use, and discuss their experiences about the services received. Other sources include the accountant and attorney for the medical group. These professionals will have had extensive experience with the banking community, and they will usually provide a list of several competent banks that can be used to gather more information.

Once several promising banks have been identified, the group administrator should contact each financial institution and request copies of their financial statements of condition and the types of loans they make to businesses. Detailed information about lenders is also available from the Federal Deposit Insurance Corporation (FDIC) on the Internet (www.fdic.gov/bankindex.html). Examination of this information will indicate the bank's financial soundness and ability to serve the medical group's credit needs.

The size and affiliation of the bank is important. Banks that are part of large national banking systems have more than adequate financial resources, but it may be difficult to deal with a top manager. On the other hand, these types of banks often have a staff of bankers who are experts in the healthcare industry. Smaller independent banks may have a more personal touch but may also lack financial resources and healthcare industry expertise.

After collecting appropriate information, introductory meetings should be set up with those who hold the most promise of being a viable lender to the group. Here are the steps:

Step 1. Interview bank officers. During meetings with bankers, the financial manager of the group should insist on meeting the banks' decision makers — those who have authority to guarantee specific services and programs. There should be a discussion of each point on the group's list of banking requirements.

Step 2. Evaluate candidate financial institutions. The final step entails careful examination and reflection of all information compiled and impressions from the interview. The bank that offers the best interest rate or the most favorable loan program may not necessarily be the best bank for the medical group. Instead, the selection should be based on whether the bank can provide most of the critical banking needs and services required by the group.

A checklist of characteristics of the top banks for the group might include:

- Competence — experience, knowledge, and interest in meeting the group's needs
- Financial and managerial strength
- Number and quality of business-oriented programs specifically geared to the healthcare industry
- Competitiveness of interest rates and loan packages
- Reputation in the community

Once a bank has been selected, the medical group should consider setting up all accounts — personal, business, savings, and pension — with the selected financial institution. This should add to the attractiveness of the medical group as a bank customer and lead to more favorable consideration in the future. Establishing a strong relationship and staying with a lender can lead to a valuable resource for the medical group.

Loan underwriting criteria — These criteria are such that small practices almost always need personal guarantees from their physicians in order to borrow. Banks are not requiring personal guarantees and require yearly updates.

Debt financing is usually categorized by the term of the loan. Short-term loans require repayment on demand or on specified terms within one year. Intermediate-term loans require repayment within one to eight years. Generally, long-term loans extend over a period greater than eight years. However, commercial banks are not in the business of providing long-term loans or a substitute for equity capital. The following paragraphs categorize the various available forms of debt financing.

Short-term loans — Short-term loans are usually obtained to provide working capital for the group practice. These types of loans finance the operating needs — payroll, supplies, utilities, rent, and other expenses — until patient charges are collected. The nature of working capital requirements may dictate that the principal of the short-term loans not have a fixed repayment schedule; payments would vary with fluctuations of working capital needs. For example, as accounts receivable balances increase, the loan balance would rise accordingly up to a predetermined maximum.

Short-term financing emphasizes the borrower's financial capacity in the near future. As such, lenders look for cash flow projections and other assurances that the indebtedness can be serviced through cash generated by operations with less emphasis on the long-run perspective of how the borrower's net worth or equity in the practice will change.

Interest rates on short-term loans are usually variable. Many lenders, especially banks, use the prime interest rate (the rate charged to a bank's most creditworthy customers) as the basis for establishing an interest rate on short-term loans.

Short-term loans take many forms. A note payable may be a demand note (subject to payment when the lender demands it) or a promissory note with a specified date for repayment. As noted earlier, principal payments may be fixed or fluctuate. Interest payments may be monthly, quarterly, or on the date the loan is due. Banks usually expect short-term debt to be paid in full periodically. This demonstrates the borrower's ability to pay off the loan and shows that the debt is not a "permanent working capital loan." Bank regulators do not normally approve of permanent working capital loans.

A line of credit establishes a predetermined dollar amount that the lender is willing to loan to a business. This is a flexible approach in that the borrower decides when to "draw" on the credit line. Interest is charged only on the amount actually borrowed.

Intermediate-term loans — Intermediate-term financing generally refers to debt instruments with maturity dates ranging from one to eight years. For the most part, these loans are asset based; that is, they are secured by specific (tangible) assets, such as equipment or leasehold improvements. The length of the loan is generally a function of the life of the asset or group of assets being financed.

Repayment is normally expected, divided in even installments over the life of the loan. However, it is often possible to match the cash flows projected for the practice with the payment schedule of the loan. Also, principal payments may be deferred; this involves interest only with a balloon payment at the maturity date. To protect the lender, most intermediate-term loan contracts include an acceleration clause providing that all installments become due upon default of any payment.

Interest rates on intermediate-term loans vary depending on the credit risk as assessed by the lender. The interest rate charged for these loans will depend on many factors including the loan amount, the borrower's credit rating, the maturity date, and the lender's relationship to the borrower. Generally, this rate is slightly higher than the rate that would be charged for a short-term loan. In addition, a compensating deposit balance of 10 to 20 percent of the outstanding loan balance may be required.

Borrowers should expect the lender to require that the assets being financed will provide collateral for the loan.

Long-term loans — Long-term loans are debt instruments with maturity dates beyond eight years. They are typically used to finance real estate and buildings or some other long-lived asset. This financing usually involves installment payments to the lender. In the negotiation of the contract terms, the lender considers the following:

- The value of the asset and its useful life
- Whether the asset is highly specialized or has more general potential uses
- The borrower's earnings and cash flow
- The medical group's management capability

- The group's track record in servicing prior long-term loans
- Prospects of the healthcare industry, both nationally and locally, and the market and the medical group's competitive position

These loans are generally in the form of mortgages, a security device allowing an individual or group to borrow money by pledging property (usually real estate) as security. The type of claim is described in the mortgage or trust deed agreements where the lender's standing relative to other creditors is summarized.

Repayment terms of mortgages require periodic installments similar to home mortgages. Alternatively, the mortgage may have lower monthly payments with a balloon payment at the end of the maturity date.

Both fixed- and variable-rate mortgage loans are available with terms of 15 to 30 years for normal mortgages. Shorter balloon-payment loans often have a shorter duration.

Leasing

Physicians, along with many other individuals and businesses, lease everything from autos to medical equipment to computers. Leasing lends itself to funding the needs of physicians and medical groups in that it taps into the medical group's or individual physician's income stream as a source of repayment. When it comes to high-tech equipment and computers, many physicians prefer leasing because it limits maintenance and repair headaches and reduces the chances of being stuck with equipment that is technologically obsolete.

Leasing is a useful component of most financing structures. However, given the magnitude of aggressive medical groups' capital needs, it is usually a small part of the total financing picture. Also, financial managers should be concerned with the large number of physicians and other individuals who do not view leases as debt, and as a result, are often lulled into a false sense of financial security.

Types of leases — Most automobile companies or equipment manufacturers or distributors will offer leasing programs to physicians and medical groups. These offers need a careful analysis of the full cost versus borrowing the money or paying for the equipment from the practice's cash flow. In other words, leasing may not be as good as it sounds. Two of the most commonly available lease arrangements are operating leases and financing leases. Operating leases (a true lease) are rental agreements that typically have a shorter term than the useful economic life of the asset leased, with ownership remaining with the lessor at the end of the lease. Operating leases usually involve office space, automobiles, or office furniture. Finance (capital) leases frequently cover periods that approximate the useful economic life of the item being leased. They are typically for a longer term than operating leases and may include a purchase option that would allow the lessee to gain ownership of the asset over the life of the lease. Financing leases are similar to conventional loans. Operating and financing leases have different tax consequences that need to be understood.

Lease versus buy — Deciding whether to lease or purchase equipment is one of the major decisions faced by a medical group. Reasons for leasing include:

- A leasing arrangement eliminates a large down payment, thereby maximizing the amount of funds available to the medical group. (Equipment loans usually entail a 10 to 20 percent down payment while leasing requires no initial payment.)

- Since the lessor retains ownership of the item being leased, it is often easier to obtain a lease than other types of financing.

- Leasing limits the risk of obsolescence for the lessee (especially important for computer equipment).

- Lease payments, which are generally larger than depreciation charges for a capital item, are 100 percent deductible for income tax purposes.

- Leases often stipulate that the lessor is responsible for servicing the leased equipment, thereby eliminating technical, financial, and administrative worries related to the equipment.

- Operating leases do not have to be reflected on the balance sheet as liabilities.

The disadvantages to leasing include:

- For lessees that can obtain other financing easily, leasing equipment is generally more costly than borrowing.

- The lessee cannot claim the tax benefits arising from depreciating the asset under the accelerated provisions of income tax laws.

Leases versus buy decisions are important and deserve careful analysis. In many cases, when initially considered, leasing may not be as good as it sounds but is more prevalent today than ever before.

Hospitals and Multihospital Systems

Along with debt financing, hospitals represent the largest source of capital for medical groups. Even for large multispecialty clinics, the hospital is a primary capital source.

There are many ways to structure financing arrangements with hospitals, many things to look out for, and much to gain. Each structure involving hospitals and physicians must be carefully crafted to avoid self-referral and other fraud and abuse legislation, anti-inurement of benefits provisions (in the case of not-for-profit hospitals), and numerous other legal concerns. Nevertheless, as a group, these options — employment models, management services organizations (MSOs), equity model MSOs, joint ventures, gainsharing — afford wide flexibility. Each of these models, of course, has positive and negative features that need to be carefully evaluated. (Fortunately, there is a substantial amount of literature available that describes the various physician-hospital equity models.)

A warning: When reviewing the performance of physician-hospital relationships, dissatisfaction on all sides is the norm. Hospital managers and boards are often disappointed in the staggering financial losses attributable to employed physicians, even when they did or should have seen them coming. Physicians are often disappointed in hospitals' slow decision making and their all-too-often fatal inability to understand when to control and when to let go.

Integrated Healthcare Systems

Most of the large integrated healthcare systems in the United States are driven by a multispecialty clinic or a large hospital system. Examples of integrated systems led by multispecialty clinics include Mayo in Minnesota, Dean in Madison, Penn State Geisinger, Fallon in Worcester, Scott & White in Texas, Carle in Illinois, and Lovelace Health Systems in New Mexico. Integrated systems largely driven by hospitals and multihospital systems include Intermountain Health Care in Utah, Baptist Health System in Birmingham, Sisters of Providence on the West Coast, Advocate in Chicago, Allina in the Twin Cities, and Sutter in California.

There are numerous advantages for physicians to access capital through an association with an integrated healthcare system. Physicians almost always lead these organizations, and there is normally a healthy respect for primary care. Many of the large integrated systems are well positioned for the future; they continue to increase market share and serve more patients. These organizations also seem to be at the cutting edge in terms of clinical information systems and the development of clinical guidelines. Both of these are, of course, critical to improving quality and controlling costs.

The key question is: How many truly integrated systems will there be? With the slow progress in hospitals' transitioning to truly integrated systems and with multispecialty groups showing less and less inclination to finance their next investments with retained earnings or debt, will the integrated healthcare system ever become the majority system?

Health Plans

Over the past decade, health plans have been in and out of financing medical groups. In the mid-1990s, it appeared that Aetna, Prudential, and CIGNA were making major moves into the delivery of healthcare. However, Aetna has sold its HealthWays Family Medical Centers to MedPartners, and Prudential disposed of its group-model clinics in several metropolitan areas.

On the other hand, several Blue Cross and Blue Shield state systems have become financial partners of medical groups (e.g., Blue Cross and Blue Shield of Minnesota and the Dakota Clinic in Fargo, Blue Cross and Blue Shield of Montana with the Great Falls Clinic, and Western Montana Clinic in Missoula). On the surface, this appears to run counter to the actions of Aetna and Prudential.

It appears that health plans are partnering with medical groups to guarantee access to patients and to maintain a distribution network for getting new products to the market. The demands placed on groups by health plans do not appear to be onerous. In most of the cases, working with a health plan may not foreclose other financing alternatives.

The biggest negative in terms of aligning with a single health plan may be the pressure, either today or in the future, for exclusivity in managed care contracting. This may not be in the best long-term interests of physicians in the group. Further, there is no strong evidence to date that most health plans understand how to work in partnership with medical groups any better than do hospitals.

PPMCs

With their promise of access to Wall Street capital, PPMCs have, for the past decade, tended to dominate physicians' discussion of capital partners. The availability of equity financing has also increased the possibility of bank credit for medical groups interested in greater use of debt financing. Equity financing comprises the selling of ownership interests in the practice through the issuance of common or preferred stock. When used, it is possible to employ different classes of stock, each having varying rights, including distributions of earnings and voting privileges.

LOOKING FOR A CAPITAL PARTNER

Where should a physician practice begin finding the right strategy and the most appropriate partner? In thinking about this question, it may be helpful to keep in mind the following general principles:

What Should a Medical Group Look for in a Capital Partner?

Keith Korenchuk, the healthcare attorney quoted early in this chapter, suggested the following:

- An operational focus — Look beyond the acquisitions phase. For example, pass over PPMCs that appear only to be concerned with turning a quick profit on Wall Street.
- Ask, "What can this organization do for my group other than provide capital?" Capital alone isn't enough. "Is there buying power, management expertise, and commitment to disease management?"
- A physician-friendly orientation — "They are run by physicians but you would never know it," Korenchuk notes about one PPMC. Sadly, the same could be said of any number of hospitals, health plans, and PPMCs.
- Ask, "Do these people have an eye to being our collaborators, or do they just want to control us?"

In addition, medical groups should consider these factors:

- A strategic opportunity — Ask, "What is our strategy for gaining a sustainable competitive advantage in our market? How risky is it? What trade-offs do we see between coming up with the needed funds ourselves and bringing in a capital partner?"

■ A match with dollars needed — As discussed previously, all groups are not equally aggressive. Also, some strategies require more dollars to implement than others. Match the funding source with the risk and the dollars needed.

What Should a Capital Partner Look for in a Medical Group?

Again, Korenchuk suggests:

■ A strategic opportunity — Look for a combination of circumstances, including a market and a capable medical group where it is possible to invest in new initiatives (including but not limited to optimizing and growing the practice, adding new profit centers, and positioning for managed care). Earn enough to sustain the group, and pay back the initial investment with a reasonable return. Check out the specifics; run the numbers.

■ Physician leadership — Determine whether there is definable leadership. If so, what is the leadership's investment philosophy? (The right answer: aggressive long-term investor.)

■ Beware of those physicians who want to do less tomorrow than they are doing today. They want your money and your capitalization rate.

■ Flexibility, or a willingness to do things in new ways — Beware of those who expect to do tomorrow what they did yesterday. They will earn what they did yesterday and split it with you, and somebody will be unhappy. Look for a genuine interest in expansion, in reducing clinical variation, in disease management, and in developing a practice information system.

■ Financial information that is accurate and communicates — This includes current income statements, comparative balance sheets, and cash flow statements. It is surprising how many medical groups cannot produce these basic financial documents that should be readily available in any business.

THE BUSINESS PLAN AND FINANCING THE MEDICAL GROUP

In obtaining any type of external financing — loans, leases, hospitals, health plans, equity capital — a business plan is essential. A business plan helps physicians and practice managers in several important ways:

■ Gain internal agreement on the goals and objectives of the organization.

■ Decide on a detailed plan of action about how to reach these goals.

■ Define the resources needed to reach the goals.

■ Project the financial resources needed to meet goals.

■ Establish a plan of action that becomes the benchmark for measuring future success.

■ Get sources of financing interested in the medical group.

Elements of a Business Plan

The contents of a typical business plan include a statement of goals and objectives, an action plan to achieve these goals, market data for the defined area of practice, a description of planned services and programs, a description of the organization and management, and projected financial statements including an income statement, balance sheet, and cash flow analysis for the practice.

Objectives and action plan — This section spells out the medical group's objectives and presents an action plan that integrates all areas of the practice. This beginning of the business plan addresses the following questions:

- What is the medical practice trying to accomplish?
- How does it propose to do so?
- What is the schedule?
- Who is responsible for what?

Levels and quality of service, targeted payer groups, and geographic areas to be served should be identified. Objectives should be stated in terms that are measurable and can be accomplished within a specific time frame.

The larger the medical group and the broader its mix of specialties, the more extensive the objectives will become. In all cases, it is important to state concisely the framework within which the practice will operate in its statement of objectives.

The action plan should explain how the objectives will be accomplished, relating them to dates, priorities, and responsibilities.

Organization and management — This section should deal with these questions:

- What management, key personnel, and professional staff are in place or available to make the practice succeed?
- What are the practice's strengths and weaknesses, and what major problems does it face?
- How much capital (in the form of equity and debt) does the practice need?
- How will the funds be used?

The names and a brief background description of the physicians and each member of the medical group's management team should be prepared. The lender or potential financial partner will not only be interested in the clinical capabilities of the practice but its business acumen.

Market data for service area — An analysis of the market for the group's services and its expected market share form the basis for determining the volume of business the group expects to achieve. Defining the market area entails the identification of service area boundaries and examining population and economic trends within the service areas. An estimate of the volume of patient visits by demographic characteristics (e.g., age, sex, family size, and income) should be included. MGMA statistical data can be valuable as a part of this analysis. Service area data form the basis for estimating service volumes and payer mix.

If new services or programs or expansion into new markets is being considered, consumer attitude surveys should be developed. These surveys, or focus group interviews, would explore interests in new programs or services and competition.

The market area data and survey results should be summarized and presented in the form of a projection of volume of business, by service and by payer.

Projected financial performance — Pro forma income statements, balance sheets, and cash flow analysis are the heart of the business plan. Financial projections integrate much of the business plan by including estimates of demand, revenues, staffing, salaries, other expenses, capital requirements, profitability, and return on investment. These projections can also be used to estimate what the medical group is worth today and in the future.

Anticipated revenue for the medical group can be estimated by multiplying projected units of service, or covered lives, by the value of units of service or capitation rates. This amount is then reduced by projected bad debts and discounts on contractual arrangements with third-party payers, such as managed care contracts and Medicare and Medicaid programs. To determine a competitive fee level and to estimate bad debts and contractual write-offs, other physicians in the market area should be informally surveyed. Financial consultants can provide databases by CPT-4 codes of charges and collected rates in the area.

Various expenses should be estimated, such as salaries and fringe benefits of physicians and support staff, rent, insurance, utilities, medical and office supplies, leased medical and computer equipment, taxes, and depreciation. Some of these expenses, such as medical supplies, are directly related to volume and will increase as volume increases. Fixed expenses, such as utilities and rent, remain constant as volumes increase.

Capital needs (e.g., equipment, furniture, office improvements, and new sites) should be projected for a three- to five-year period and should indicate the year of acquisition or construction. Also, required principal and interest payments have to be factored into the financial model.

Revenue and expense projections are included in the projected income statement. Generally, lenders like to see a projected income statement for a three- to five-year period, depending on the size and nature of the loan and the scheduled payback period.

The balance sheet reflects the financial status of the practice at a particular point in time. The balance sheet should show all assets, such as accounts receivable and obligations due, both short and long term. A note to the financial statement should describe any contingent liabilities.

A cash flow statement presents the timing of the receipt and payment of cash, including operations, capital investments, and debt repayments. Cash flow analysis is valuable in identifying potential problem areas. Most cash flow models include assumptions about the minimum amount of cash that will be kept on hand.

To the Point

- Most medical groups do, or will, need capital. How much capital and for what purposes is often determined by how aggressive the group is or plans to become. Those groups with an aggressive long-term orientation are almost certain to need substantial amounts of capital, and those that are aggressive but with a shorter-term perspective will also benefit from outside financing. Retained earnings, debt financing, and leasing are often insufficient for the more aggressive types of medical groups.

- There are 10 common needs for capital:
    1. Growing and optimizing the existing practice
    2. Adding primary care physicians and sites
    3. Investing in new profit centers
    4. Adding next-generation facilities and equipment
    5. Adding next-generation information systems
    6. Developing single-specialty networks
    7. Accepting and managing medical risk
    8. Providing an exit strategy for older physicians
    9. Covering cash flow shortages
    10. Insulating against risk

  Most groups will focus on two or three reasons why they need capital. For example, geographic expansion and IT may be the most important. For some groups, positioning for managed care, including the acceptance of financial risk, will be critical.

- There are seven general sources of capital — (1) retained earnings, (2) borrowing, (3) leasing, (4) hospitals, (5) integrated systems, (6) health plans, and (7) PPMCs. Each of these needs to be carefully evaluated against the type of group and its strategic objectives. A well-constructed capital plan can also be helpful in selecting from among the various alternative sources of capital.

- A detailed business plan is essential for any medical group, whether it needs outside capital or not. For those groups seeking outside lending or a capital partner, a business plan is an essential document.

- A business plan includes:
  - Statement of goals and objectives
  - Action plan
  - Market data
  - Description of planned services and programs
  - Description of the organization and its management
  - Projected financial statements

CHAPTER 16

Focus on Accountability to Achieve Quality Results

Edited by Owen Dahl, FACHE, CHBC, LSSMBB

After completing this chapter, you will be able to:

- Define the word "accountability" in general terms and more specifically as it is used in the healthcare setting.

- Explain the elements comprising a generalized model of accountability that shows the nature and workings of accountable relationships in any setting.

- Apply the accountability model to the operations of a medical group, particularly from the viewpoint of the financial manager, and gain insights into ways to increase results and enhance productivity.

- Engage in a dialogue about current industry and government efforts to address issues of accountability that emphasize fraud and abuse among all players.

- Recognize potential situations in medical practice activities that tend to foster employee theft and fraud, then determine how to minimize their occurrence, including developing a corporate compliance program.

- Act in a leadership role to use the principles of accountability and decide how they can be adapted to the medical practice environment to produce more efficient operations and greater successes in delivering patient care.

Today's financial manager of medical groups supports all operational aspects of the practice. In addition to the traditional accounting, billing, receivables/payables, and reporting/analysis functions of the finance area, it is not unusual for financial managers to be responsible for health information systems, materials management, and telecommunications, among other duties. Physicians are expecting medical group administrators and financial managers to look at the big picture and take a proactive role in managing the practice through involvement in strategic planning, systems development, and operational management.

The increasing breadth and complexity of the financial manager's areas of focus require a central theme of integration. This integration can be provided by understanding the concepts and using the elements of accountability. The call for accountability prevails throughout our society. In government, the issue of governmental officials and politicians — elected and appointed — being accountable for the use of taxpayer funds has always been foremost in voters' minds. Corporate accountability has emerged as a prominent requirement for boards of directors and members of management, as they must report how they have used stockholders' and creditors' resources. However, this view of accountability goes well beyond financial statements. It embraces other forms of reporting, such as disclosure of the board and management's performance on the use of an organization's resources and the efficiency and effectiveness of operations.

We see increasing demands for members of the healthcare industry to be more accountable for what they do when treating and caring for the ill. Pressures are mounting for providers, purchasers, insurers, and patients to conduct themselves in more accountable modes so that the total care system can produce quality results at affordable prices to payers and underwriters of the cost of delivery. As these demands on medical practices increase, the role of the financial manager will be central to ongoing success.

In order for group administrators and financial managers to understand and use elements of accountability, this chapter treats the subject of accountability in some depth. It explains what it is, how it functions, and how it can be useful to a medical practice. We will take a brief look at the current treatment of accountability within the healthcare industry as a whole. Emphasis will be placed on fraud and abuse practices that seem to be widely prevalent.

DEFINITION

The simplest definition of *accountability* is individuals accepting the consequences of their actions. In order to understand accountability, it is necessary to break it down into three aspects. In Exhibit 16.1, we have identified the organizational level, a model, and the individual/team level of accountability. Each of these aspects require a detailed review.

ORGANIZATIONAL LEVEL

Culture

Each organization has a culture that has grown over the years based on experiences, leadership, and decisions that help identify how "it" will deal with activities, from daily routines to crises. Employees share their common experiences, identify basic beliefs, and make assumptions based on those experiences. This culture may be openly stated, covertly functional, or implied, each of which dictates actions taken by an employee. The key stakeholders help form the culture through leadership, directions, and actions. Cultures are formed based on crisis situations that may occur and how the organization responds to those crises. Or a culture may be formed through evolution, as decisions are made, actions occur, and patterns emerge that indicate expected

EXHIBIT 16.1 ■ **Accountability Flow Chart Including Organizational Level, Model, and Individual/Team Level**

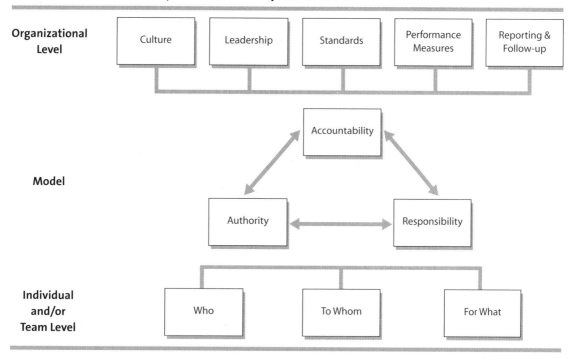

behaviors. The organization will set standards through language, attitude, and expected actions.

The level of accountability in the organization is then related to how "compliant" the employees are to internal policies and procedures as well as to federal, state, and local laws. The organization will have a "risk tolerance" position as it considers compliance or lack of compliance. Adherence to policies and procedures will directly result in the level of performance by the employee. It is assumed that the more compliant, the better the outcome. Likewise, the more "accountable" the employee, the better the outcome.

Accountability within an organization's culture can come from open discussion or thoughts. In today's healthcare environment, there are significant external factors that must be considered and that lead to actions taken. These will be reviewed in greater detail later in this chapter.

In terms of accountability, we can look at an organization's culture as a continuum. On the left side is a defensive position, the right side is a chosen position, and in the middle is a position of compliance. The defensive accountability position means that little action is taken unless there is an occurrence that requires a response. This response will be one of denial, or "I/ We didn't do it." The compliant position suggests that we will comply with the direction given, or "Okay, I'll do it but with no more effort than is necessary to achieve compliance." The choice position is a proactive role: "Not only will I do it, but I will also do it well and fully within the selected guidelines."

Leadership

Today's healthcare leaders must understand the culture of the organization, its mission, and its strategic objectives. Leadership will set the tone for accountability through establishing guidelines, setting priorities and standards, and identifying performance measures. Leadership has the responsibility to develop or provide tools and establish processes. *What leadership pays attention to is what gets done.*

Leadership must communicate effectively to all employees. A leader will be a role model, teacher, or coach to the employees for whom he or she is responsible. Effective delegation will follow with the expectation that the employee will be accountable for his or her actions. The leader then establishes a level of trust with each employee. The leader who micromanages the employee has not effectively delegated and holds himself or herself fully accountable for his or her actions. Culture, therefore, is set through the leadership actions of delegation or micromanagement.

The leader will enforce or change the accountability culture through the assignment of tasks or as problems or issues are resolved. When a problem arises, it is human nature to deny that there was a problem or that you caused the problem when in fact that may not be true. The next step is to attempt to repair the problem and/or support the denial. Eventually the truth will come out, and you may suffer the consequences of your actions. Often times, the denial is greater than the problem itself. Witness many politicians! Thus, the culture of accountability is defined by the actions of the leader.

It is also essential that the leader recognize the organization's subcultures. These may be different office locations, specialties, or even a difference in how Dr. A deals with a patient when compared with Dr. B.

An aspect of leadership is also the role of the *stakeholder*, or a person of interest.[1] This implies a potential for direct involvement with a project or a relationship to the outcome without directly influencing the actions taken. Employees are afraid of the concept of accountability since they see it as potentially being blamed for something that they may not have done or punishment that may result in the wrong action being taken.

To be successful, the leader must recruit the right employee and follow through with adequate orientation and ongoing training. Often it is the first impression that results in the subsequent actions taken. Therefore, today's healthcare leader sets the tone for the quality of care and patient outcomes. The financial leader may seem removed since there is little direct contact with the patient. The role of leadership crosses every department and location, and therefore the financial leader contributes to the success of the organization through employee selection and actions taken.

Standards

Goals, objectives, values, and beliefs must be clearly understood in order to ensure sufficient outcomes. Standards are based on these key items and may come from internal actions as well as external dictates. Standards set the criteria for rewards as well as punishment for actions taken. Standards set a clear focus for what is expected and for what actions individuals are held accountable. Standards set the boundaries for decisions made and actions taken.

These standards should be based on the mutual goals and objectives set and should refer directly back to these directives. Since the specifics of the standards must be developed and jointly agreed upon by stakeholders and accountable parties, in a sense, they constitute a definable contract used to determine the adequacy of performance. In some instances, these standards may be articulated by some external authority, such as statutes, contracts, or agreements. Furthermore, standards, for the most part, are specific and unique for each accountability relationship. To determine possible types of standards, the following examples are provided:

■ **Financial managers** — Standards of accountability for the financial manager with regard to the stakeholder — governing board — would be the quality, completeness, relevancy, and timeliness of reports that the board requires from the financial manager to monitor practice activities and plan future strategic directions. Concerning the physician compensation, the financial manager must comply with the agreed-upon formula and concept of fairness determined by the physician group in distributing practice profits.

▪ **Physicians** — When the physician group is addressed for standards of accountability, the task becomes much more complex. For example, the medical director and the physicians might develop clinical practice guidelines. While there are recognized protocols that physicians generally agree on in treating specific cases, standards need greater specification than a mere listing of steps to perform. There needs to be explicit criteria to evaluate the technical quality of care rendered, such as the appropriateness of various interventions. Further, explicit criteria also need to be established to assess the skill of the healthcare professional in carrying out a particular procedure or treatment regimen.[2] The recent emphasis on pay-for-performance (P4P) and value-based purchasing is an example of what the outcomes of compliance with standards can yield. Additional reimbursement, recognition, or the ability to continue with a managed care plan make the effort to understand and accept P4P as a strategy for the medical practice a valid concept.

▪ **Chief administrator, medical director, and board of directors** — Different types of standards are required when the chief administrator, medical director, and the board of directors must answer for the overall performance of the medical group. Here, two industry accountability standards growing in importance are accreditation and data reporting of provider performance. Accreditation is a formal process involving peer examination of practices to differentiate qualified performers from those who do not meet accreditation standards. Accreditation of the medical practice is recognized by The Joint Commission (TJC) and the Accreditation Association for Ambulatory Health Care (AAAHC). Another form of market competition of accountability — data reporting — seems to be dominated by Health Plan Employer Data and Information Set (HEDIS). HEDIS continually develops and publishes common performance measured that are used by purchasers, business coalitions, and others to evaluate the performance of practices and to make contracting decisions.

Performance Measures

The companion element to accountability standards are indicators to measure the performance of accountable parties. These measures provide the means to verify whether actions taken meet the agreed-upon standards. If the results fall short of standards, corrective action needs to be taken to get performance back on track. To determine any kind of performance for any type of accountable party, two elements must be measured:

1. What is done
2. How well it is done

Beyond these two factors, "good" measures should possess some or all of the following attributes:[3]

▪ **Significance** — The measures should evaluate something that is relevant to the task, the object of activity, the patient, or the practice.

- **Range and scope of services** — The measure should be applicable to a wide range of services or activities being performed.

- **Reliability and validity** — The measure should be accurate and reproducible.

- **Cost effectiveness** — The measure should provide enough benefit to justify the cost of collection and analysis.

- **Discrimination ability** — The measure should be sensitive and specific, identifying "all and only" true positives and avoiding false negatives.

- **Controlled by the entity being measured (individual or group)** — It serves no useful purpose to measure something that cannot be influenced by those who are being measured.

- **Ease of establishment and comprehension** — The measure should be easily developed and clearly understood by all parties.

For nonclinical performance measures within a medical practice, individuals in the roles of accountable party and stakeholder must reach a mutual understanding of what will constitute acceptable performance measures to evaluate each person's work. These generally relate to written work, interpersonal communications, and interfacing with patients and other external parties. Although it may be somewhat difficult in nonclinical matters to reach these types of consensus, they seem reasonably achievable if efforts are conscientiously made to develop them. Judging the adequacy of physician technical performance, however, is extremely difficult; only peers can reach these determinations. The use of provider profiles and outcomes measurement are two approaches that are currently being considered as ways to evaluate physician performance. In the area of measuring physician treatment of patients from a patient (stakeholder) perspective, patient survey data are perhaps the best tool to use.

Holding the staff accountable for their decisions or actions will:

- Improve accuracy of the work performed
- Provide adequate response to requests made
- Improve problem solving
- Ensure better decisions are made
- Improve cooperation with others

Reporting and Follow-up

The nature of reporting by accountable parties can take one of several forms. Generally, the most common types are oral communication, visual observation, and written reports. The output of the financial managers' activities — operating reports, budget documents, financial statements, and compliance reports to various authorities — are examples of this element. The issuance of these documents will depend on the established needs of group management and legal requirements, and they will be accompanied by analysis, discussion, and follow-up actions. Similarly, feedback by other accountable parties, such as the chief administrator, board members, and administrator staff members, will generally comprise written reports and oral communications.

Nonfinancial metrics such as patient volume, new patients, and referring source activities are also critical to the measurement of success. Individual actions such as collections at the time of visit by the check-out staff are reported daily. One of the critical points that happens to the busy financial manager is a lack of follow-up. A decision is made to change a procedure, training occurs, and it is then assumed that staffers will follow the new procedure. But what typically happens is that there is no follow-up, and the staffers revert to the way they have always done things. Therefore, it is as important to make the change and report on it as it is to ensure that the change worked by following up and reviewing it later.

Physicians' reporting includes documentation of patients' histories, diagnoses, treatments, patient reactions and recovery patterns, and future prognosis to form a complete record for each patient. Referred physicians, as accountable parties, will render written documents summarizing their diagnoses, treatment protocols, and patient responses.

For the practice as a whole, purchasers of health services, employer coalitions, and to some extent consumers and beneficiaries are demanding reports that show in detail providers' performance — including individual physicians, hospitals, and medical groups, especially those comprised of specialists — so that comparisons with other providers can be made. A popular type of report for this purpose is the "report card" found on the Internet. A report card is any type of report containing performance data of a specific provider for particular disease treatments and procedures. These report cards serve in a similar capacity to grading a group's efforts through comparison with other groups or based on some standard or measure of acceptability. An increasingly popular form of report card is the HEDIS system of performance measures.

ACCOUNTABILITY REDEFINED — MODEL

Our initial definition that individuals accept consequences for their actions needs to be broadened based on the previous discussion. Staff members are expected to contribute to the fulfillment of the overall organizational mission. They do that based on the tasks assigned. However, they cannot be successful unless they assume the responsibility for their actions and have the authority to take the necessary steps to accomplish the tasks assigned. These can be simple routine daily tasks or more broad in scope. In any event, staffers must have the authority and assume responsibility for their actions.

A task is accomplished by deciding to do it and taking the action necessary. This requires authority. The employee also must accept responsibility, which means he or she accepts the reward or consequences for his or her action. The employee's manager or stakeholder is ultimately responsible and must provide the guidance and support necessary to ensure that the desired results are achieved. The stakeholder may be the immediate supervisor, a management committee, the board, or some other entity of authority.

Thus, the definition of accountability must include the sufficient delegation of authority from the stakeholder and the acceptance of responsibility by the employee to take the action necessary.

INDIVIDUAL/TEAM LEVEL

The model can be applied to any environment — business, government, personal, and healthcare. To start the analysis of accountability issues in any situation, these three key questions should be answered:

1. Who should be held accountable? The one who acts
2. To whom should the accountable party answer? The stakeholder(s)
3. For what should the accountable party be held to account? The activity, standards, or measures

Who Should Be Held Accountable?

All members of a medical group can be held accountable for their actions. These include physicians, clinical staff persons, the medical director, the chief administrator, administrative personnel, and, of course, the financial manager. If physicians and nonphysicians serve on the board of directors, they are accountable for their performance in that capacity. Another important accountable party is the individual patient. External to the medical group, all others having some form of relationship to the practice are also accountable for carrying out designated activities. For example, nongroup physicians to whom the practice's patients are referred are accountable. Other entities, such as hospital staff members, health plan administrators, vendors who provide equipment and supplies, and lessors of facilities and equipment, are some of the major players who can be accountable for providing services to the practice.

To Whom Should the Accountable Party Answer?

Stakeholders are the parties who have a stake in the outcome since they are recipients of actions performed by individuals who are accountable. In most circumstances, every party mentioned in the preceding paragraph can be a stakeholder. For example, a patient is normally a stakeholder when treated by a physician. And a patient can become an accountable party when he or she is called to account for carrying out the care instructions of the attending physician. The model enables us to place an individual or group in changing roles of accountable party and stakeholder. In another example, the financial manager is accountable for conducting the financial affairs of the practice and can be a stakeholder when an HMO administrator responds to claims for payments for medical services rendered by the practice. It is possible when considering the model that many other reciprocal accountability roles are played by every member of the medical group.

For What Should the Accountable Party Be Held to Account?

The answer to this question flows from the objectives established by the parties who form an accountability relationship. These "what" elements should be the parties' continued focus in carrying out activities related to their respective roles. For example, the financial manager's objective is to provide leadership and know-how in structuring an information system that captures financial and clinical data to be integrated into meaningful sets of operating reports for making practice decisions. Thus, this objective becomes the "what" for which the financial manager is held to account. When the medical director of the group has the responsibility of providing leadership to the physicians in the group, he or she is held accountable for the effectiveness with which leadership traits are displayed and how well the physicians conduct their professional activities within the group environment.

Let's combine these three key questions of accountability relationships for a typical medical group and illustrate a variety of combinations to illustrate how these elements interrelate.

Exhibit 16.2 shows the reciprocal accountability relationship; that is, the stakeholder becomes the accountable party, and the accountable party assumes the role of the stakeholder. However, the objective or the focus of accountability would differ for each role.

ADVANTAGES OF ACCOUNTABILITY

You might conclude that the workings of the accountability model and its principles within a medical practice are interesting and seem to make sense. But how can they help financial managers perform their roles and carry out their responsibilities more effectively? The following are the advantages of adopting an accountability perspective:

- **Focuses on problems** — When objectives are clearly and fully articulated between the stakeholders and those accountable, these become the center of attention in taking action and measuring results. When results are less than satisfactory, the focus of the problem is more clearly identified and stands out as the area to be addressed. **Example:** When physician coding errors cause over-reporting of values for services rendered, actions can be taken to improve the coding process.

- **Identifies doers** — Once work activities related to objectives have been established for those accountable, everyone is aware of who is responsible for accomplishing certain tasks. The more definitive and complete these specifications are, the greater the clarity of doer identification. **Example:** When the financial manager has been assigned the task of ensuring that all new clinical staffers complete an orientation class on the group's financial information system, he or she becomes the individual responsible for centering groupwide efforts to determine whether an adequate knowledge base among staff is maintained.

- **Results in self-regulating conduct** — There is a part of the human psyche that drives individuals to conduct their actions and report results truthfully when others are aware of their responsibilities and they know they will be held accountable for what they do. Accountable parties, thus, are likely to carry out their activities in ways to preclude producing unfair

EXHIBIT 16.2 ■ **Examples of Accountability Relationships**

Accountable Party	Stakeholder	Objective
Financial manager	Governing board	Accounting and reporting
Financial manager	Physicians	Accurate cash distributions
Financial manager	Chief administrator	Budget preparation
Physicians	Medical director	Adhering to practice guidelines
Physicians	Patients	Quality care
Physicians	PPO	Meeting standards
Patient	Physicians	Following treatment directives
Patient	Financial manager	Satisfying payment obligations
Patient	HMO	Complying with contract provisions
Chief administrator	Governing board	Overall management of practice
Chief administrator	Medical director	Supporting all clinical activities
Chief administrator	Financial manager	Providing resources to carry out role
Members of the board	Medical director and physicians	Policymaking, leadership, and sound governance
Members of the board	Local community	Delivering healthcare services to the community
Clinical staff members	Physicians	Supporting care treatments
Clinical staff members	Patients	Patient care
Administrative staff	Chief administrator and financial manager	Carrying out assigned responsibilities
Health plans and insurers	Chief administrator and financial manager	Prompt and accurate payment for service claims
Referred physicians	Referring physicians	Quality care in accordance with established protocols
Suppliers of equipment	Chief administrator, physicians, and financial manager	Efficient and effective functioning of purchased equipment

outcomes. **Example:** When physicians within the practice are informed that the renewal of a large contract with an HMO is pending and meeting the profit plan for the group is contingent upon retaining this contract, the physicians may carefully and diligently prescribe and treat patients in accordance with agreed-to practice guidelines.

▪ **Encourages planning** — The entire process involving identifying and defining clearly stated objectives between the parties fosters thoughts prior to action-taking and requires open communication among everyone. Results are more likely to be productive and contribute to the overall goals and objectives of the practice. **Example:** When physicians in the group are aware that their profit distributions depend on a substantial increase in practice revenue for next year, the physicians will likely respond positively for setting aside time to engage in operational planning for the following year.

▪ **Establishes meaningful benchmarks** — Developing accountability standards that are related to the relationship objective(s) serve as meaningful benchmarks or standards of excellence for the employees to aspire to in conducting their activities. These standards can be continuously reviewed and adjusted to meet the growth and development of those accountable. **Example:** An accounting staff person can be motivated when he or she has been assigned to learn and implement a new software package to handle billings and collections for the practice and is informed that successful implementation will be rewarded with a specified salary increase and promotion in responsibilities. A precise definition of "success" would be developed to measure the outcome.

▪ **Avoids excuses** — The clear delineation of responsibilities that constitute the objectives of an individual's job description provides the foundation for accounting for results. The more specific and clear these areas are stated, the more difficult it is for individuals to cop out of admitting their shortcomings and blame others or circumstances for those failures. **Example:** The chief administrator has been assigned by the board of directors the responsibility of meeting the practice operating budget each year, which is stated clearly in the chief administrator's job description and in the board minutes. To avoid allowing this individual to blame others, "meeting the budget" must be carefully and specifically described and closely monitored by the board.

▪ **Enables productive improvement objectives** — Implementing an air of accountability throughout the medical practice can instill a continuing sense of improvement. When viewed from an accountability perspective, nearly all aspects of individuals' work promote positive attitudes and establish a climate for continuous improvement. Exhibit 16.3 supplies a list of examples of how medical practice operations can incorporate accountability concepts for the betterment of productivity and a more successful group practice.

THOUGHTS ON THE BOARD OF DIRECTORS' ACCOUNTABILITY

Much of this narrative about accountability principles applies equally to members of medical group governing boards. An accountability perspective provides a similar all-encompassing framework for visualizing board members' duties and responsibilities more clearly. When interpersonal relations among

EXHIBIT 16.3 ■ Application of Accountability Concepts to Medical Groups

The following examples represent how medical practice operations can incorporate accountability concepts:

- Establish periodic opportunities for staff members to share innovations or improved ways to carry out their activities and to indicate what specific aspects of these changes they will be accountable for.

- Improve claims processing by getting the physicians to agree they will learn more accurate coding procedures to speed up timely reimbursement from third-party payers.

- Obtain an agreement with insurers and third-party payers to provide timely reimbursement of the group's medical claims, or if not paid by the agreed-upon date, have the payer call the group administrator explaining the reason for the delay.

- Conduct timely performance reviews of staff members whereby staff members take the leadership role in presenting their appraisal of their performance before management provides their feedback; then have agreement on new postures of accountability in carrying out future job responsibilities.

- Provide a daily and weekly summary of the significant financial and nonfinancial indicators of the practice to all physicians and encourage them to raise questions for items not clear.

- Arrange with outside service vendors, such as equipment manufacturers and key suppliers, to contact the group administrator on a regular basis, such as quarterly, to determine whether any problems exist or if any new services or products are available to increase productivity and improve operations.

- Optimize communications between patient and physician by establishing a routine practice whereby patients are asked to keep diaries of their symptoms, feelings, reactions, and complications between office visits to share during their next visit.

- Focus on finding solutions to problems when they occur rather than trying to place blame or accuse others of not doing their job; the emphasis should be on results and how best to achieve them at all times.

- Establish clear and unequivocal performance standards in all job descriptions for all members of the group and have an understanding that the expectations are the minimum levels of acceptable performance, with everyone encouraged to exceed these standards frequently.

members become strained or impeded and when results are not obtained, the accountability model sets forth a mechanism to analyze working interfaces and relationships and a structure for addressing ways to improve the conditions. When new board members are appointed, a document that defines board members' roles and responsibilities couched with principles of accountability will likely ensure proper behavior of members, including full and complete answering for their performance. Similarly, this role doubles as a stakeholder.

ACCOUNTABILITY IN HEALTHCARE INDUSTRY — A MACRO VIEW

Let's turn the spotlight on the healthcare industry and take a macro view of accountability. Financial managers must understand this broader perspective since forces are mounting and calling for all players in the healthcare industry to be held accountable for their performance.

In demanding assurance that the delivery system meets the expectations for cost, quality, access, and patient satisfaction, healthcare purchasers are seeking accountability. They recognize large discrepancies in performance and want to ensure that the needs of the consumer are served well by the healthcare system. These purchasers and others have found that if sophisticated information systems coupled with new analytical methods are applied to healthcare, appropriate information can be generated to evaluate performance meaningfully.

In the 1990s under the Clinton administration, the effort at healthcare reform was centered on "managed competition," which addressed accountability through networks of payers and providers using the concept of competition. As part of the model, there was a national board that would help determine and define standards of quality to be included in any aspect of the competitive marketplace under the federal government. Voters' influence emboldened Congress to lay aside the president's plan as too complex and too centered on federal government controls. This decision thrust the issue of accountability into the marketplace, the courts, and state legislatures.

Today the concepts described in "Obama Care," or the Affordable Care Act (ACA), emphasize the idea of quality and holding the provider accountable to patient outcomes and satisfaction. The program includes several federal government agencies that will "regulate" care provided. Again, a national board will identify evidence-based care models. The concept of managing quality while managing costs (defined as payer costs) is believed to be central to the future.

The key point is that with or without the actual ACA provisions, there are many key changes coming to the healthcare industry. These changes are asking for accountability on the part of the provider through use of evidence-based care and comparative effectiveness.

The financial manager will not only have to understand this macro view of what the payers are controlling, rewarding, and thus paying to the internal aspects of what it really costs to deliver services. This aspect of accountability is a true measure of what will lead to success in the future.

As we look to the future, the increase in government regulations at the federal and state levels as well as what continues in the market through managed care regulations will be the financial manager's accountability model.

Case Law and Regulations

Case law has been limited to largely holding the physician and managed care organizations (MCOs) liable for bad patient outcomes. Who is liable for the outcome is often settled through contract terminology and the courts. There is too much time lag between the harm suffered by the patient and the filing of the lawsuit to the determination of the preliminary issues and the trial (if the case survives a motion of summary judgment) and then finally to appellate court decisions to provide real guidance to the industry. Given this extraordinary delay, regulation has emerged as a more significant force promoting managed care accountability for quality.

At the state regulatory level, the most fundamental accountability technique has been the establishment of basic requirements for a managed care organization to be licensed to do business. The state departments of insurance and insurance commissioners' offices are primarily responsible for dealing with health insurance issues. But states vary greatly in regulating quality. Methods include access and availability requirements for clinicians, external quality audits by recognized accrediting agencies, and the reporting of relevant data. The most aggressive effort in regulatory accountability has been the so-called anti-managed care laws. These statutes result from concerted lobbying efforts by aggrieved parties seeking redress for perceived inequities or, in some cases, direct injury. Other recent laws address concerns over secrecy, which has become a characteristic of the business of managed care. Examples of this type of law are the anti-gag clause provisions — requirements to disclose to patients physician financial incentives, utilization review criteria, and clinical practice guidelines.

The exception to the above jurisdictional approach to regulating health insurance is the Employee Retirement Income Security Act (ERISA), which impacts the financial manager with employer self-funded plans regulated by the federal-level Department of Labor, as opposed to the individual state insurance commissioner.

At the federal regulatory level, where Medicare and Medicaid populations are at issue, the record of government requiring plan accountability for quality has been spotty. Some early quality controls were imposed through federal qualifications, but they have not been enhanced. The peer review program has been the principal federal approach to quality control in Medicare hospitals and Medicare HMOs. Federal efforts have recently shifted into concerns over fraud and abuse. There are also recently enacted programs for ePrescribe, PQRI, EHRs, meaningful use, and resource-use reporting. This area will likely continue to grow.

Market Competition

The second driving force — market competition — has as one form, accreditation, as a technique to differentiate qualified performers from those who do not meet the accreditation standards. These initiatives are usually self-regulatory and emerge from the industry itself. They may relate to accrediting hospitals or healthcare professionals. The power of accreditation is its link to purchasing opportunities. When employers or state agencies on behalf of their employees mandate accreditation for a plan to be offered to the subscriber population, plans move to make themselves accountable by seeking accreditation.

Another form of market competition force of accountability is data reporting of provider performance. As stated previously, two organizations are currently dominant in pushing this approach —HEDIS and Foundation for Accountability (FACT). One of the most prominent users of HEDIS data is the National Committee for Quality Assurance (NCQA), which issues report cards indicating the performances of HMOs and health insurance plans. NCQA also offers certification of several programs including patient centered medical homes (PCMH).

A third form pertains to how plans relate to their network of contracted providers by efforts to hold them accountable while enhancing the plan's position in a competitive environment. Issues currently of concern are credentialing of physicians and other providers and selection and then termination of providers based on quality factors. Two important mechanisms are the use of physician profiling and clinical practice guidelines as techniques for monitoring quality.

The combination of law and market forces appears to hold promise for the ultimate development of relevant and workable standards of accountability for the major players in healthcare. Although present indicators seem basic, we are beginning an evolutionary process that should lead to the development of more refined sets of standards for each type of player.

FEDERAL LEGISLATION RESPONSES TO FRAUD AND ABUSE

Recently, several new federal laws have been enacted to combat the growing amount of fraud and abuse in healthcare. This legislation coupled with increased funding for the investigation of physicians, clinics, and other medical providers by the Department of Justice make the likelihood of audits and possible felony convictions a grim reality. The Office of Inspector General (OIG) has received broader authority, and the creation of a national data bank has enabled state agents to share records of licensure revocations and criminal offenses that assists in detecting fraudulent billing patterns. In addition, citizens and beneficiaries outside of enforcement agencies are being offered significant incentives to help fight medical fraud. Whistle-blowers have received millions of dollars in rewards from litigation they have instigated against fraud practitioners. *Qui tam* or "whistle-blower" lawsuits are an increasing source of leads for federal investigators and have played key roles in many high-profile cases.

The emphasis on enforcement has been on Medicare and Medicaid billing practices. The intention is to identify physicians and administrators who are "knowingly and willingly" committing billing and coding frauds. However, honest billing mistakes can be under scrutiny, as well.

The OIG under CMS and the Department of Justice has joined to create the Health Care Fraud Prevention and Enforcement Action Team (HEAT). This joint team shows the emphasis and effort being expended by the federal government to deal with fraud and abuse.

Stark Law

In general terms, the Stark Law prohibits physicians referring Medicare or Medicaid patients to entities with which they (or family members) have a "financial relationship" for the delivery of designated health services, unless an exception applies. A "financial relationship" may be of two types: (1) an ownership or investment interest by the physician in the entity or (2) a compensation arrangement between the physician and the entity. Several exceptions to the law apply to both types. A violation of the Stark Law can result in severe economic penalties, including significant fines, potential loss of Medicare and Medicaid reimbursement, and exclusion from participating in these government programs.

When Stark was first enacted, it applied to referrals by physicians for clinical laboratory services. On January 1, 1995, the list of services to which the self-referral ban applied was expanded to include the following:[4]

- Clinical laboratory services
- Physical therapy services
- Occupational therapy services
- Radiology services (including MRI, CAT, and ultrasound)
- Radiation therapy services and supplies
- Durable medical equipment and supplies
- Parenteral and enteral nutrients, equipment, and supplies
- Prosthetics, orthotics, and prosthetic devices and supplies
- Home health services
- Outpatient prescription drugs
- Inpatient and outpatient hospital services

In 2007, nuclear medicine was added to the list of designated health services affecting any nuclear scanning including positron emission tomography, or PET.

Anti-kickback Statute

The Medicare/Medicaid statute prohibits specific categories of referral payments, including kickbacks, bribes, or rebates. Specifically, the law forbids any act involving the solicitation, receipt, offer, or payment of any remuneration in return for referring an individual or arranging the purchase, lease, or ordering of an item or service that may be wholly or partially paid for under a federal healthcare program.

As in Stark, protection is available under the anti-kickback statute if a physician is an employee of a group practice or another healthcare organization — the so-called safe harbor rule. Physicians may have similar "safe harbor" protection when they are compensated under independent contractor agreements for personal services and management contracts under specific circumstances. This statute should be consulted for more detailed coverage of this important legislation.

Health Insurance Portability and Accountability Act (HIPAA)

This act formally establishes a federal fraud and abuse control program to better coordinate federal, state, and local investigations and enforcement by federal agencies, including the Federal Bureau of Investigation, the Postal Inspection Service, and Office of Veterans Affairs, among others. The major provisions of the act include:[5]

- Established reporting and disclosure mechanisms that create a new data bank for fraud and abuse investigators to access

- Increased staff in the Health and Human Services (HHS) OIG from fewer than 800 to nearly 2,000 over the next few years, with offices in every state and major city to carry out investigations and audits

- Established a Medicare integrity program in which HHS can assign the task of utilization and fraud review of providers to outside contractors other than its Medicare carriers that will likely spur the carriers to carry out more aggressive review efforts

- Extended federal oversight activities and penalties to private health plans, including ratcheting up the penalties for false claims, expanding the use of whistle-blowers, and lowering the standard of proof required for assessing various civil and criminal penalties

- Made the liability provisions of the law applicable to administrators, billing agents, and other officer(s) or managing employee(s) for various civil and criminal penalties

- Extended mandatory exclusions to include all other federal health programs in addition to Medicare, thus placing a premium on providers "getting it right the first time" because cleaning it up later will make the matter much messier

The Balanced Budget Act of 1997

Certain provisions in this act make it easier for the government to exclude individuals from Medicare and extend the grounds for exclusion to include family members of the excluded persons. Other provisions establish civil penalties and possible exclusion for anyone who knows or should have known that they were contracting for services with an individual excluded from the program.

The False Claims Act

This act is the federal government's primary civil remedy for improper or fraudulent claims. It applies to all federal programs, from military procurement contracts and welfare benefits to healthcare benefits. Individuals who "knowingly" submit false claims may be found liable under the act for penalties of between $5,000 and $10,000 for each false claim up to three times the amount of damages caused to the federal program. Specific intent to defraud the government is not required; the government need only establish that the claim submitted was false and that it was submitted knowingly, as defined by the statute.

Each U.S. attorney's office now has a healthcare fraud coordinator, and there is increasingly close coordination among the Department of Justice, the Federal Bureau of Investigation, state Medicaid fraud units, and other federal agencies. The False Claims Act has been applied to cases of improper billing practices; claims for services not rendered; provision of medically unnecessary services; misrepresenting eligibility or credentials; and most recently, substandard quality of care.

DEFINITIONS OF FRAUD AND ABUSE UNDER THE FEDERAL ACTS

The above acts cited fraud and abuse extensively. What do these terms mean related to healthcare? *Fraud* is defined as:[6]

> *Knowingly and willfully making or causing to make any false statement or representation of a material fact, in an application for a Medicare/Medicaid benefit or payment, or for use in determining the right to any such benefit or payment; or having knowledge of a right to receive a benefit (on the part of the party under consideration) or affecting the right of another individual in whose behalf the party under consideration receives such benefit, and failing to disclose such event with the intent to secure either a greater amount or quantity than is due or to receive benefit when none is due.*

Abuse is defined as "incidents and practices, which although not considered fraudulent acts, may directly or indirectly cause financial losses to the Medicare/Medicaid program or to beneficiaries and their families."[7]

Specific Instances of Law Infractions

The following list indicates practices for which physicians and medical providers have been fined, sanctioned, or convicted:[8]

- Billing/Medicare/Medicaid X-rays, blood tests, and other procedures that were never performed or falsifying a patient's diagnosis to justify unnecessary tests
- Ordering excessive tests that are performed by practices in which there is a financial interest, that are pay-based on referrals, or that are tenants in a building owned by the referring physician
- Giving a patient a generic drug and billing for a name-brand version of the medication and giving a patient an over-the-counter drug and billing for the prescription drug

- Billing Medicare/Medicaid for care not given, for care given to patients who have died or who are no longer eligible, or for care given to patients who have transferred to another facility
- Requiring vendors to "kickback" part of the money received for rendering services to Medicare/Medicaid patients
- Billing patients for services already paid for by Medicare/Medicaid
- Falsifying credentials and double billing
- Billing a service in disguise as another service so that it falls under Medicare/Medicaid coverage
- Changing codes to "get a claim paid"
- Downcoding to maximize reimbursement

COMPLIANCE PROGRAMS FOR MEDICAL PRACTICES

With the proliferation of federal and state fraud and abuse legislation and the enforcement activities aimed at the healthcare industry, implementation of a tailored compliance program is recommended not only to prevent violations but also to reduce the potential for liability should violations occur. The HHS OIG believes significant reductions in fraud and abuse liability can be accomplished through the use of compliance plans. An effective compliance plan can minimize the consequences resulting from a violation of the law and may, in some cases, convince a prosecutor not to pursue a criminal action. Sentencing guidelines and the U.S. Department of Justice provide for lesser criminal sanctions for companies that have effective compliance plans in operation.

In addition, a compliance program provides other valuable benefits to healthcare organizations. Such a program permits outside counsel to ensure that an organization's documentation and communications procedures make maximum use of the important attorney-client and attorney-work product privileges. A compliance program also establishes a mechanism for employee training on how to handle search warrants and unannounced searches by investigators. The program also sets up a relationship with outside counsel who thereafter is familiar with the practice's corporate structure, document system, and general operations. Finally, a compliance program promotes a law-abiding corporate ethos and discourages wrongdoing, and it provides some protection for officers and directors from individual criminal and civil liability.

What Is a Corporate Compliance Program?

The term *corporate compliance program* is designed to standardize and increase the predictability of the medical practice through the use of guidelines. These were designed to encourage the implementation of internal mechanisms to prevent, detect, and report criminal conduct by providing that the organization will be determined by the steps it has taken prior to the offense to achieve these goals. A corporate compliance program refers to the internal mechanisms or steps that an organization takes to prevent and detect violations of law. It is more than a document and embraces a set of procedures, responsibilities, and activities that must be operationalized and continuously maintained.

Designing a Corporate Compliance Program

Prior to the actual design of a corporate compliance program, a practice should have board authorization and commitment to the program. The corporate compliance program reflects upper management's intent to comply with federal regulations and indicates a culture of compliance. Employees need to know and support the compliance initiative, understand the reasons for compliance, view the program as fair and flexible, and see senior management as complying fully with the tenets of the program. The compliance program includes seven components:

1. The practice must establish a written plan with compliance standards and procedures to be followed by its employees and other agents that are reasonably capable of reducing the prospect of criminal or wrongful conduct.

2. An effective compliance program must address oversight responsibilities. This involves appointment of a compliance officer and committee. The officer should report to the "board" and not the practice administrator to maintain as much independence as possible.

3. Once the above has been established, an adequate enforcement and discipline procedure should be set to ensure consistent enforcement of the compliance standards via an appropriate disciplinary mechanism.

4. The practice is responsible for maintaining the plan with regularly scheduled reviews and updates as well as monitoring changes in regulations to ensure that the plan itself is fully compliant.

5. Employees have eyes and ears that will benefit the compliance program. Encouraging them to monitor and giving them a vehicle with which they can report suspicious items that they feel may be noncompliant is a key step in the plan.

6. The practice should develop a monitoring and auditing system to detect criminal and other wrongful conduct by its employees and other agents; the practice should also have in place and publicize a reporting system whereby employees and other agents can report criminal and other wrongful conduct by others within the practice without fear of retribution.

7. The practice must take all reasonable steps to respond to detected offenses and to prevent further similar offenses, including any necessary modifications to its program.

With the implementation of the Affordable Care Act (ACA), there is greater emphasis on internal compliance programs. The increased use of the electronic health record and enhancements in the meaningful use application will provide ample opportunities for the government to access practice information. This "window" will put more and more individual practices at risk for noncompliance. This adds to the importance of establishing an effective compliance program.

MGMA COMPLIANCE TOOLS

To assist medical groups in complying with the federal regulatory requirements and to assist them in developing formal compliance programs, MGMA has three types of tools available: (1) education programs, (2) publications, and (3) consulting services.

Education programs include audio recordings of conferences covering compliance subjects, live courses dealing with compliance programs and fraud and abuse, and turnkey programs involving national subject matter experts.

Publications include a small group practice resource guide on compliance programs, *The Physician Practice Compliance Report* newsletter, and information exchanges on Medicare compliance plans and Medicare corporate compliance plans.

For complex and larger practices, expert consultants within the MGMA Health Care Consulting Group are available to assist organizations in assessing their compliance needs and providing guidance in compliance plan development.

Since governmental emphasis is being placed on fraud and related abuses, financial managers must lead an overall effort to address these problems and design systems and practical processes to preclude their occurrence.

What Should Practice Administrators Do?

The scope and seriousness of these new federal efforts to combat fraud and abuse require physicians and practice administrators to be proactive in searching out and eliminating possible fraudulent situations. The following list of steps indicate "imperative" actions for management to undertake:

1. Even if there is full compliance with Medicare/Medicaid requirements, conduct a review and develop a quality control system to ensure continued compliance and any indicated improvement.

2. Physicians should ensure that patients' medical records are complete and accurate. It is important for physicians to recognize that when a payer questions a claim, the first step is to send the payer a copy of the medical record for examination, comparison, and clarification. If discrepancies exist between the record and a claim, a delay in payment, further investigation, and a possible audit of other claims may be the result. Thus, care must be taken to ensure that there is complete and sufficient medical record information. Patient records must be able to stand alone in any subsequent review or dispute.

3. Coding must be proper and accurate. Providers are the best people to determine which services are actually performed and that codes are correct. The burden of proof is on the physicians to validate that services

were performed and at the level of care billed. Thus, an extensive internal comparative review of the offices' coding patterns should be done to identify potential problems. A certified procedural coder (CPC) could assist in this process, relieving some of the tension felt by the provider.

4. As part of an internal compliance program, arrange for an "off the record" audit, which, based on confidential attorney-client privilege, allows physicians to safely explore any potential problem areas. If any fraudulent practices are found, the employee(s) can reveal his or her wrongdoing with the assurance that the company will not be prosecuted criminally. During this process, pay close attention to licensure, Medicare certification, utilization, reimbursement, billing and coding matters, and relationships between physicians and other contractors and vendors.

5. Consider revising patient education materials to better explain procedures and the billing process, thus avoiding confusion and unnecessary complaints.

6. Review human resource procedures to identify disgruntled employees. Employee training programs and effective communication efforts will assist in dealing with this type of issue.

FRAUD AND THEFT

Why do employees steal? While experts say that reasons for economic crime in the workplace are numerous, most agree that human greed is at the heart of the problem. Also, the combination of temptation and opportunity offers a formula that can translate to significant losses. The problem probably goes much deeper. These other factors seem to play a role, too: (1) lax hiring policies, (2) allowing long-time employees easy access to money and products, (3) a corporate attitude that appears resigned to a certain amount of crime, and (4) executives who project a callous and uncaring attitude toward employees. Virtually all individuals who steal from an employer feel that the company is big and profitable and can afford the loss. If you factor in the ease with which employees can manipulate and remove information from a computer, then the potential for loss is enormous.

Some Precursors of Fraud and Theft

Certain conditions within medical groups could lead to employee theft and fraud. Recognizing and altering these conditions can deter abusive practices and strengthen the overall framework of control and ethical behavior. Some include:

Accounting systems and procedures — Many potential trouble spots arise with handling cash, inventory control, supply rooms, and tampering with the accounting system. Here are some samples of poor procedures:

■ The same person handles cash receipts and has access to accounts receivable records. In some cases, this individual also deposits the checks at the bank.

■ The individual who writes checks for payments also reconciles the bank statements.

- Incomplete documentation of the purchase of goods and services such as purchase authorizations, receiving slips, and vendor invoices and a failure to independently verify the transaction by examining these documents before payment is made

- Poor physical safeguards and no limitations on persons who can access drugs and medical supplies

- Failure to require an annual audit of the financial statements and underlying accounting records by an independent auditor or failure to have at least one independent review annually

- Access to credit card information that the patient has provided for regular payments on their accounts

Operations — Several areas involving the staffing and implementation of group activities may indicate ethical weaknesses, such as the following:

- Heavy employee turnover, particularly at the financial manager position. For example, if there have been three or four different financial managers over a two- or three-year period, it could be a sign that senior management is manipulating the books.

- Any large payments made for "miscellaneous purposes or services" or unusual patterns in employee expense claims, such as travel or expenditures of a personal nature

- Employees not taking vacations or time off, especially the financial manager or staff working in finance

Management caricatures — Certain characteristics about physician managers and nonphysician managers might provide an indication of possible misconduct, such as the following:

- The setting of unrealistic performance goals of performance, such as large increases in net income, that drive financial managers to fraudulent practices. These might include creating fictional financial reports, collusion with outside payers, and falsifying records to support erroneous transactions.

- Managers assuming clerical functions, such as insisting on personally reconciling all bank statements

- Managers who are unable to find "missing" records that document large transactions or a series of relatively small transactions

- A lackadaisical attitude or uncaring concern by physician-owners for anything financial or financially related to the practice

Measures to Prevent Theft and Fraud

Faced with the increase in unethical conduct, healthcare entities are taking many preventive measures to deter fraudulent activities. These measures include:

Tightening the hiring process — The effort to decrease employee theft begins with the hiring process. Medical groups can weed out potential thieves in these ways:

- Conduct a complete and probing personal interview of each applicant.

- Contact previous places of employment to verify dates of employment and positions held.

- Check with the candidate's university or professional school to see if the person actually graduated.

- Interview personal references very thoroughly by asking tough follow-up questions.

- If appropriate, administer pencil-and-paper honesty tests to screen out potentially untrustworthy employees. These tests predict future behavior based on the applicant's attitudes and admissions of past conduct. Handwriting analysis is also a useful purveyor of personal traits. (Care must be taken in this regard to ensure that these tests meet the professional standards of reliability and validity; otherwise, they may open the door to lawsuits against the user and the test publisher.)

- Conduct complete background checks on physicians and higher-level managers to be hired.

- Develop your own references for candidates for high-level positions.

Strengthening deterrents — Every business, including medical groups, should have an ethical policy, and if necessary, a published and prominent standard of conduct for all group members to follow. The policy and code should stipulate what constitutes illegal and irregular activities as well as the consequences of such actions. Furthermore, the physician-owners and top management should set the example by displaying proper behavior that typifies ethical conduct. With this proper overall framework, other deterrent actions might consist of the following:

- Establish a strong system of accountability among the members of the governing body in which they must answer fully for their actions and the fulfillment of their responsibilities. Such a requirement can thwart the development of absolute power and domination among one or a few members of the governing group.

- Devise methods to keep all members of the governing body informed in a clear, concise, and current manner about the activities of the medical group. Make sure those with less training or experience understand the financial impacts of all decisions on the organization.

- Designate certain members of the governing body who have some financial experience to be the prime monitors of the financial statements and reports prepared by the financial manager and/or the staff.

- Set up a budgetary control system that physicians and other managers can understand. The system should embrace the operating budget and long-term capital budget. Both budgets should be subject to the scrutiny of top management and the governing body of the medical group.

- Insist that professional service contracts be explicit as to what is to be provided, how it is to be paid for, and what supporting documentation will be part of the contract. Do not permit the submission of documents "for X hours of service" as the only support for payment.

- Encourage a positive attitude toward the medical group by treating all employees fairly and openly and making sure that human relations policies are supportive of employee rights and concerns.

- Provide adequate compensation levels and employee benefits comparable to other healthcare entities in the local area.

Establishing conflict-of-interest restrictions — Many practices today require all employees to sign conflict-of-interest statements promising they will not take advantage of an outside interest to profit illegally from the company. While this may not yet be a practice followed by medical groups, the time has arrived to consider such a policy for the physicians and managers of the group. For example, if someone in the group has an interest in an outside business not necessarily connected with direct medical care services but that provides a service to the group, that relationship is immediately suspect, especially if it is not openly revealed. Also, when a member of the group — physician or manager — is doing business with a longtime friend or relative, the group member should remain objective and insist on having detailed contracts and underlying documentation. These data should be scrutinized by other members of the group to ensure that transactions are appropriate and sanctioned by group management.

Installing and continuously updating computer security systems — A growing proportion of business fraud is committed via the computer. Management must be alert and should use the latest electronic security tools. The most important preventive controls are those that limit access to computers, data files, programs, and system documentation to a minimum number of persons. Methods of limiting access include defining employee duties, segregating functional responsibilities, dual-person access, enforced vacations for personnel, physical security, and electronic surveillance and security including access-code passwords. Governing bodies of medical groups should use outside consultants who specialize in security password control, networking security, and other key elements of computer security to establish and make sure the latest measures are in effect.

Protecting the medical group itself — Usually as part of the standard business insurance package, dishonesty insurance protects the business against losses from employee theft. Medical groups can add this coverage to their policies, which will require the insurer to check the group's hiring procedures and theft-prevention efforts.

In addition, employers can buy fidelity bonds to cover all employees or only certain positions, such as bookkeepers or financial managers or specifically named employees.

Confronting and prosecuting offenders — In carrying out policies and procedures aimed at stopping theft and fraud, medical group management must confront violators openly and in a straightforward manner. Ignoring these violations or excusing such actions sends the wrong message to other employees and destroys the tone that top management should be setting for all to act honestly and legally. There must be strong and visible evidence of a commitment to ethics and moral behavior in all aspects of the group's activities. Some helpful hints to reinforce these ideas include:

- Do not tolerate harassment at any level of the organization, particularly at the top. There should be no bending of the rules or ignoring them since such action will likely lead to a degeneration of the rules of proper conduct.

- Pay attention to stress factors that key staff members may exhibit. To avert possible misappropriation by stressed individuals, intervene when it is in the best interest of the group by offering assistance to the person in whatever manner is deemed necessary.

- Do not compromise on carrying out professional and personal ethics. If a problem exists with an individual, assist in finding a solution even if there is some discomfort experienced by the participants.

While it seems humane to refrain from prosecuting violators of ethical conduct, aggressive prosecution can also send a strong warning to anyone else who is stealing or conspiring with others. Medical group managers must be determined to reduce theft with a broad program of surveillance, security, and, where necessary, prosecution of offenders.

In the final analysis, financial decision making depends on the integrity of the financial manager. Groups must have in place management and staff with ethical and moral values and the strength necessary to act within a defined set of rules that are appropriate in our society. Leadership is needed to exhibit personal character and courage because, without it, we will not have ethical behavior in any of our institutions.

FUTURE HORIZONS FOR ACCOUNTABILITY

The healthcare industry's response to the call for greater accountability has moved beyond the fraud and abuse area. Two significant developments are (1) outcomes-based research and (2) measuring, reporting, and improving the quality of care. Let's examine these movements briefly.

Outcomes-based Research

In the context of healthcare, outcomes refer to the results of medical interventions. They include health outcomes and/or cost outcomes. Thus, outcomes-based research is the assessment of the effect of a given product, procedure, or medical technology on health and/or cost outcomes. This research focuses on outcomes measurements — that is, collecting data and evaluating the extent to which individual providers meet the health and/or cost outcome goals of their patients and/or their institutions.

Outcomes data derived to date promise to impact many participants of the healthcare industry and many of its activities. These include:

- **Medical professionals and physicians** — Outcomes data can be used to develop practice guidelines that can then be used in selecting care protocols that have proven to bring about good outcomes. Physicians can use outcomes data feedback to continually improve their delivery system to enhance appropriateness, effectiveness, and efficiency.

- **Patients** — The public availability of outcomes data outlining the prognosis and success likelihoods of alternative medical interventions can significantly elevate the role of the patient in the decision-making process for treatment. Ultimately, such data can help patients, families, and physicians to jointly make sound decisions.

- **Payers** — Payers want to use outcomes data to reduce cost of care and to have better criteria to select physicians and other providers for their clients. Also, this data can benefit payers by leading to the reduction of defensive medicine whereby physicians supporting their decisions with outcomes data will feel less pressured to order tests on a just-in-case basis.

- **Employers** — Employers also envision outcomes data as a way to reduce costs. Information that couples the status of outcomes from medical treatments with associated costs will be revealing and will help in choosing the best plan for employees.

- **Physician profiling** — After outcomes management systems are widely implemented in hospitals, clinics, and health plans, the process of granting physician privileges and credentials will likely become largely outcomes-data driven.

- **Publication of outcomes data for public use** — As data such as hospital mortality rates, length of stay, charges, and so on become more widespread, employer coalitions are campaigning to collect them in order to rate institutions and physicians on the basis of quality care.

Measuring, Reporting, and Improving Quality of Care

The quality-of-care issue has been addressed elsewhere in this text. Here, we want to summarize some specific methods the industry is currently using to measure quality. Initially, improving quality of care involved utilization review and utilization management techniques. Today, the following four approaches seem to be dominant:

1. **Benchmarking databases and physician profiling** — Databases collecting the protocols and operations of providers form the basis for benchmark-setting practices that allow groups to compare their internal performance to that of their competitors or "best practice" sites around the country. When data indicate areas of underperformance, efforts can be initiated for improvement using a method called "drill down" to precisely identify problem areas. Physician profiling is an analytic tool that uses epidemiological methods to compare practiced patterns of providers on dimension of cost, service, use, and/or quality (process and outcomes of care).

2. **Customer-focused continuous quality improvement (CQI)** — This approach focuses on the customer or patient. Data compiled in benchmarking and physician profiling are used to improve quality of care delivery to the patient. The goal of CQI is to improve customer satisfaction with additional aims being customer retention and an increase in market share. Practice leadership must be the driver of this process, as recounted in our earlier discussion of this topic.

3. **Standardized measurement systems** —HEDIS has become the standardized performance measurement system of choice for many medical practices. HEDIS has evolved into a measurement tool capable of assessing how effectively health plans treat acute and chronic illnesses, as well as member satisfaction and health plan stability.

4. **Clinical practice guidelines** — These guidelines can be used to improve upon HEDIS performance. They are an important tool ensuring that physicians do not over- or underutilize treatments and procedures. Practice guidelines are available from the American Medical Association. Specialty societies and other organizations or medical groups may develop their own set based on the collective experience of the group's physicians.

As accountability becomes recognized as an overriding focus for healthcare delivery, both outcomes data and quality measures will be important tools that the financial manager must use to stay abreast of healthcare industry developments. These efforts offer sound bases for measuring performance as physicians, medical groups, and other entities in the industry are called to account in larger ways in the future. Continued monitoring of these initiatives must become an important element in the manager's arsenal of knowledge to guide the practice successfully.

To the Point

■ Accountability is accepting the consequences of actions taken. One party, the accountable party, has an obligation to answer or report actions taken on behalf of the other party, the stakeholder, in striving to achieve practice objectives.

■ The accountability model identifies three levels:

- The organization must have a culture of accountability with the leadership, standards, performance measures, and reports to ensure that it stays true to its accountable culture.

- There is a distinction between accountability, responsibility, and authority. Responsibility is the obligation to act and a willingness to see oneself as the principal source of the results produced by actions taken. Accountability is the obligation to answer and willingness to claim ownership for results of actions. Authority enables the employee to accomplish the task in a responsible and accountable manner.

- — At the individual and team level, the assignments are made to determine who will do the work, to whom are they accountable, and what exactly will be done.

■ The enabling activities and processes include:
  - — Intentions of action plans
  - — Resources or authorizations to act
  - — Standards of accountability reporting
  - — Performance measures
  - — Accountability reports
  - — Balance of power and level of trust

■ To start an analysis of accountability issues in any environment — business, government, personal, and healthcare — three key questions should be answered:

  1. Who should be held accountable?
  2. To whom should the accountable party answer?
  3. For what should the accountable party be held to account?

■ Standards of accountability reporting relate to the norms or standards of acceptable performance that accountable parties and stakeholders agree to use in measuring performance.

■ Performance measures are the companion element to accountability standards and are indicators to measure the performance of accountable parties; they should describe what is done and how well it is done.

■ Accountability reports can take myriad forms depending on the parties involved; generally, they include oral communication, visual observations, and written reports prepared by the accountable party.

■ The advantages of adopting an accountability perspective for a financial manager as a focal point for approaching his or her major responsibilities include:

- Helps focus on the problem
- Identifies clearly the doers of activities
- Results in self-regulating conduct
- Encourages planning throughout the medical group
- Establishes meaningful benchmarks for doers to aspire to
- Avoids excuses for failures by clearly delineating responsibilities
- Enables the setting of productive improvement objectives

■ Managed care and the emphasis on quality service are driving forces for greater accountability in the healthcare industry. To date, holding parties accountable has centered on efforts grounded in law and market competition.

■ Five major federal legislative acts addressing fraud and abuse in healthcare are the (1) Stark Law, (2) Anti-kickback Statute, (3) Health Insurance Portability and Accountability Act (HIPAA), (4) Balanced Budget Act of 1997, and (5) False Claims Act.

■ To prevent fraud and abuse and to ameliorate any wrongdoing discovered, most medical practices should establish a corporate compliance program following the seven components.

■ In responding to the call for greater accountability, the healthcare industry is developing two additional approaches: (1) outcomes-based research and (2) measuring, reporting, and improving quality of care.

REFERENCES

1. "Stakeholder." Wikipedia. Retrieved from http://en.wikipedia.org/wiki/Stakeholder. Accessed October 1, 2012.

2. McGlynn, E. A. 1997, May/June. "Six Challenges in Measuring the Quality of Health Care." *Health Affairs*, 14.

3. Ibid., 14–15.

4. Sandrick, K. M. 1993, March. "Ethical Misconduct in Health Care Financial Management." *Health Care Financial Management*, 35.

5. Ibid.

6. Britton, W. 1997, December 1. "Health Care Providers Beware — And Be Prepared." *Medical Group Management Update*, 1.

7. Ibid.

8. Ibid., 4.

CHAPTER 17

An Era of Reform

Deborah Walker Keegan, PhD, FACMPE

Each chapter in this book has been devoted to a key aspect of financial management in today's medical practices. Financial management for the future is expected to be more complex as we proceed through an era of healthcare reform. While healthcare reform is a continuous journey rather than a turnkey event, there is sufficient evidence to support the assertion that financial management for the future will require new skill sets and new metrics and will be situated and aligned within new structural models of care.

THE NEW FINANCIAL MANAGEMENT

The "new financial management" will require an expansion of data metrics and new skill sets among practice leaders, accountants, financial analysts, and revenue cycle managers.

Expenditure Management

Measuring the cost of a medical practice today involves a careful analysis of revenue and expenditures, processes that have been described in many of the chapters in this book. These measures will continue to have relevancy in the future, as medical practices work to align business operations with clinical operations.

However, a new measure related to the cost of practice will be its value proposition. Value-based purchasing is expected to overtake fee-for-service reimbursement in the near future.[1] Medical practices will be required to demonstrate their value, defined as high quality at low cost. This extends beyond common data metrics, such as cost per visit or cost per work relative value unit (wRVU). It will be necessary to develop the infrastructure to report and manage the cost per diagnosis, per procedure, per episode of care, and across the transitions of care, with linkages to the outcomes of that care.

As we transition to value-based purchasing, each and every diagnosis, each and every service, and each and every procedure will be parsed to an unprecedented level of detail. In the future, medical practices will be evaluated on their interventions and the cost and outcomes of those interventions, not only at the level of the individual patient, but also at the level of the patient population served by the medical practice.

For many medical practices, such an undertaking will not be easy. Data mining and data analytics skills are required for these measurements. Business intelligence must also be coupled with clinical intelligence, an advanced understanding of the clinical diagnoses and the impact of care and service interventions provided by the practice's care team.

Supportive infrastructures are just now being readied to facilitate these new value metrics. These include ICD-10 codes that offer a level of specificity heretofore not even imagined, with the diagnosis code beginning the algorithm for differential reimbursement. A differential diagnosis code specific to the patient and the patient's condition will permit individualized care, with the addition of value-based modifiers providing variable payment based on quality and cost between and among medical practices. EHRs are also instrumental in measuring value. As improvements are made to EHRs, data mining and reporting are becoming increasingly sophisticated to permit data analysis at a more refined level.

Revenue Cycle Management

Reimbursing medical practices for value rather than service volume will also tax current revenue cycle management. The revenue cycle of the future will be more complex as it transitions from fee-for-service to newer reimbursement models. We do not currently know the end-state reimbursement model; however, each of the following payment reform strategies is currently in process or is in a demonstration project state.

Payment for New Systems Adoption

The Medicare and Medicaid EHR Incentive programs for the meaningful use of electronic health records provide financial incentives for physicians to adopt EHRs.[2] These programs serve as levers to ensure that medical practices adopt new technologies.

Payment for Geographic Location

Beyond the geographic price cost index (GPCI) that is applied in the calculation to determine procedural reimbursement for the Medicare Part B fee schedule, differences in reimbursement exist due to the demographic classification of the medical practice and the location where a service is provided. For example, rurally qualified healthcare centers receive cost-based reimbursement at a level that differs from traditional fee-for-service reimbursement. Similarly, payment differentials based on the location where a service is performed are likely to continue to serve as a steerage mechanism to lower cost care venues.

Payment for Reducing the Cost of Care

Shared savings programs — most notably, the CMS Shared Savings Program to create or participate in ACOs — provide incentives to coordinate care and to reduce the cost of care.[3] These programs encourage a new structural reform agenda. Today's commercial payers are ahead of or aligning with this trend.

Payment for Care Coordination

Two models have emerged as likely alternatives to fee-for-service reimbursement. These include fixed fee arrangements and bundled payment models, both of which encourage coordination of care. Many large systems and early entrants to accountable care are in the planning phases or have already adopted risk-based reimbursement for a defined patient population using one or both of these models.

Fixed fee arrangements are akin to a global capitation payment to manage the full continuum of care. Bundled payments are a type of fixed fee arrangement and involve a fixed fee payment for Part A and Part B services for a defined episode of care. The CMS bundled payment demonstration project has proven so successful that it has recently been expanded from the Acute Care Episode (ACE) Demonstration Program that was focused on orthopedic surgery and cardiovascular services to a Bundled Payments for Care Improvement Initiative (BPCII) involving four bundled payment models.[4]

Payment for Value

Value-based payment modifiers (VBPM) are expected to be applied to the Medicare Physician Fee Schedule (MPFS) and will differentiate reimbursement based on value as part of the Physician Feedback/Value-Based Modifier Program.[5] This program will likely have interruption effects on current pay-for-performance reimbursement schemes since the value-based modifiers are expected to differentiate quality and cost differences in care delivery at a refined level, above and beyond current pay-for-performance programs.

No Payment for Errors

The National Quality Forum continues to refine its list of "serious reportable events" for which many payers will not be reimbursing in the future.[6] It is difficult to make the case that these errors should continue to be funded, and it is likely that the list of serious reportable events will be longer in the future. This essentially creates a "warranty" for many procedures and services with no additional reimbursement paid to rectify preventable or possibly preventable errors.

Nonparticipation Penalties

Over the past few years, we have witnessed CMS's approach toward steerage to new technology and quality reporting. The approach typically involves a voluntary opportunity to participate, coupled with a small incentive to recognize the learning curve required for change. Once positive change has been demonstrated, the voluntary program essentially becomes mandatory as nonparticipation penalties are applied.

This carrot-and-stick approach is likely to continue and is currently in evidence with the PQRS program, the Electronic Prescribing (e-RX) Incentive Program, and the Medicare EHR Incentive Program. Financial planning is needed to develop the infrastructure for these programs within a medical group and to ensure appropriate outcomes reporting and receipt of incentive payments.

The above examples of payment reform strategies signal the need to alter the financial management systems of a medical practice. To ensure that the practice receives an appropriate amount of a fixed fee payment, it will be necessary to develop a deeper understanding of the individual costs that comprise a service delivered by the practice's physicians. Equally challenging is the financial management that will need to occur between and among a practice's physicians. Parsing out a fixed fee payment across specialists and across locations of service will require skill and detailed financials. It will also require new models to recognize not only productivity, but also quality, cost, and outcomes of work conducted by the care team.

Picture a new revenue cycle that does not involve the submission of individual claims for each service provided to the patient. Instead, a per-member per-month fee or a bundled payment — or these reimbursement methodologies in combination — will determine the revenue of the medical practice. A per-member per-month fee will reduce the many steps in the billing and collection process of the revenue cycle, and a bundled payment (similar to the current method by which transplant services are reimbursed to medical practices) essentially collapses all of the services into a single claim. A renewed focus on financial management, not billing and collection per se, is likely, ensuring that the medical practice and its physicians receive sufficient reimbursement from a fixed payment model that is characteristic of many of these payment reform strategies.

New health plan products within the fee-for-service arena will require medical practices to "front-load" their revenue cycle management. Many medical practices today are working with significant volumes of patients who have high-deductible health plans. Patients with high-deductible health plans are insured patients, but for a significant portion of their care, they pay out of pocket until their deductible is met. This requires a change in the revenue cycle management of a medical practice to conduct more of its billing at the point of care (provided contracts permit).

Patient financial clearance conducted prior to the patient being seen by the medical practice will require not only an understanding of insurance verification, but also an understanding of the type of plan the patient has, its eligibility requirements, and the amount to collect from the patient at the point of care and/or prior to rendering elective services. Patient payment obligations collected at the point of care will be the norm as patients assume greater out-of-pocket financial responsibility for their healthcare services.

During this important transition period when the reimbursement models are being tested, advocated, and debated, the medical practice will be required to manage its finances in two worlds — the fee-for-service world and the newer payment-reform world, signifying a significant challenge beyond today's financial and revenue cycle management.

Work Relative Value Units

We have discussed in this book the importance of wRVUs and their ability to permit a comparison of work and effort among physicians. Work relative value units are used by many medical practices as key components of their physician compensation plans. They are also used to analyze the cost of a medical practice and to make changes to its staffing deployment model. It is likely that with newer payment models, the usefulness of wRVUs will diminish.

If a medical practice is paid a portion of a bundled rate for a procedure, the wRVU may still be used as an internal distribution vehicle to allocate the bundled payment to the appropriate physicians based on work effort. More likely, we will witness a transition away from production-oriented physician compensation models that often rely on wRVUs to base-plus-incentive models that recognize the base level of work required of all physicians coupled with incentives for quality, outcomes, and patient experience of care. In fact, increasing work volume (and wRVUs) runs counter to the value equation of providing the appropriate care with high quality at low cost.

General Accounting

General accounting will continue to be important, due to the tax and legal structure of medical practices and healthcare systems. However, budgeting revenue based on trend data will continue to be a frustrating exercise in the near term. Financial analysts will be vexed as they work to answer the following questions in a new healthcare reform environment:

- Will the changes in high-deductible healthcare plans lead patients to postpone or even elect not to pursue costly intervention strategies?
- Will greater patient involvement in care decision making lead to lower demand for elective procedures?
- How much will the online patient portal and EHR reduce face-to-face visits?
- What is the volume of virtual medicine performed, and at what level will it be reimbursed?
- Will the sustainable growth rate (SGR) be repealed, or do we need risk modeling in preparation for a significant revenue reduction?
- What projections should be used for state Medicaid programs, and what will be our share of these patients?

The budgeting process today is challenging for financial experts, and this will continue in the near term. It is hoped that the budgeting process will be less complex once the payment, structure, and delivery system reform strategies have been tested and clear winners emerge.

Health Plan Products

New benefit plans are emerging, and the introduction of state insurance exchanges will likely also add a new level of complexity. Beyond high-deductible health plans coupled with health savings accounts, we are witnessing stratification of patient payment levels based on type of service and location of service. Examples include variable copayment and deductible levels based on type of service such as no or low out-of-pocket payment for preventive care, and variable payment levels based on location of service such as a higher copayment if nonurgent care is sought in a hospital's emergency room.

FUTURE OF MEDICAL PRACTICES

Emerging Models

Payers, hospitals, and medical practices are now merging or aligning to create accountable care organizations and to integrate the financing and delivery of healthcare.[7] Payment reform is driving structural reform, and structural reform is in turn driving delivery system reform. Each of the disparate entities — payer, hospital, and medical practice — brings a different lens with which to view an integrated system.

From the payer's perspective, the hospital is viewed as a cost center. Horizontal integration or the merging of hospitals will do little to reduce the cost of care unless there are significant economies of scale or leverage to close hospitals within a community or region where redundancies exist. Some payers have therefore determined that their "best" option is to align with medical practices whose physicians have direct control of the cost of care and are integral to effective coordination of care along the continuum of primary, specialty, hospital, post-acute care facility, and home care venues.

A hospital generally makes money by filling its beds with high-margin procedures and services. From the hospital's perspective, a payer's lead in the new structural models translates to reduced admissions and lengths of stay. Many hospitals are therefore attempting to simultaneously execute two integration strategies:

▪ Horizontal integration or merging with other hospitals to build market share

▪ Vertical integration involving closer linkages with medical practices and their physicians

Some medical practices are also taking the lead to integrate financing and delivery. From the physician's perspective, it is the physician who controls much of the resource utilization involved in care delivery. For medical practices that have sufficient access to capital, it is a natural step to take the lead in aligning the hospital and payer in a new structural or contractual relationship that furthers the demonstration of accountable care. Medical group mergers and clinically integrated networks are therefore being pursued.

Systems that integrate financing and delivery are emerging in many markets today. Let's take a look at some of the models already emerging as forerunners in this area.

Payer-Led Integration

CMS's Medicare Shared Savings Program, Pioneer ACO Model, and Advance Payment Model are examples of payer-led integration strategies. Each of these programs provides for a financial incentive to encourage integration between hospitals and physicians as they collectively manage Medicare beneficiaries.[8]

Other payers are also taking the lead and implementing similar strategies. For example, Blue Cross Blue Shield of Massachusetts contracts with medical groups and hospitals via its Alternative Quality Contract (AQC), with a goal of reducing annual health spending growth. With the AQC, the medical group or hospital has an annual risk-adjusted global budget based on historical spending. Though fee-for-service payments are made throughout the year, these payments are debited against the budget, with a year-end financial reconciliation determining if a surplus is to be paid or if the medical group or hospital needs to repay the payer. The hospitals and medical groups are essentially "on a budget" when it comes to providing care to a defined patient population.[9]

An important payer strategy not to be overlooked is the increasing volume of payer acquisitions of medical practices. Recent acquisitions of large medical groups by payers (with many of these models designed to grow a payer's Medicare or Medicaid patient base) have demonstrated that integration of financing and delivery can occur in a material way and essentially overnight.[10]

Hospital-Led Integration

CMS has a number of initiatives in place that encourage hospitals to develop collaborative models with their physicians to achieve long-term financial success. These initiatives typically involve a reduction in revenue to the hospital if it is not able to demonstrate value (the Hospital Value-Based Purchasing Program), demonstrate appropriate levels of hospital-acquired conditions (the Hospital Acquired Conditions expansion program involving Medicare and Medicaid), and meet new measures for hospital quality reporting (the Hospital Inpatient Quality Reporting Program and the Readmissions Reduction Program).[11] These initiatives are serving as steerage mechanisms to more closely align hospitals with physicians in their communities. It will be difficult for a hospital to achieve the new targets and goals without physician cooperation and active engagement.

As a consequence, hospitals are adopting a number of structural models to foster enhanced coordination with physicians. These include "loose" integration models, including service line co-management agreements and pay-for-quality programs, to tighter collaborative models involving professional services agreements or direct physician employment.[12]

Some of today's hospitals look as though they are "one stop" delivery systems, having employed a multispecialty group of physicians to provide inpatient and outpatient services to the community. They have expanded their direct employment models to extend along the full continuum of physicians from primary care to specialist to subspecialist.

Medical Group-Led Integration

Many medical groups have pursued clinical integration as a method of aligning and coordinating care. Not surprisingly, the Federal Trade Commission has exercised an active voice regarding this method of integration, stating that the network clinical integration program must be "real," that joint contracting is "reasonably necessary" to achieve the efficiencies of the clinical integration program, and that initiatives of the program must be designed in such a way to achieve likely improvements in quality and efficiency.[13]

Examples of clinically integrated networks include Atrius Health based in Massachusetts, which is currently the largest independent, nonprofit physician-based accountable care organization,[14] and Advocate Physician Partners in the Chicago area, which was an early entrant to clinical integration, aligning multiple physician-hospital organizations and contracting for pay-for-performance with payers.[15] Clinically integrated networks are currently transitioning from a contracting vehicle to an ACO, as they work to expand patient access, reduce unnecessary care, and manage care transitions.

Financial Integration

To foster integration among payers, hospitals, and medical groups, a financial model is required. Without such a financial model, there is insufficient capital to develop the required infrastructure and insufficient incentive for the parties to develop collaborative ties. CMS estimates that an ACO in its Shared Savings Program will likely need start-up costs of $580,000 and ongoing annual operating costs of $1.27 million.[16]

Certainly many of the ACOs that are being developed at the present time are not of this magnitude; however, capital is needed to develop new infrastructures, adopt evidence-based clinical guidelines, create new staffing deployment models, and expand patient access to care and services, which are only some of the many delivery system changes adopted by organizations as they work to demonstrate accountable care.

There are a number of capitalization strategies that are under way. These include:

- Additional fee-for-service reimbursement, fixed fee payment, or per-member per-month payment for a defined period to develop new infrastructure
- Grant or seed money paid by a payer or payer foundation
- Loans to be repaid via subsequent cost savings
- Investment incentives for successful targets and goals
- Development of management services organizations or other entities[17]

Importantly, the initial financial model likely will not be the end-state financial model. The initial financial model's usefulness is to foster collaboration, infrastructure development, trust, and other similar requirements to promote close alignment of previously disparate entities. For example, pay-for-performance programs serve to align disparate entities and focus efforts on improving quality and efficiency. Yet, beyond additional reimbursement to achieve targets and goals, there is a need to expand these models to achieve the goals of accountable care and patient population management. Similarly, a shared savings program may serve to align hospitals, payers, and medical practices; however, once the savings have been wrung out of the system, a point of diminishing return is reached.

As these examples illustrate, pay-for-performance and shared savings financial models are likely intermediate vehicles to foster integration, rather than end-state models. The current payment reform experiments under way are expected to help define the future state of payment reform and a number of leading experts are weighing in.

A group of Harvard academicians, for example, has postulated different reimbursement models based on service type.[18] Based on their research:

- "Intuitive medicine" involving the determination of a differential diagnosis should be reimbursed on a fee-for-service basis

- ■ "Precision medicine" involving a procedure or treatment should be reimbursed based on outcomes (such as via a bundled payment or fixed fee reimbursement)
- ■ Health maintenance and prevention involving facilitated networks should be paid on a membership basis (such as via a per-member per-month reimbursement)

We do not yet know the end-state payment reform model. It may be that fully integrated systems are paid a fixed fee to manage the full continuum of care for the patient or via a hybrid model involving multiple payment methods.

Patient Engagement in Financial Management

Throughout this chapter we have discussed the changes in financial management for medical practices and the new structural models that are emerging that integrate financing and delivery of healthcare. An important stakeholder in all of these discussions should not be overlooked — that of the patient. How are patients being engaged in their care and with the finances necessary for that care?

High-deductible health plans coupled with health savings accounts are one of the vehicles being used to financially and clinically engage patients. With more out-of-pocket payment requirements, the data suggest that patients are changing their utilization patterns, at least in the near term. When high-deductible health plans enter a market, studies suggest a reduction in elective procedure volume. Whether this is simply a near-term strategy — with patients postponing elective procedures until their deductible has been met or until they qualify for Medicare, for example — has yet to be seen. However, there are data to suggest that patients are "shopping" for lower cost venues of care when a significant portion of the cost is paid out of pocket.

Beyond high-deductible health plans, there are new benefit redesigns emerging. Some of these new benefit designs include:

- ■ Higher premiums
- ■ Higher out-of-pocket payments
- ■ Steerage mechanisms for treatment type and facility
- ■ Incentives for health prevention and maintenance

The delivery system itself is changing to encourage patient activation and engagement. Examples include:

- ■ Streamlined patient access involving virtual medicine, essentially taking care out of the physical facility and placing it directly with the patient
- ■ Shared decision making for preference-sensitive conditions
- ■ Care and case outreach
- ■ Supportive self-management
- ■ Individualized care and treatment plans
- ■ Streamlined transitions of care

While the jury is still out on the final outcome of healthcare reform, it is clear that medical practices will be challenged internally, in terms of financial management, revenue cycle, and general accounting, and externally, in terms of structural models of care and their level of participation in these new models. As we learn lessons from healthcare reform, financial management for the future is in for a bumpy ride. Prepare for the future now by developing new skills, data metrics, and strategies to align your medical practice with the changing healthcare environment and ensure you are well positioned for success.

REFERENCES

1. Centers for Medicare & Medicaid Services. n.d. "Medicare FFS Physician Feedback Program/ Value-Based Payment Modifier." *CMS.gov*. Retrieved from www.cms.gov/PhysicianFeedback-program/02_Background.asp. Accessed October 1, 2012.

2. Centers for Medicare & Medicaid Services. n.d. "EHR Incentive Programs." *CMS.gov*. Retrieved from www.cms.gov/EHRIncentivePrograms. Accessed October 1, 2012.

3. Centers for Medicare & Medicaid Services. n.d. "Shared Savings Program." *CMS.gov*. Retrieved from www.cms.gov/sharedsavingsprogram. Accessed October 1, 2012.

4. Center for Medicare & Medicaid Innovations. n.d. "Bundled Payments for Care Improvement." Retrieved from innovations.cms.gov/initiatives/bundled-payments/index.html. Accessed October 1, 2012.

5. Centers for Medicare & Medicaid Services. "Medicare FFS Physician Feedback Program/ Value-Based Payment Modifier." *CMS.gov*. Retrieved from www.cms.gov/PhysicianFeedback-program/02_Background.asp. Accessed October 1, 2012. CMS is expected to define measures for value-based payment in 2012, with impact on some physicians' payment levels in 2015 based on 2014 performance.

6. National Quality Forum. n.d. "Serious Reportable Events." Retrieved from www.qualityfo-rum.org/Topics/SREs/Serious_Reportable_Events.aspx. Accessed October 1, 2012.

7. Mathews, A. W. 2011, December 12. "The Future of U.S. Health Care." *The Wall Street Journal*, p. B1.

8. Centers for Medicare & Medicaid Services. "Shared Savings Program." *CMS.gov*. Retrieved from www.cms.gov/sharedsavingsprogram. Accessed October 1, 2012.

9. Song, Z., Safran, D. G., et al. 2011, July 13. "Health Care Spending and Quality in Year 1 of the Alternative Quality Contract." *New England Journal of Medicine, 365*, 909–918.

10. Mathews, A. W. 2011, December 12. "The Future of U.S. Health Care." *The Wall Street Journal*, p. B1.

11. Healthcare.gov. 2011, July 27. "Better Health, Better Care, Lower Costs: Reforming Health Care Delivery." Retrieved from www.healthcare.gov/news/factsheets/deliverysys-tem07272011a.html. Accessed October 1, 2012.

12. Johnson, B. A., and Anderson, J. 2011. *Hospital and Independent Physician Alignment: Structural Options, Business and Compliance Considerations*. Polsinelli Shughart White Paper.

13. Federal Trade Commission. 2009. Staff Letter Regarding Tri-State Health Partners, Hagerstown, MD. Retrieved from www.ftc.gov/os/closings/staff/090413tristateaoletter.pdf. Accessed October 1, 2012.

14. Atrius Health. 2011. *A Model for Health Care Reform*. ACO Bloginar. Retrieved from www.atriushealth.com.

15. Advocate Health. n.d. Search for "value report." Retrieved from www.advocatehealth.com.

16. Centers for Medicare & Medicaid Services. n.d. "Shared Savings Program." *CMS.gov.* Retrieved from www.cms.gov/sharedsavingsprogram. Accessed October 1, 2012.

17. Author discussions with Bruce A. Johnson, senior healthcare attorney, Polsinelli Shughart. 2011, October.

18. Christensen, C. M., Grossman, J. H., and Hwang, J. 2009. *The Innovator's Prescription: A Disruptive Solution for Health Care.* Columbus, OH: McGraw-Hill.

Appendices

Appendix 1
Transaction information — accrual basis

The Denell Group, PC
Marcia, Janis, and Paul Denell, MDs

($000s)

Month 1 Transactions	Assets		Liabilities		Capital		+Revenues		−Expenses	
1. Marcia, Janis & Paul start a group practice; invest $100K	Cash	100			Capital stock	100				
2. Purchase equipment – $25K cash and 5-year, 12% note for $100K	Equipment Cash	125 (25)	Notes payable	100						
3. Purchase one-year liability insurance policy ($12K)	Prepaid insurance Cash	12 (12)								
4. Purchase supplies from vendors on credit - $10K due in 30 days	Supplies	10	Accounts payable	10						
5. Deliver patient services - receive $5K cash, $20K due from insurance companies	Cash Accounts receivable	5 20					Patient revenue	25		
6. Pay rent - $3K cash	Cash	(3)							Rent expense	3
7. Receive bills due in 30 days: lab services ($2K); utilities ($2K); telephone ($1K)			Accounts payable	5					Lab service expense Utilities expense Telephone expense	2 2 1
8. Pay nurse and reseptionist salaries ($3K); withholding taxes ($1K)	Cash	(2)	Withholding taxes	1					Salary expense	3
9. Marcia, Janis, and Paul withdraw salary ($2K each)	Cash	(6)	Withholding taxes	2					Physician salary expense	8
Adjustments										
10. Record depreciation on equipment ($2K)	Equipment	(2)							Depreciation expense	2
11. Amortize liability insurance prepaid ($1K)	Prepaid insurance	(1)							Insurance expense	1
12. Record supplies used during month ($2K)	Supplies	(2)							Supplies expense	2
13. Record accural of interest on 5-year note ($1K)			Interest payable	1					Interest expense	1
Balances		**219**		**119**		**100**		**25**		**25**

Appendix 2
Transaction information — accrual basis

The Denell Group, PC
Marcia, Janis, and Paul Denell, MDs

($000s)

Month 2		Assets	=	Liabilities		+			Stockholders' Equity		
Transactions						Capital		+Revenues		−Expenses	
Balance forward		219			119		100		25		25
1. Collect receipts from insurance companies - $10K	Cash Accounts receivable	10 (10)									
2. Pay accounts payable - $15K	Cash	(15)		Accounts payable	(15)						
3. Deliver patient services - receive $5K cash, $25K due from insurance companies	Cash Accounts receivable	5 25						Patient revenue	30		
4. Pay rent - $3K	Cash	(3)								Rent expense	3
5. Pay payroll taxes withheld during Month 1 - $3K	Cash	(3)		Withholding taxes	(3)						
6. Receive bills due in 30 days; lab services ($3K); utilities ($2K); telephone ($1K)				Accounts payable	6					Lab service expense Utilities expense Telephone expense	3 2 1
7. Pay nurse and receptionist salaries ($3K); withholding taxes ($1K)	Cash	(2)		Withholding taxes	1					Salary expense	3
8. Marcia, Janis, and Paul withdraw salary ($3.33K each)	Cash	(7)		Withholding taxes	3					Physician salary expense	10
Adjustments											
9. Record depreciation on equipment ($2K)	Equipment	(2)								Depreciation expense	2
10. Amortize liability insurance prepaid ($1K)	Prepaid insurance	(1)								Insurance expense	1
11. Record supplies used during month ($3K)	Supplies	(3)								Supplies expense	3
12. Record accrual of interest on 5-year note ($1K)				Interest payable	1					Interest expense	1
Balances		213			112		100		55		54

Appendix 3
Transaction information — accrual basis

The Denell Group, PC
Marcia, Janis, and Paul Denell, MDs

($000s)

Month 3		Assets	=	Liabilities		+		Stockholders' Equity			
Transactions						Capital		+Revenues		−Expenses	
Balance forward		213			112		100		55		54
1. Collect receipts from insurance companies - $15K	Cash Accounts receivable	15 (15)									
2. Pay accounts payable - $6K	Cash	(6)		Accounts payable	(6)						
3. Deliver patient services - receive $10K cash, $25K due from insurance companies	Cash Accounts receivable	10 25						Patient revenue	35		
4, Purchase supplies from vendors on credit - $8K due in 30 days	Supplies	8		Accounts payable	8						
5. Pay rent - $3K	Cash	(3)								Rent expense	3
6. Pay payroll taxes withheld during Month 2 - $4K	Cash	(4)		Withholding taxes	(4)						
7. Receive bills due in 30 days; lab services ($4K); utilities ($2K); telephone ($1K)				Accounts payable	7					Lab service expense Utilities expense Telephone expense	4 2 1
8. Pay nurse and receptionist salaries ($3K); withholding taxes ($1K)	Cash	(2)		Withholding taxes	1					Salary expense	3
9. Marcia, Janis, and Paul withdraw salary ($367K each)	Cash	(11)		Withholding taxes	5					Physician salary expense	16
10. Pay principle amount on note payable ($5K) and interest for 3 months ($3K)	Cash	(8)		Notes payable Interest payable	(5) (2)					Interest expense	1
Adjustments											
11. Record depreciation on equipment ($1K)	Equipment	(2)								Depreciation expense	2
12. Amortize liability insurance prepaid ($1K)	Prepaid insurance	(1)								Insurance expense	1
13. Record supplies used during month ($4K)	Supplies	(4)								Supplies expense	4
Balances		216			116		100		90		91

Appendix 4
Balance sheet — accrual basis

The Denell Group, PC
Marcia, Janis, and Paul Denell, MDs

($000s)

	End of Month 1	End of Month 2	End of Month 3
Assets			
Cash	$ 57	$ 42	$ 33
Accounts receivable	20	35	45
Supplies	8	5	9
Prepaid insurance	11	10	9
Equipment	125	125	125
Accumulated depreciation	(2)	(4)	(6)
Total	$ 219	$ 213	$ 215
Liabilities & Stockholders' Equity			
Accounts payable	$ 15	$ 6	$ 15
Interest payable	1	2	0
Payroll withholdings	3	4	6
Notes payable	100	100	95
Capital stock	100	100	100
Retained earnings	0	1	(1)
Total	$ 219	$ 213	$ 215

Appendix 5
Income statement — accrual basis

The Denell Group, PC
Marcia, Janis, and Paul Denell, MDs
For the first three-month period

($000s)

	Month 1	Month 2	Month 1 & 2	Month 3	Month 1, 2 & 3
Revenue	$ 25	$ 30	$ 55	$ 35	$ 90
Expenses					
Non-physician salary	$ 3	$ 3	$ 6	$ 3	$ 9
Rent	3	3	6	3	9
Utilities	2	2	4	2	6
Supplies	2	3	5	4	9
Lab service	2	3	5	4	9
Depreciation	2	2	4	2	6
Telephone	1	1	2	1	3
Insurance	1	1	2	1	3
Interest	1	1	2	1	3
Total	$ 17	$ 19	$ 36	$ 21	$ 57
Income before physician salaries	$ 8	$ 11	$ 19	$ 14	$ 33
Physician salaries	8	10	18	16	34
Net Income	$ 0	$ 1	$ 1	$ (2)	$ (1)

Appendix 6
Cash flow statement — accrual basis

The Denell Group, PC
Marcia, Janis, and Paul Denell, MDs
For the first three-month period

($000s)

	Month 1	Month 2	Month 1 & 2	Month 3	Month 1, 2 & 3
Operating activities					
Collections for services	$ 5	$ 15	$ 20	$ 25	$ 45
Pay various expenses	(17)	(21)	(38)	(12)	(50)
Pay interest	—	—	—	(3)	(3)
Salary distributions to physicians	(6)	(9)	(15)	(14)	(29)
Cash used by operations	$ (18)	$ (15)	$ (33)	$ (4)	$ (37)
Investing activities					
Purchase equipment	$ (125)	—	$ (125)	—	$ (125)
Cash used by investing	$ (125)	—	$ (125)	—	$ (125)
Financing activities					
Invest in practice	$ 100	—	$ 100	—	$ 100
Increase long-term debt	100	—	100	—	100
Reduce long-term debt	—	—	—	(5)	(5)
Cash provided (used) by financing	$ 200	—	$ 200	$ (5)	$ 195
Increase (decrease) in cash	$ 57	$ (15)	$ 42	$ (9)	$ 33
Beginning balance — cash	0	57	0	42	0
Ending balance — cash	$ 57	$ 42	$ 42	$ 33	$ 33

Appendix 7
Transaction information — modified cash basis

The Denell Group, PC
Marcia, Janis, and Paul Denell, MDs

($000s)

Month 1	Assets		=	Liabilities		+				Stockholders' equity			
Transactions							Capital		+Revenues		−Expenses		
1. Marcia, Janis & Paul start a group practice, invest $100K	Cash	100					Capital stock	100					
2. Purchase equipment - $25K cash & 5-year, 12% note for $100K	Equipment Cash	125 (25)		Notes payable	100								
3. Purchase one-year liability insurance policy ($12K)	Cash	(12)									Insurance expense	12	
4. Purchase supplies from vendors on credit - $10K due in 30 days													
5. Deliver patient services - receive $5K cash $20K due from insurance companies	Cash	5							Patient revenue	5			
6. Pay rent - $3K cash	Cash	(3)									Rent expense	3	
7. Receive bills due in 30 days; lab services ($2K); utilities ($2K); telephone ($1K)													
8. Pay nurse and receptionist salaries ($3K); withholding taxes ($1K)	Cash	(2)		Withholding taxes	1						Salary expense	3	
9. Marcia, Janis, and Paul withdraw salary ($2K each)	Cash	(6)		Withholding taxes	2						Physician salary expense	8	
Adjustments													
10. Record depreciation on equipment ($2K)	Equipment	(2)									Depreciation expense	2	
Balances		**180**			**103**			**100**		**5**		**28**	

Appendix 8
Transaction information — modified cash basis

The Denell Group, PC
Marcia, Janis, and Paul Denell, MDs

($000s)

Month 2	Assets		=	Liabilities		+				Stockholders' equity		
Transactions						Capital		+Revenues		−Expenses		
Balance forward		180			103		100		5			28
1. Collect receipts from insurance companies - $10K	Cash	10						Patient revenue	10			
2. Pay accounts payable - $15K	Cash	(15)								Supplies expense Lab service expense Utilities expense Telephone expense		10 2 2 1
3. Deliver patient services - receive $5K cash, $25K due from insurance companies	Cash	5						Patient revenue	5			
4. Pay rent - $3K cash	Cash	(3)								Rent expense		3
5. Pay payroll taxes withheld during Month 1 - $3K	Cash	(3)		Withholding taxes	(3)							
6. Receive bills due in 30 days; lab services ($3K); utilities ($2K); telephone ($1K)												
7. Pay nurse and receptionist salaries ($3K); withholding taxes ($1K)	Cash	(2)		Withholding taxes	1					Salary expense		3
8. Marcia, Janis, and Paul withdraw salary ($3.33K each)	Cash	(7)		Withholding taxes	3					Physician salary expense		10
Adjustments												
9. Record depreciation on equipment ($2K)	Equipment	(2)								Depreciation expense		2
Balances		**163**			**104**		**100**		**20**			**61**

Appendix 9
Transaction information — modified cash basis

**The Denell Group, PC
Marcia, Janis, and Paul Denell, MDs**

($000s)

Month 3		Assets =	Liabilities		+	+Revenues		−Expenses	
Transactions					Capital				
Balance forward		163		104	100		20		61
1. Collect receipts from insurance companies - $15K	Cash	15				Patient revenue	15		
2. Pay accounts payable - $6K	Cash	(6)						Lab service expense / Utilities expense / Telephone expense	3 / 2 / 1
3. Deliver patient services - receive $10K cash, $25K due from insurance companies	Cash	10				Patient revenue	10		
4. Purchase supplies from vendors on credit - $8K due in 30 days									
5. Pay rent - $3K cash	Cash	(3)						Rent expense	3
6. Pay payroll taxes withheld during Month 1 - $4K	Cash	(4)	Withholding taxes	(4)					
7. Receive bills due in 30 days; lab services ($4K); utilities ($2K); telephone ($1K)									
8. Pay nurse and receptionist salaries ($3K); withholding taxes ($1K)	Cash	(2)	Withholding taxes	1				Salary expense	3
9. Marcia, Janis, and Paul withdraw salary ($3.67K each)	Cash	(11)	Withholding taxes	5				Physician salary expense	16
10. Pay principal amount on note payable ($5K) and interest for 3 months ($3K)	Cash	(8)	Notes payable	(5)				Interest expense	3
Adjustments									
11. Record depreciation on equipment ($2K)	Equipment	(2)						Depreciation expense	2
Balances		152		101	100		45		94

Appendix 10
Balance sheet — modified cash basis

The Denell Group, PC
Marcia, Janis, and Paul Denell, MDs
At the end of the first three months

($000s)

	End of Month 1	End of Month 2	End of Month 3
Assets			
Cash	$ 57	$ 42	$ 33
Equipment	125	125	125
Accumulated depreciation	(2)	(4)	(6)
Total	$ 180	$ 163	$ 152
Liabilities & Stockholders' Equity			
Payroll withholdings	$ 3	$ 4	$ 6
Notes payable	100	100	95
Capital stock	100	100	100
Retained earnings	(23)	(41)	(49)
Total	$ 180	$ 163	$ 152

Appendix 11
Income statement — modified cash basis

The Denell Group, PC
Marcia, Janis, and Paul Denell, MDs
For the first three-month period

($000s)

	Month 1	Month 2	Month 1 & 2	Month 3	Month 1, 2 & 3
Revenue	$ 5	$ 15	$ 20	$ 25	$ 45
Expenses					
Non-physicial salary	$ 3	$ 3	$ 6	$ 3	$ 9
Rent	3	3	6	3	9
Utilities	—	2	2	2	4
Supplies	—	10	10	—	10
Lab service	—	2	2	3	5
Depreciation	2	2	4	2	6
Telephone	—	1	1	1	2
Insurance	12	—	12	—	12
Interest	—	—	—	3	3
Total	$ 20	$ 23	$ 43	$ 17	$ 60
Income before physician salaries	$ (15)	$ (8)	$ (23)	$ 8	$ (15)
Physician salaries	8	10	18	16	34
Net Income	$ (23)	$ (18)	$ (41)	$ (8)	$ (49)

Appendix 12
Cash flow statement — modified cash basis

The Denell Group, PC
Marcia, Janis, and Paul Denell, MDs
For the first three-month period

($000s)

	Month 1	Month 2	Month 1 & 2	Month 3	Month 1, 2 & 3
Operating activities					
Collections for services	$ 5	$ 15	$ 20	$ 25	$ 45
Pay various expenses	(17)	(21)	(38)	(12)	(50)
Pay interest	—	—	—	(3)	(3)
Salary distributions to physicians	(6)	(9)	(15)	(14)	(29)
Cash used by operations	$ (18)	$ (15)	$ (33)	$ (4)	$ (37)
Investing activities					
Purchase equipment	$ (125)	—	$ (125)	—	$ (125)
Cash used by investing	$ (125)	—	$ (125)	—	$ (125)
Financing activities					
Invest in practice	$ 100	—	$ 100	—	$ 100
Increase long-term debt	100	—	100	—	100
Reduce long-term debt	—	—	—	(5)	(5)
Cash provided (used) by financing	$ 200	—	$ 200	$ (5)	$ 195
Increase (decrease) in cash	$ 57	$ (15)	$ 42	$ (9)	$ 33
Beginning balance — cash	0	57	0	42	0
Ending balance — cash	$ 57	$ 42	$ 42	$ 33	$ 33

Index